# Veterinary epidemiology

**Michael Thrusfield**

*Department of Animal Health*
*Royal (Dick) School of Veterinary Studies*
*University of Edinburgh*

**Butterworths**
London  Boston  Durban  Singapore  Sydney  Toronto  Wellington

First published 1986

© **Butterworth & Co. (Publishers) Ltd, 1986**

---

**British Library Cataloguing in Publication Data**

Thrusfield, Michael
    Veterinary epidemiology.
    1. Communicable diseases in animals
    I. Title
    636.089′44          SF781
    ISBN 0–408–10861–4

---

**Library of Congress Cataloging in Publication Data**

Thrusfield, M. V.
    Veterinary epidemiology.

    Bibliography: p.
    Includes index.
    1. Veterinary epidemiology.   I. Title.
  SF780.9.T48   1986      636.089′4       86-11758
    ISBN 0–408–10861–4

---

Photoset by Scribe Design, Gillingham, Kent
Printed and bound in Great Britain by Robert Hartnoll (1986) Limited, Bodmin, Cornwall

# Preface

The common aim of the many disciplines that comprise veterinary medicine is an increase in the health of animal populations, notably of domestic livestock and companion animals. This goal traditionally has been achieved by individual diagnosis and treatment: procedures that evolved contemporaneously in veterinary and human medicine when infectious diseases, which had predominantly single causes and clearly identifiable signs, were commonplace.

Four major changes in the veterinarian's appreciation of and approach to disease have occurred over the past 20 years. First, despite traditional control techniques, for example slaughter and vaccination, some diseases remain at refractory levels and now require continuous scrutiny to detect changing levels of occurrence associated with ecological and management factors. An example is the detection of 'pockets' of bovine tuberculosis in England in areas where infection of badgers is recorded. Secondly, the control of infectious disease has freed animals from major causes of death, thereby facilitating the emergence of non-infectious diseases as major problems: examples are the cardiac, dermal and renal diseases of dogs. Many of these diseases have a poorly understood, often complex (i.e. multifactorial) cause. Thirdly, the intensification of animal industries has highlighted new 'diseases of production', often manifested as poor performance rather than clinical disease, and frequently with multifactorial causes. Fourthly, economic evaluation has become important: the economic advantages of disease control, which are obvious with the major animal plagues such as rinderpest, can be difficult to identify when overt disease and dramatic changes in levels of performance are not involved. These four changes in the approach to and appreciation of disease have added momentum to the emergence of veterinary epidemiology as a discipline concerned with the measurement of the amount of disease and its economic effects, the identification and quantification of the effects of factors associated with disease, and the assessment of the effects of prevention and treatment of disease in groups of animals.

This book is designed as an introduction to veterinary epidemiology for the veterinary undergraduate, for the graduate student who later wishes to study more advanced texts, and for those from other disciplines who have an interest in veterinary epidemiology. It is hoped that the book will be of value to any veterinarian, whether he or she is concerned with farm or companion animals and whether working in a developed or a developing country.

A knowledge of elementary statistics is essential for an understanding of the full range of epidemiological techniques. Hitherto, most epidemiology books either have assumed a knowledge of statistics or have avoided a description of the mathematical manipulations that are commonly used in epidemiology. However, the extent of statistical teaching varies widely between veterinary schools. Chapters 12 and 13 therefore are included as an introduction to basic statistics, and are intended to make this book statistically self-sufficient (though not comprehensive). Similarly, Chapter 11 includes an introduction to computers which are now used widely in the recording and analysis of epidemiological data.

I am indebted to the colleagues who gave advice during the writing of this book. Gareth Davies, Tom Farver, Mark Felton, David Finney FRS, Nancy Hebert, Pat Imlah, Tony Luckins, Gordon Scott, Jill Smith, David Whitaker and Tony Woods criticized various parts of the text. Many hours were spent with Colin Aitken and George Gettinby discussing the chapters relating to statistics and modelling; their comments have been invaluable. Keith Howe, similarly, gave indispensable advice on the writing of Chapter 18: 'The economics of disease'. I am also grateful to David Blackmore for his involvement in the writing of this book. John Cuthbertson and Alex Russell scrutinized most of the chapters and helped to clarify many of the ideas presented therein. Helen London, librarian at the University of Edinburgh's Veterinary Field Station, rapidly acquired many of the publications cited in the text. Jane Connel, Anne Frost and Lida Newell typed parts of the manuscript. I am particularly indebted to Rona Hunter who enthusiastically typed the majority of the manuscript and all of its many revisions; her contribution to the rapid completion of this book, which involved many long hours, has been considerable. Sue Deeley, commissioning editor of Butterworth Scientific Limited, has given much support and guidance during the period of writing. I offer my warmest thanks to all of these people. Finally, I am grateful to the Literary Executor of the late Sir Ronald A. Fisher, FRS, to Dr Frank Yates, FRS, and to the Longman Group Limited, London, for permission to reprint Tables III, IV, V and VII from their book, *Statistical Tables for Biological, Agricultural and Medical Research* (6th edition, 1974).

Michael Thrusfield
*Edinburgh*

# Contents

**CHAPTER 1: THE DEVELOPMENT OF VETERINARY MEDICINE     1**

**Historical perspective     1**
Domestication of animals and early methods of healing     1
Changing concepts of the cause of disease     2
Impetus for change     5
**Contemporary veterinary medicine     6**
Current and emerging problems: new crises     6
The fifth period     8
Emerging trends     9

**CHAPTER 2: THE SCOPE OF EPIDEMIOLOGY     11**

Definition of epidemiology     11
**The uses of epidemiology     11**
**Types of epidemiological investigation     14**
**Components of epidemiology     14**
Qualitative investigations     14
Quantitative investigations     14
**Is epidemiology a science?     17**
The interplay between epidemiology and other sciences     17
The relationship between epidemiology and other diagnostic disciplines     18

**CHAPTER 3: SOME GENERAL EPIDEMIOLOGICAL CONCEPTS     20**

Endemic, epidemic, pandemic and sporadic ocurrence of disease     20
**The cause of disease     22**
Koch's postulates     22
Evans' postulates     22
Variables     23
Types of association     23
Causal models     25
Confounding     26
Formulating a causal hypothesis     27

**CHAPTER 4: DESCRIBING DISEASE OCCURRENCE     30**

**The structure of animal populations     30**
Contiguous populations     30
Separated populations     31
**Measures of disease occurrence     31**
Prevalence     31
Incidence     31
The relationship between prevalence and incidence     33
Application of prevalence and incidence values     34
Ratios, proportions and rates     35
Life tables     39
Displaying morbidity and mortality values and demographic data     40
**Mapping     40**
Geographic base maps     41
Demographic base maps     44

**CHAPTER 5: DETERMINANTS OF DISEASE     46**

Classification of determinants     46
**Host determinants     48**
Age     48
Sex     49
Species and breed     51
Other host determinants     52
**Agent determinants     52**
Virulence and pathogenicity     52
Gradient of infection     53
Outcome of infection     54
Microbial colonization of hosts     55
**Environmental determinants     56**
Location     56
Climate     56
Husbandry     57
Stress     57

Interaction    58
Biological interaction    59
Statistical interaction    59
The cause of cancer    60

CHAPTER 6: THE TRANSMISSION AND
MAINTENANCE OF INFECTION    63
Horizontal transmission    63
Types of host and vector    64
Factors associated with the spread of
infection    65
Routes of infection    67
Methods of transmission    69
Vertical transmission    70
Types and methods of vertical transmission    70
Immunological status and vertical
transmission    72
Transovarial and trans-stadial transmission in
arthropods    72
Maintenance of infection    72
Hazards to infectious agents    72
Maintenance strategies    73

CHAPTER 7: THE ECOLOGY OF
DISEASE    76
Basic ecological concepts    76
The distribution of populations    76
Regulation of population size    78
The niche    81
Some examples of niches relating to disease    82
The relationships between different types of animals
and plants    83
Ecosystems    86
Types of ecosystem    86
Landscape epidemiology    88
Nidality    88
Objectives of landscape epidemiology    89

CHAPTER 8: PATTERNS OF DISEASE    91
Basic epidemic theory    91
Epidemic curves    91
Epidemic waves    93
Trends in the temporal distribution of disease    94
Short-term trends    94
Cyclical trends    94
Long-term (secular) trends    95
True and false changes in morbidity and
mortality    96
Detecting temporal trends: time series
analysis    96
Trends in the spatial and temporal distribution of
disease    100
Spatial trends in disease occurrence    100
Time-space clustering    100

CHAPTER 9: THE NATURE OF DATA    101
Data elements    101

Nomenclature and classification of disease    101
Diagnostic criteria    103
Sensitivity and specificity    104
Accuracy, refinement, precision, reliability and
validity    104
Bias    106
Representation of data: coding    107
Code structure    107
Numeric codes    107
Alpha codes    109
Alphanumeric codes    109
Symbols    110
Choosing a code    110
Error detection    111
Measurements    112
Discrete measurements    112
Continuous measurements    112

CHAPTER 10: SOURCES OF DATA    114
Some general considerations    114
Nature of data    114
Cooperation    114
Trace-back    114
Bias    115
The cost of data collection    115
Problems unique to developing countries    115
Sources of epidemiological data    115
Government veterinary organizations    115
Veterinary practices    115
Abattoirs    117
Poultry packing plants    118
Knacker yards    118
Serum banks    118
Registries    118
Pharmaceutical and agricultural sales    119
Zoological gardens    119
Agricultural organizations    119
Commercial livestock enterprises    119
Non-veterinary government departments    119
Farm records    119
Veterinary schools    119
Other sources    119

CHAPTER 11: DATA STORAGE AND
RETRIEVAL    121
Data base models    121
Non-computerized recording techniques    122
Longhand recording techniques    122
Punched card recording techniques    123
Computerized recording techniques    125
Structure of computers    125
Languages    126
Changing approaches to computing    127
Accessing computerized data    128
Veterinary data bases    129
Scales of project recording    129
Some examples of veterinary data bases    130

**CHAPTER 12: PRESENTING NUMERICAL DATA 132**
**Some basic definitions 132**
**Some descriptive statistics 133**
Measures of position 133
Measures of spread 134
Interval estimation 134
**Statistical distributions 135**
The Normal distribution 135
The binomial distribution 135
The Poisson distribution 136
Other distributions 136
Transformations 137
Normal approximations to the binomial and Poisson distributions 137
**Displaying numerical data 137**

**CHAPTER 13: DEMONSTRATING ASSOCIATION 141**
**Some basic techniques 141**
The principle of a significance test 141
The null hypothesis 142
Errors of inference 142
Student's $t$-test 143
The $\chi^2$-test of association 144
Estimation of risk 145
Measuring interaction 147
Correlation 149
Non-parametric tests 150
**Multivariate analysis 151**
**Statistical packages 151**

**CHAPTER 14: SURVEYS 153**
Sampling: some basic concepts 153
Types of sampling 154
**Surveys 155**
What sample size should be selected? 156
Estimation of disease prevalence 156
Detecting the presence of disease 157
The cost of surveys 159
**Collecting information: questionnaires 159**
Structure of a questionnaire 159
Designing a questionnaire 163
Mailed and self-completed questionnaires 164
Interviews 164
Testing a questionnaire 164
Criteria for success of a questionnaire 164

**CHAPTER 15: OBSERVATIONAL STUDIES 166**
The three types of observational study 166
Nomenclature of observational studies 167
Measures of association used in observational studies 167
Interpreting results 168
Bias in observational studies 168
Controlling bias 170

Selection of sample size in cohort and case-control studies 171
Multivariate techniques 171
Comparison of the types of observational study 171

**CHAPTER 16: SEROLOGICAL EPIDEMIOLOGY 175**
**Assaying antibodies 175**
Methods of expressing amounts of antibody 175
Quantal assay 176
**Serological estimations and comparisons in populations 178**
Detecting the presence of antibody 178
Comparison of antibody levels 178
**Interpreting serological tests 179**
Refinement 179
Accuracy 180
The relationship between sensitivity and specificity 181
The predictive value of serological tests 182
Antibody prevalence 184
**Serum banks 184**
Applications of serum banks 185
Sources of serum 185
Collection and storage of serum 185

**CHAPTER 17: MODELLING 187**
**Types of model 187**
**Forecasting systems 188**
Empirical models 188
Explanatory models 189
**Deterministic population models 189**
Deterministic models using differential calculus 190
Deterministic matrix models 192
**Stochastic population models 193**
Stochastic models using differential calculus 193
Stochastic network models 194
**Further veterinary applications of modelling 194**

**CHAPTER 18: THE ECONOMICS OF DISEASE 199**
Production as an economic process 199
The nature of economic decisions 199
The economic analysis of animal disease 200
The need for economic assessment of disease control 200
Methods of financial evaluation 200
**Assessing the cost of disease 200**
**Cost-benefit analysis of disease control 202**
Principles of CBA 202
An example of CBA 204
Some problems associated with CBA 205

**CHAPTER 19: HEALTH AND PRODUCTIVITY SCHEMES 206**
The development of health and productivity schemes 206

Structure of health and productivity
schemes    206
**Dairy health and productivity schemes    208**
Targets    208
Routine visits    208
**Pig health and productivity schemes    209**
Targets    209
Routine visits    209
**Sheep health and productivity schemes    211**
Targets    211
Routine visits    211
**Beef health and productivity schemes    213**
Targets    213
Routine visits    213
**Companion animal health schemes    213**

**CHAPTER 20: THE CONTROL OF
DISEASE    215**

**Disease control and eradication    215**
Definition of 'control' and 'eradication'    215
Strategies of control and eradication    216
Important factors in control and eradication
programmes    220
**Veterinary medicine towards the end of this
century    223**
Livestock medicine    223

Companion animal medicine    224

**GENERAL READING    225**

**APPENDICES    227**
Appendix I: Glossary of terms    229
Appendix II: Basic mathematical notation and
terms    233
Appendix III: Student's *t*-distribution    235
Appendix IV: The $\chi^2$-distribution    236
Appendix V: The correlation coefficient    237
Appendix VI: Technique of selecting a simple
random sample    238
Appendix VII: Sample sizes    240
Appendix VIII: The probability of detecting a small
number of cases in a population    247
Appendix IX: The probability of failure to detect
cases in a population    249
Appendix X: The variance-ratio (*F*)
distribution    250

**REFERENCES    253**

**INDEX    273**

# 1

# The development of veterinary medicine

Although man's association with animals began in prehistoric times, the development of scientific veterinary medicine is a comparatively recent event. A milestone in this growth was the establishment of the first permanent veterinary school at Lyons, France, in 1762. Early developments were governed largely by commercial rather than humanitarian motives, associated with the importance of domestic stock as a source of food and as working animals. Later, with the advent of the industrial revolution and the invention of the internal combustion engine, the importance of draft animals declined in the developed countries. Although dogs and cats have been companion animals for several thousand years, it is only recently that they and other pets have increased in importance as components of human society.

Until recently the emphasis of veterinary medicine has been put on the treatment of individual animals suffering from clearly identifiable diseases or defects. Apart from routine immunization programmes and prophylactic treatment of internal parasites, restricted attention has been given to herd health and comprehensive preventive medicine which give proper consideration to both infectious and non-infectious diseases.

Currently, the nature of traditional clinical practice is changing in all developed countries. The stock owner is better educated and the value of individual animals relative to veterinary fees has decreased. Therefore, contemporary large animal practitioners, if they are to meet modern requirements, must increase their knowledge of and expertise in herd health programmes that are designed to increase production by preventing disease, rather than just dispensing traditional treatment to clinically sick animals.

In the developing countries, the infectious diseases still cause considerable loss of animal life and production. Traditional control techniques, based on identification of recognizable signs and pathological changes, cannot reduce the level of some diseases to an acceptable degree. Different techniques, based on the study of patterns of disease in groups of animals, are needed.

Similarly, contemporary companion animal practitioners, like their medical counterparts, are becoming increasingly involved with chronic and refractory diseases that can be understood better by an investigation of the diseases' characteristics in populations.

This chapter outlines the changing techniques of veterinary medicine by tracing man's attempts at controlling disease in animals, and introduces some current problems of animal disease that can be solved by an epidemiological approach.

## Historical perspective

### Domestication of animals and early methods of healing

The importance of animal healers has been acknowledged since animals were initially domesticated. The dog, naturally a hunter, was probably the first animal to be domesticated over 14 000 years ago when it became the companion of early hunters. Sheep and goats were domesticated by 9000 BC in the fertile Nile valley and were the basis of early pastoral cultures. A few of these societies have lasted, for example the Jews, but many were superseded by cattle cultures; in some the pig

1

increased in importance (Murray, 1968). An Egyptian cattle culture evolved from 4000 BC; there is archaeological evidence of cattle shrines in Anatolia dating back to 6000 BC (Mellaart, 1967). This record illustrates that animals had a religious as well as an economic significance in early civilizations. The aurochs was central to the religion of the Sumerians, who migrated throughout Asia, North Africa and Europe in the third millennium BC taking their animals and beliefs with them. India is the largest cattle culture that remains. Cattle cultures also persist in NE Africa, the result of interaction between the Ancient Egyptians and early Nilotic tribes. Cattle still play important roles in these cultures: they are food, companionship, and status and religious symbols to the Suk (Beech, 1911) and Dinka tribes (Lienhardt, 1961) of the Sudan.

Later, a Eurasian horse culture, associated with warrior tribes, developed. Some of these tribes overran the older cattle cultures. The horse is represented in Iranian, Greek and Celtic pantheons. It has become a symbol of veterinary medicine in the form of a centaur, one of which, Chiron, was considered to be the mythological founder of Greek medicine.

There have been several movements of animals with concomitant social and agricultural modifications since the early changes. The Spanish introduced cattle, sheep, pigs and goats to North America in the 16th century. Haired sheep were introduced to Africa by European slave traders. The Spanish brought turkeys to Europe from North America.

The early Egyptian healers combined religious and medical roles by being priest-healers, often associated with temples. Their therapeutic techniques are recorded in the veterinary *Papyrus of Kahun* (*c*.1900 BC). Literary records of similar age, describing veterinary activities, are extant from other parts of the world, such as Indian Sanskrit texts from the Vedic period (1800–1200 BC).

## Changing concepts of the cause of disease

A method of treatment used by early Egyptians was incantation. This was partly ritual, but also reflected their belief in supernatural spirits as a possible cause of disease. Approaches to treatment and prevention are the direct result of theories of cause. There have been five main theories up to the middle of this century. One theory was often superseded by another, but traces of each can still be seen in different parts of the world.

### Demons

Early man attributed disease to supernatural powers, the product of animism which imbued all moving things with a spirit. In this 'spirit-world' disease could be produced by witches, superhuman entities and spirits of the dead. Treatment therefore included: placation, for example by sacrifice; exorcism (forcible expulsion); evasion, for example scattering millet seeds to avoid vampires (Summers, 1961); and transference, the best known example of which is the Gadarene swine (the *Bible*: Mark 5, i–xiii). The techniques included: ritual ceremonies; material objects that could be suspended (amulets), carried (talismans), hung in a building (fetishes and icons) or displayed in the community (totems); the use of special people such as witch doctors; and incantations. The meaning of the Indian word 'brahmin' originally was 'healer' because the brahmin were a class of healers. The African Nuer tribe still uses incantations during ritual sacrifice when cattle epidemics occur (Evans-Pritchard, 1956), and sacrifice was practised in England as late as the 19th century (Baker, 1974).

### Divine wrath

The demonic theory involved many spirits; the next development, monotheistic in origin, argued that disease was the product of a displeased supreme being: disease was punishment. This belief is prominent in the Old Testament, for example the animal plague of Egypt (the *Bible*: Exodus 9, iii), and is also evident in Persian and Aztec writings. The only effective treatment of disease induced in this way was placation because exorcism and evasion would not be effective against a supreme being. Traces of this belief have persisted until recent times. The English veterinary surgeon William Youatt, writing in 1835, supported the practice of burning crosses on the heads of cattle to cure and prevent disease. In 1865, Queen Victoria, recognizing that the current British rinderpest outbreak was the result of divine displeasure, ordered that a prayer should be used in each church in England while the epidemic continued.

### Metaphysical medicine

The next development did not assume the existence of a supreme being, either demonic or divine, but presumed the presence of occult forces beyond the physical universe. This 'metaphysical' medicine embodied a theory of natural laws but excluded scientific principles such as observation and the repeatability of phenomena. The moon, stars and planets were considered to affect health, these concepts being obvious predecessors of astrology. Several outbreaks of rinderpest in Dark Age Europe were ascribed to earthquakes, floods and comets.

Treatment frequently included particularly foul medicines and practices that persisted for many centuries. A recommended 17th century cure for broken wind in horses comprises toads, swallows and moles roasted alive and mixed with shoe soles. Divination, practised by the Babylonians using sheep livers, and the 'Doctrine of Signatures' that suggested a similarity between the disease and its cure—for example using toads to treat warts—were notable metaphysical developments.

## The universe of natural law

A major intellectual revolution began in Greece in the sixth century BC in which the universe was rationalized without either demonic or metaphysical influences. The Greeks thought that disease was the result of derangement of four **humours** of the body that were associated with four properties (heat, moisture, dryness and cold) and with four elements (air, earth, water and fire) (*Figure 1.1*).

| CHARACTERISTIC | | Moisture | Dryness |
|---|---|---|---|
| **Heat** | | Humour = Blood<br>Associated element = Air<br>Source = Heart<br>Excess → Sanguine temperament | Humour = Yellow bile<br>Associated element = Fire<br>Source = Liver<br>Excess → Choleric (bilious) temperament |
| **Cold** | | Humour = Phlegm<br>Associated element = Water<br>Source = Pituitary gland<br>Excess → Phlegmatic temperament | Humour = Black bile<br>Associated element = Earth<br>Source = Spleen<br>Excess → Melancholic temperament |

**Figure 1.1** Components of humoral pathology.

Diseases were considered to be caused by external forces, including climatic and geological changes, that affected the population. Local outbreaks of disease were thought to be the result of local eruptions of noxious air: the **miasma**. The word 'malaria' literally means 'bad air' and hints at the 19th century belief that the disease was caused by stale air around swamps. The popularity of the miasmatic theory fluctuated in Europe until the beginning of the 20th century, by which time the microbial theory of infectious disease was adequately supported.

The Greek idea of disease was susceptible to scientific investigation. Careful observation and the identification of specific causes became the hallmarks of the fifth century BC school of medicine at

Cos, and were refined by Hippocrates whose text *Discourse on airs, waters and places* (Jones, 1923) dominated medicine for many centuries. Therapy was consistent with causal concepts, and included alterations in diet and purges.

## Contagion

The idea that some diseases can be transmitted from one animal to another has its ubiquitous origins in antiquity. The Romans, Galen and Lucretius, believed that disease could be spread by airborne **seeds** or **animalculae** (not necessarily living) that were taken in through the nose and mouth. The Jewish Talmud describes demons as hiding 'everywhere'—in water, crumbs and air—implying contagiousness. The primitive Hindus associated sick rats with human plague, the first suggestion of a zoonosis. The Veronan Fracastorius, writing in the early 16th century, argued that diseases were transmitted by minute, invisible particles. Lancisi, physician to Pope Clement XI, freed Rome from rinderpest by using a slaughter policy to prevent infection of unaffected animals.

The main advances in the identification of microbes as causes of infectious diseases occurred in the 19th century, although the concept of a living contagious agent, **contagium animatum**, was founded in the 17th century. Edward Jenner's development of a smallpox vaccine using cowpox infective material, and early biological warfare conducted by American settlers who gave blankets belonging to smallpox victims to Indians as presents, implicitly recognized contagion.

Louis Pasteur's investigation of anthrax and rabies, and Robert Koch's discovery of the bacteria causing tuberculosis and cholera, firmly established microbiology and marked the downfall of the miasmatic theory. The set of postulates formulated by Koch to define causal agents has been used to identify many microbial diseases since those early days of bacteriology (*see* Chapter 3).

Viruses were also discovered in the late 19th century, although not actually 'seen' until the invention of the electron microscope in the 1930s. In 1892, Iwanowsky demonstrated that tobacco mosaic disease could be transmitted by sap that had been filtered through bacteria-proof filters. Beijerinck serially transmitted the disease using bacteria-free filtrates, and coined the term **contagium vivum fluidum** to describe the infectious 'living' agent. In 1898–99 Loeffler and Frosch discovered the first animal virus, foot-and-mouth disease virus, and in 1911 Rous reported the first virus-induced transmissible tumour.

Towards the end of the 19th century, the first arthropod carrier (a tick) of an infectious disease was identified by Kilborne, Smith and Curtis, investigating Texas fever of cattle in the USA.

**Table 1.1 Some dates of occurrence of animal plagues. (Most dates extracted from Smithcors, 1957)**

| Date | Animal plagues | | | | | | |
|---|---|---|---|---|---|---|---|
| | Rinderpest | Pleuropneumonia | Canine distemper | Anthrax | Foot-and-mouth disease | Equine influenza | Ill-defined diseases |
| 500 BC | | | | | | | Egypt 500 BC —time of Christ Egypt 278 BC abortion |
| AD | | | | Rome AD 500 | | | Rome 4th century AD (cattle) France 6th century AD (cattle) Ireland 8th century AD France 820 850 940–43 (cattle) England 1314 (cattle) |
| AD 1400 | | | | | Italy 1514 | England 1688 | |
| AD 1700 | France 1710–1714 Rome 1713 England 1714 England 1745–46 France 1750 France 1774 | Europe 18th century | USA 1760 Spain 1761 England 1763 | | | England 1727 Ireland 1728 England 1733 England 1737 England 1750 England 1760 England 1771 England 1788 | |
| AD 1800 | England 1865 | England 1841–1898 | | | England 1839 England 1870–72 1877–85 | England 1837 North America 1872 England 1889–90 | |
| AD 1900 | Belgium 1920 | | | | England 1922–25 1942 1952 1967–68 | Czechoslovakia 1957 Britain 1963 USA 1963 Europe 1965 | |

## *Impetus for change*

Changing attitudes towards the cause of disease and the concomitant alterations in techniques of treatment and prevention are a small part of shifts in overall scientific thought. These changes have not taken place gradually but have occurred as distinct 'revolutions' (Kuhn, 1970) that terminate periods of stable science, characterized in the applied sciences by similar attitudes towards the nature of a subject and the methods employed in its investigation (Nordenstam and Tornebohm, 1979). When application of these attitudes ceases to solve problems associated with the discipline (i.e. some problems— 'anomalies'—remain), a crisis occurs that stimulates new ideas and methods: the 'revolution'.

Veterinary medicine has experienced five stable periods and revolutions up to the middle of the 20th century relating to disease control (Schwabe, 1982) that stimulated the changes in the causal concepts that have been described. The major problem that persisted during these periods, precipitating crises, was large-scale outbreaks of infectious disease: the classical animal plagues (*Table 1.1*).

### The first period: until the first century AD

The initial domestication of animals brought man into close contact with animals and therefore with their diseases. The demonic theory was prevalent. However, despite the use of control techniques consistent with the theory, draft animals continued to die and a crisis arose when urbanization increased the importance of animals as food resources. This resulted in the development of the first stable phase of veterinary medicine. This was characterized by the emergence of veterinary specialists such as the early Egyptian priest-healers and the Vedic **Salihotriya** who founded the first veterinary hospitals. Humoral pathology developed and the miasmatic theory of cause evolved. Techniques of treatment required careful recognition of clinical signs following the Greek Coan tradition. Quarantine (derived from the Italian word meaning 'forty'—the traditional length, in days, of isolation in the Middle Ages) and slaughter became preventive strategies. These local actions, which lasted until the first century AD, were incapable of solving major problems in the horse which was becoming an important military animal. This crisis resulted in the second phase: that of military healers.

### The second period: first century AD until 1762

Veterinarians specialized in equine medicine and surgery. A major veterinary text, the *Hippiatrika*, comprising letters between veterinarians, cavalry officers and castrators, dates from early Byzantine times. The major contributor to this work was Apsyrtus, chief *hippiatros* to the army of Constantine the Great. This phase lasted until the mid-18th century and was marked by a continuing interest in equine matters. Several important texts were written, including Ruini's *Anatomy of the Horse* (published in 1598). Some interest was taken in other animals. John Fitzherbert's *Boke of Husbandrie* (published in 1523) included diseases of cattle and sheep. The horse, however, was pre-eminent. This bias survived in Europe until early this century when equine veterinary medicine was still considered to be a more respectable occupation than the care of other species.

Varying emphasis was placed on the miasmatic and metaphysical theories of cause and on humoral pathology. The Arabians, for example, based their medicine largely on the metaphysical theory.

### The third period: 1762–1884

The animal plagues, especially those of cattle, became particularly common in Europe in the mid-18th century with the introduction of rinderpest from Asia. They provided the next major crisis involving civilian animals. The miasmatic theory persisted but the miasma were thought to originate from filth generated by man, rather than from natural sources. A third stable phase developed, characterized by improvement of farm hygiene, slaughter and treatment as control techniques. When rinderpest entered England from Holland in 1714, Thomas Bates, surgeon to George I, advocated fumigation of buildings, slaughter and burning of affected animals, and resting of contaminated pasture as typical tactics. Cattle owners also were compensated for loss.

Half of the cattle in France were destroyed by rinderpest between 1710 and 1714. The disease occurred irregularly until 1750 when it again became a serious problem. Little was known about the disease. This provided impetus for the establishment of the first permanent veterinary school at Lyons in 1762. Alfort was founded in 1766, Hannover in 1778, London in 1791, Edinburgh in 1823 and Toulouse in 1825.

The lifting of animal importation restrictions in England in 1842 increased the risk of disease occurring in Britain. Sheep pox entered Britain in 1847 from Germany, and pleuropneumonia became a serious problem. Public concern, highlighted by the rinderpest outbreak of 1865, was responsible for the establishment of the British State Veterinary Service in the same year. Similar services were founded in other countries. The legislature continued to strengthen the power of the veterinary services by passing Acts relating to the control of animal diseases.

## The fourth period: 1884–1960

The animal plagues continued despite sanitary campaigns. This crisis coincided with the inception and acceptance of the microbial theory which, epitomized by Koch's postulates, defined a specific single cause of an infectious disease and therefore implied a suitable control strategy directed against the causal agent.

This fourth stable phase of campaigns or mass actions began in the 1880s. Treatment of disease was based on laboratory diagnosis involving isolation of agents and identification of lesions followed by therapy. Control of disease by prevention and, subsequently, eradication involved mass testing of animals and immunization when an increasing number of vaccines became available. The discovery of disease vectors facilitated prevention by vector control. An improved understanding of infectious agents' life histories enabled their life-cycles to be broken by manipulating the environment; the draining of land to prevent fascioliasis is a good example. Bacterial diseases remained as major clinical problems until the discovery and synthesis of antibiotics in the 20th century which increased the therapeutic power of the veterinarian.

## Contemporary veterinary medicine

### Current and emerging problems: new crises

#### The animal plagues

The mass infectious diseases still pose problems. They remain as major disruptive diseases in the developing countries. There have been some recent successes, for example the JP15 campaign against rinderpest in Africa (Lepissier and MacFarlane, 1966), although the effects of this campaign have subsequently been negated by civil strife. Several vector-transmitted diseases with complex life-cycles, including haemoprotozoan infections such as trypanosomiasis, have not been controlled satisfactorily. More than half of the world's livestock are located in developing countries (*Table 1.2*) and therefore are exposed to these disease problems. The techniques of the microbial revolution have enabled these diseases to be identified. However, accurate means of assessing the extent and distribution of the diseases are also necessary in order to plan control programmes.

**Table 1.2 World livestock populations 1982 (1000s of animals). (From FAO, 1983)**

|  | Cattle | Sheep | Goats | Pigs | Horses | Chickens | Buffaloes |
|---|---|---|---|---|---|---|---|
| World | 1 226 432 | 1 157 690 | 472 784 | 763 813 | 65 044 | 6 578 483 | 122 053 |
| USA and Canada | 128 210 | 13 441 | 1 417 | 67 949 | 10 525 | 474 921 | |
| Central America | 58 523 | 9 319 | 9 474 | 19 503 | 9 051 | 270 054 | 8 |
| South America | 218 132 | 108 213 | 19 641 | 53 046 | 13 038 | 700 890 | 570 |
| Europe | 133 248 | 142 852 | 12 347 | 177 442 | 5 273 | 1 230 150 | 440 |
| Africa | 173 387 | 186 167 | 152 178 | 10 298 | 3 666 | 620 388 | 2 447 |
| Asia | 365 578 | 343 053 | 271 207 | 357 617 | 17 292 | 2 219 938 | 118 257 |
| Oceania | 33 435 | 212 287 | 397 | 4 656 | 649 | 56 144 | |
| USSR | 115 919 | 142 358 | 6 123 | 73 302 | 5 570 | 1 006 000 | 330 |
| All developed countries | 427 190 | 542 923 | 25 681 | 332 963 | 22 160 | 3 110 166 | 770 |
| All developing countries | 799 243 | 614 767 | 447 103 | 430 850 | 42 884 | 3 468 318 | 121 283 |

Many infectious diseases were either effectively controlled or eradicated between the latter part of the 19th century and the middle of the 20th century in the developed countries using the new techniques of the microbial revolution and older techniques including quarantine, importation restrictions, slaughter and hygiene. In 1892, pleuropneumonia in the USA was the first disease to be regionally eradicated after a campaign lasting only 5 years. Notable British successes included rinderpest, eradicated in 1877, pleuropneumonia in 1898, glanders in 1928 and equine parasitic mange in 1928.

Some infectious diseases, for example brucellosis and tuberculosis, persist at low levels in developed countries, despite the application of traditional control methods. This problem can result from inadequate survey techniques and insensitive diagnostic tests (Martin, 1977). In some cases, an infectious agent may have a more complex natural history than initially suspected. For example, continued outbreaks of bovine tuberculosis in problem herds in England (Wilesmith *et al.*, 1982) recently have been shown to be associated with pockets of infection in wild badgers (Little *et al.*, 1982).

**Table 1.3 The livestock population of Great Britain 1866–1981 (1000s of animals). (From HMSO, 1968, 1982)**

| Year | Cattle | Sheep | Pigs | Horses (agricultural use) | Fowls | Turkeys |
|------|--------|-------|------|---------------------------|-------|---------|
| 1866 | 4 786 | 22 048 | 2 478 | — | — | — |
| 1900 | 6 805 | 26 592 | 2 382 | 1 078 | — | — |
| 1925 | 7 368 | 23 094 | 2 799 | 910 | 39 036 | 730 |
| 1950 | 9 630 | 19 714 | 2 463 | 347 | 71 176 | 855 |
| 1965 | 10 826 | 28 837 | 6 731 | 21 | 101 956 | 4 323 |
| 1981 | 11 701 | 30 952 | 7 201 | — | 111 279 | 8 202 |

— Indicates data not available.

The effective control of the animal plagues has allowed an increase in both animal numbers (*Table 1.3*) and productivity (*Table 1.4*) in the developed countries (mechanization making draft horses the exception). There has been an increase in the size of herds and flocks, notably in dairy, pig (*Table 1.5*) and poultry enterprises. Intensification of animal industries is accompanied by different animal health problems.

**Table 1.4 World cattle productivity 1981. (From FAO, 1983)**

| | Number of animals slaughtered (1000s of animals) | Carcass weight (kg/ animal) | Milk yield (kg/ animal) | Milk production (1000 metric tons) |
|------|------|------|------|------|
| World | 233 861 | 195 | 1 935 | 437 909 |
| USA | 39 175 | 266 | 5 637 | 61 553 |
| South America | 34 816 | 196 | 1 028 | 24 062 |
| Asia | 30 586 | 140 | 699 | 40 321 |
| Africa | 20 822 | 140 | 473 | 10 269 |
| Europe | 47 006 | 217 | 3 583 | 181 573 |
| USSR | 38 000 | 174 | 2 052 | 89 600 |
| Oceania | 11 995 | 175 | 3 027 | 11 908 |
| Developed countries | 144 373 | 217 | 3 185 | 362 651 |
| Developing countries | 89 488 | 160 | 669 | 75 258 |

## Complex infectious diseases

The animal plagues are caused by 'simple' agents, that is their predominant causes can be identified as single infectious agents. Diseases caused by single agents still constitute problems in developed countries. Examples include salmonellosis, leptospirosis, babesiosis and coccidiosis. However, diseases have been identified that are produced by simultaneous infection with more than one agent (mixed infections), and by interaction between infectious agents and non-infectious factors. These are common in intensive production enterprises. Diseases of the body surfaces—enteric and respiratory diseases—are particular problems. Single agents alone cannot be incriminated in the pathogenesis of these 'complex' diseases.

## Subclinical diseases

Some diseases do not produce overt clinical signs. These are called **subclinical** diseases. They often affect production. Helminthiasis and marginal mineral deficiencies, for example, decrease liveweight gain. Porcine adenomatosis decreases weight gain in piglets, although there may be no clinical signs (Roberts *et al.*, 1979). Infection of pregnant sows with porcine parvovirus in early pregnancy destroys fetuses, the only sign being small numbers of piglets in litters. These diseases are major causes of production loss; their identification often requires laboratory investigations.

**Table 1.5 Pig herd structure in England and Wales (June). (From Muirhead, 1978a)**

| | 1965 | 1971 | 1975 |
|------|------|------|------|
| Number of farms with pigs | 94 639 | 56 900 | 32 291 |
| Total sows (1000s) | 756.3 | 791 | 686 |
| Average herd size (sows) | 10.4 | 18.5 | 27.6 |
| Herd size: | | | |
| 1–49 | 56 560 (75.4%) | 39 000 (90.9%) | 20 873 (84%) |
| 50–99 | 10 445 (13.9%) | 2 700 (6.3%) | 2 401 (9.7%) |
| 100–199 | 8 034*(10.7%) | 1000 (2.3%) | 1 141 (4.6%) |
| 200–499 | — — | 200 (0.5%) | 372 (1.5%) |
| 500 and over | — — | — — | 54 (0.2%) |
| Total | 75 039 | 42 900 | 24 841 |

*Reported only as 100.

## Non-infectious diseases

Non-infectious diseases have increased in importance following control of the major infectious ones. They can be predominantly genetic (e.g. canine hip dysplasia), metabolic (e.g. bovine ketosis) or neoplastic (e.g. canine mammary cancer). Their cause may be associated with several factors; for example, feline urolithiasis is associated with diet, age, sex and breed (Willeberg, 1977).

Some of these conditions, such as ketosis, are particularly related to increased levels of production; ketosis is more likely in cows with high milk yields than in those with low yields. Intensive production systems may also be directly responsible for some conditions, for example foot lesions in individually caged broilers (Pearson, 1983).

## Diseases of unknown cause

The cause of some diseases has not been elucidated despite intensive experimental investigation. Equine grass sickness, a fatal disease of British horses, and the recently identified feline dysautonomia, initially called the Key-Gaskell syndrome (Gaskell, 1983), are examples that pose challenges to veterinary research.

In some situations, infectious agents have been isolated from cases of a disease but cannot be unequivocally associated with the disease. An example is *Pasteurella haemolytica* in relation to 'shipping fever' (Martin *et al.*, 1982). This syndrome occurs in cattle soon after their arrival at feedlots. Post-mortem examination of fatal cases has revealed that fibrinous pneumonia is a common cause of death. Although *P. haemolytica* is frequently isolated from lungs, it is not invariably present. Attempts to experimentally reproduce the disease using the bacterium alone have failed (Jericho, 1979). Other factors also seem to be involved, including mixing animals and then penning them in large groups, the feeding of corn silage, dehorning, and, paradoxically, vaccination against agents that cause pneumonia, including *P. haemolytica*.

Management and environment also appear to play significant, although often not clearly defined, roles in other diseases. Examples include enzootic pneumonia and enteritis in calves (Roy, 1980), enteric disease in suckling pigs, porcine pneumonia, bovine mastitis associated with *Escherichia coli* and *Streptococcus uberis* (Francis *et al.*, 1979) and mastitis in intensively housed sows (Muirhead, 1976).

In some instances, the infectious agents that are isolated are ubiquitous and can also be isolated from healthy animals, for example, enteric organisms (Isaacson *et al.*, 1978). These are 'opportunistic' pathogens, only causing disease when other detrimental factors are also present.

In all of these cases, attempts to identify a causal agent by fulfilling Koch's postulates frequently fail, unless unnatural techniques, such as abnormal routes of infection and the use of gnotobiotic animals, are applied.

## Economics

Owners of companion animals (cats, dogs, other small animals and leisure horses) are usually willing to pay for any veterinary treatment, within reasonable limits. However, farm animals are reared as economic units and so the cost of their treatment and of preventive measures needs to be considered in relation to any financial benefits that would accrue. This is true both on the individual farm and at the national level. One reason for the subsequent recrudescence of rinderpest in Africa following the JP15 campaign was a lack of appreciation of the long-term value of continued vaccination of calves because of the seemingly high cost (Rossiter *et al.*, 1983). The microbial revolution did not provide animal owners and government decision-makers with the means of economically evaluating disease and its control.

# The fifth period

These 20th century animal health problems and anomalies stimulated a change in attitude towards disease causality and control which began in the 1960s.

## Causality

The inappropriateness of Koch's postulates as criteria for defining the cause of some syndromes suggested that more than one factor may operate in producing disease. A **multifactorial** theory of disease has developed, equally applicable to non-infectious and infectious diseases. Interest in human diseases of complex and poorly understood cause grew after the Second World War and was responsible for the development of new methods for analysing risk factors, for example smoking in relation to lung cancer (Doll, 1959). These epidemiological techniques are also being applied in veterinary medicine.

## New control strategies

Two major strategies have been added to the earlier techniques (Schwabe, 1980a,b):

(1) the structured recording of information on disease;
(2) the analysis of disease in populations.

The collecting of disease information is not new; the ancient Japanese reported outbreaks of animal disease and in the 17th century John Graunt collected human mortality data in England. The newer methods, however, involve two complementary approaches: the continuous collection of data on disease, termed **surveillance** and **monitoring**, and the intensive investigation of particular diseases. A further technique, used at the individual farm level, is the recording of information on both the health and productivity of each animal in a herd, as a means of improving production by improving herd health.

## Emerging trends

Diseases of food animals are being considered directly in relation to their effect on production. Reduced levels of production can be used as 'diagnostic indicators'. For example small litter size as an indicator of infection with porcine parvovirus. More significantly, veterinary emphasis has shifted from disease as a clinical entity in the individual animal to disease assessed in terms of suboptimal health, manifested by decreased herd performance: disease is being defined as the unacceptable performance of groups of animals. There is thus a need to identify all factors that contribute to the occurrence of disease, to select suitable 'performance indicators' (e.g. 'calving to conception interval'), and to define normal production targets for these indicators in herds under a particular system of husbandry. It is then possible to identify those herds that fall short of the targets. This is called **performance related diagnosis**. It includes not only the measurement of overt indicators, such as liveweight gain, but also estimation of covert biochemical values, such as metabolite levels in serum. Although these techniques are being applied mainly to food animals such as dairy cattle, there is an increasing interest in biochemical changes as performance indicators in other animals such as racehorses (Dant and Blackmore, 1981).

The veterinarian therefore is becoming more involved in husbandry, management and nutrition than previously, and less involved in traditional 'fire brigade' treatment of clinically sick animals. The livestock owner frequently still regards the veterinarian solely as a dispenser of treatment (Goodger and Ruppanner, 1982), relying on feed representatives, dairy experts and nutritionists for advice on breeding, nutrition and management. The extent of this problem varies from one country to another, but indicates that the veterinarian's evolving involvement in animal production requires a change not only in veterinary attitudes but also sometimes in those of animal owners.

The diseases associated with intensive animal production currently are essentially major problems in developed countries that have intensive animal industries (although some developing countries also have intensive enterprises, such as poultry and pig units in Malaysia and the Philippines). These diseases will become increasingly significant in developing countries when the mass infectious diseases are controlled.

There is also a requirement for improved disease-reporting systems at farm, national and international level to identify problems, define research and control priorities and assist in the prevention of spread of infectious agents from one country to another. Established organizations, such as the *Office International des Epizooties*, are modifying their goals and techniques, taking account of these new requirements (Blajan, 1982).

Government veterinary services will probably become more concerned with investigations of specific animal health problems of complex cause, thereby extending their role beyond the traditional control of mass infectious diseases.

The advent of low cost computing following the microelectronic revolution offers powerful means of storing and analysing data. Also, information can be transported rapidly using modern communications systems. These developments increase the scope for efficient disease-reporting and analysis of the many factors that contribute to clinical disease and suboptimal production, both of which require increased statistical acumen among veterinarians. Epidemiology has developed to supply these contemporary veterinary requirements.

## Further reading

BRITISH VETERINARY ASSOCIATION TRUST PROJECT (1982) *Future of Animal Health Control—The Control of Infectious Diseases in Farm Animals*. Report of a symposium, University of Reading, 14–16 December 1982. British Veterinary Association, London

DAVIES, G. (1985) Art, science and mathematics: new approaches to animal health problems in the agricultural industry. *Veterinary Record*, **177**, 263–267

MELBY, E.C. (1985) The veterinary profession: changes and challenges. *Cornell Veterinarian*, **75**, 16–26

MINISTRY OF AGRICULTURE, FISHERIES AND FOOD (1965) *Animal Health: A Centenary 1865–1965*. Her Majesty's Stationery Office, London

MORRIS, R.S. (1982) New techniques in veterinary epidemiology—providing workable answers to complex problems. In: *Epidemiology in Animal Health*. Proceedings of a symposium held at the British Veterinary Association's Centenary Congress, Reading, 22–25 September 1982. Pp. 1–16. Society for Veterinary Epidemiology and Preventive Medicine

PENNY, R.H.C. (1976) Preventive medicine: the science and

art. In: Proceedings of the International Pig Veterinary Society, 4th Congress, June 22–24, 1976. Opening session (unpaginated). Ames, Iowa

SCHWABE, C.W. (1978) *Cattle, Priests and Progress in Medicine*. The Wesley W. Spink lectures on comparative medicine, Vol. 4. University of Minnesota Press, Minneapolis

SMITHCORS, J.F. (1957) *Evolution of the Veterinary Art*. Veterinary Medicine Publishing Company, Kansas City

WINSLOW, C.E.A. (1944) *The Conquest of Epidemic Disease*. Princeton University Press, Princeton

# 2

# The scope of epidemiology

Many contemporary disease problems can be solved by an investigation of animal populations rather than the individual. The natural history of infectious diseases can be understood by studying their amount and distribution in different populations. The measurement of the amount of infectious and non-infectious diseases in a population assists in determining their importance and the efficacy of control campaigns. Complex and unknown causes of diseases can be elucidated by studying the diseases in various groups of animals. The effects of diseases on production can be realistically estimated only in relation to decreased production in the herd or flock rather than in a single animal. The economic impact of disease and of attempts at its control similarly are evaluated best in groups of animals, ranging from the individual farm to the national level. The investigation of disease in **populations** is the basis of epidemiology.

## Definition of epidemiology

Epidemiology is **the study of disease in populations and of factors that determine its occurrence**, the key word being **populations**. Veterinary epidemiology involves observing animal populations and making inferences from the observations.

A literal translation of the word 'epidemiology', based on its Greek roots επι- (*epi-*)=upon, δημο- (*demo-*)=people, and λογο- (*logo-*)=discoursing, is 'the study of that which is upon the people' or, in modern parlance, 'the study of disease in populations'. Traditionally, epidemiology related to studies of human populations, and epizootiology, from the Greek ζωο- (*zoo-*)=animal, to studies of animal (excluding human) populations. Outbreaks of disease in human populations were called epidemics, in

animal populations were called epizootics and in avian populations were called epornitics, from the Greek ορνιθ- (*ornith-*) = bird (e.g. Montgomery *et al.*, 1979).

The various derivatives can be used in different contexts. A study of a disease that is present only in an animal population, such as *Brucella ovis* infection of sheep, would not involve a simultaneous study of disease in humans; the term 'epizootiology' might then be used by some to indicate that the study was confined to animals other than man. Many diseases, called **zoonoses**, may be shared by man and lower animals. Thus, when studying diseases such as bovine brucellosis and leptospirosis, both of which are zoonoses, mechanisms of transfer of disease between human and non-human populations have to be considered. An important factor that determines the occurrence of such occupationally acquired zoonoses (in veterinarians, abattoir workers and farmers in these examples) is the amount of disease in domestic animals. The 'epidemiology' of brucellosis and leptospirosis in dairy farmers is therefore closely associated with the 'epizootiology' of these diseases in cattle. The semantic differentiation between studies involving human diseases and those concerned with animal diseases therefore is considered neither warranted nor logical. Throughout this book, the word epidemiological is used to describe any investigation relating to disease in a population, whether the population consists of humans, domestic animals, or wildlife.

## The uses of epidemiology

There are five objectives of epidemiology:

(1) determination of the origin of a disease whose cause is known;

(2) investigation and control of a disease, whose cause initially is unknown;

(3) acquisition of information on the ecology and natural history of a disease;

(4) planning and monitoring of disease control programmes;

(5) assessment of the economic effects of a disease and analysis of the costs and economic benefits of alternative control programmes.

## Determination of the origin of a disease whose cause is known

Many diseases with a known cause can be diagnosed precisely by the signs exhibited by the affected animals, by appropriate laboratory tests and by other clinical procedures such as radiological investigation. For instance, the diagnosis of salmonellosis in a group of calves is relatively straightforward (the infection frequently produces distinct clinical signs). However, determining why an outbreak occurred and using the correct procedures to prevent recurrence can be difficult. For example, the outbreak may have been caused either by the purchase of infected animals or by contaminated food. Further investigations are required to identify the source of infection. When the food is suspected, the ration may consist of several components. Even if a sample of each component is still available, it would be expensive and possibly uneconomic to submit all of the samples for laboratory examination. Consideration of the risk associated with the consumption of each component of the ration may narrow the field of investigation to only one or two items.

There are many examples of the investigation of diseases with known causes that involve answering the questions: 'why has an outbreak occurred?' or 'why has the number of cases increased?'. For instance, an increased number of actinobacillosis cases in a group of cattle might be associated with grazing a particular pasture of 'burnt off' stubble. Such an occurrence could be associated with an increase in abrasions of the buccal mucosae which could increase the animals' susceptibility to infection with *Actinobacillus lignieresi*. An increased number of cases of bone defects in puppies might be due to local publicity given to the use of vitamin supplements, resulting in their administration to animals that were already fed a balanced diet, with consequent hypervitaminosis D and osteodystrophy (Jubb and Kennedy, 1971). An increase in the number of lamb carcasses with high ultimate pH values could be associated with excessive washing of the animals prior to slaughter (Petersen, 1983). These possible explanations can be verified only by epidemiological investigations.

## Investigation and control of a disease whose cause initially is unknown

There are many historical instances of disease control based on epidemiological observations before a cause was identified. Examples include contagious bovine pleuropneumonia, which was eradicated from the USA by an appreciation of the infectious nature of the disease before the causal agent, *Mycoplasma mycoides*, was isolated (Schwabe, 1984). Lancisi's slaughter policy to control rinderpest, mentioned in Chapter 1, was based on the assumption that the disease was infectious, even though the causal agent had not been discovered. Similarly, Edward Jenner's classical observations on the protective effects of cowpox virus against human smallpox infection in the 18th century (Fisk, 1959), before viruses were isolated, laid the foundations for the global eradication of smallpox.

Although the exact cause of 'blood splash' (ecchymoses in muscle) in carcasses is still not known, observations have shown that there is a correlation between this defect and electrical stunning by a 'head only' method (Blackmore, 1983). The occurrence of this condition can be reduced by either stunning animals with a captive bolt or by using a method of electrical stunning that causes concurrent cardiac dysfunction.

The cause of squamous cell carcinoma of the eye in Hereford cattle ('cancer eye') is not known. Epidemiological studies have shown that animals with unpigmented eyelids are much more likely to develop the condition than those with pigment (Anderson *et al.*, 1957). This information can be utilized by cattle breeders to select animals with a low susceptibility to this neoplasm.

## Acquisition of information on the ecology and natural history of a disease

An animal that can become infected with an infectious agent is a **host** of that agent. Hosts and agents exist in communities that include other organisms, all of which live in particular environments. The aggregate of all facts relating to animals and plants is their **natural history**. Related communities and their environments are termed **ecosystems**. The study of ecosystems is **ecology**.

A comprehensive understanding of the natural history of infectious agents is possible only when they are studied in the context of their hosts' ecosystems. Similarly, an improved knowledge of non-infectious diseases can be obtained by studying the ecosystems and the associated physical features with which affected animals are related. The geological structure of an ecosystem, for example, can affect the mineral content of plants and therefore can be an important factor in the occurrence of mineral deficiencies and excesses in animals.

The environment of an ecosystem affects the survival rate of infectious agents and of their hosts. Thus, infection with the helminth *Fasciola hepatica* is a serious problem only in poorly drained areas, because the parasite spends part of its life-cycle in a snail which requires moist surroundings.

Each of the 200 antigenic types (serovars) of *Leptospira interrogans* is maintained in one or more species of hosts. Serovar *copenhageni*, for instance, is maintained primarily in rats (Babudieri, 1958). Thus, if this serovar is associated with leptospirosis in either man or domestic stock, then part of a disease control programme must involve an ecological study of rat populations and control of infected rats. Similarly, in Africa, a herpesvirus that produces infections without signs in wildebeeste is responsible for malignant catarrhal fever of cattle (Plowright *et al.*, 1960). Wildebeeste populations, therefore, must be investigated when attempting to control the disease in cattle.

An ecosystem's climate is important because it limits the geographical distribution of infectious agents that are transmitted by arthropods by limiting the distribution of the arthropods.

Infectious agents may extend beyond the ecosystems of their traditional hosts. This has occurred in bovine tuberculosis in the UK, where the badger population appears to be an alternative host for *Mycobacterium tuberculosis* (Little *et al.*, 1982; Wilesmith *et al.*, 1982). Similarly, in certain areas of New Zealand, wild opossums are infected with this bacterium and can therefore be a source of infection to cattle (Thorns and Morris, 1983). Purposeful routine observation of such infections provides valuable information on changes in the amount of disease and relevant ecological factors and may therefore indicate necessary changes in control strategies.

Infectious diseases that are transmitted by insects, ticks and other arthropods, and which may be maintained in wildlife, present complex ecological relationships and even more complex problems relating to their control. Comprehensive epidemiological studies of these diseases help to unravel their life-cycles, and can indicate suitable methods of control.

## Planning and monitoring of disease control programmes

The institution of a programme to either control or eradicate a disease in an animal population must be based on a knowledge of the amount of the disease in that population, the factors associated with its occurrence, the facilities required to control the disease, and the costs and benefits involved. This information is equally important for a mastitis control programme on a single dairy farm and for a national brucellosis eradication scheme involving all the herds in a country. The epidemiological techniques that are employed include the routine collection of data on disease in populations (monitoring and surveillance) to decide if the various strategies are being successful.

Surveillance is also required to determine whether the occurrence of a disease is being affected by new factors. For example, during the eradication scheme for bovine tuberculosis in New Zealand, opossums became infected in certain areas. New strategies had to be introduced to control this problem (Julian, 1981). During the foot-and-mouth disease epidemic in the UK in 1967 and 1968, surveillance programmes indicated the importance of wind-borne virus particles in the transmission of the disease (Smith and Hugh-Jones, 1969). This additional knowledge was relevant to the establishment of areas within which there was a restriction of animal movement, thus facilitating eradication of the disease.

## Assessment of the economic effects of a disease and of its control

The cost of the control of disease in the livestock industry must be balanced against the economic loss attributable to the disease. Economic analysis is therefore required. This is an essential part of most modern planned animal health programmes (exceptions are found in diseases of companion and sacred animals). Although it may be economic to reduce a high level of disease in a herd or flock, it may be uneconomic to reduce even further the level of a disease that is present at only a very low level. If 15% of the cows in a herd were affected by mastitis, productivity would be severely affected and a control programme would be likely to reap financial benefit. On the other hand, if less than 1% of the herd were affected, the cost of further reduction of the disease might not result in a sufficient increase in productivity to pay for the control programme.

This introduction to the uses of epidemiology indicates that the subject is relevant to many areas of veterinary science. The general agricultural practitioner is becoming increasingly concerned with herd health. The companion animal practitioner is faced with chronic refractory diseases, such as the idiopathic dermatoses, which may be understood better by an investigation of the factors that are common to all cases. The state veterinarian cannot perform his routine duties without reference to disease in the national animal population. The diagnostic pathologist investigates the associations between causes and effects (i.e. lesions); this approach is epidemiological when inferences are made from groups of animals. The veterinarian in abattoirs and meat-processing plants attempts to reduce the occurrence of defects and contamination by identifying and eliminating their causes. Similarly, industrial veterinarians, concerned with the design of field trials, compare disease rates and response to treatment in various groups of animals that are treated or managed differently (e.g. drug trials).

## Types of epidemiological investigation

There are four approaches to epidemiological investigation that traditionally have been called 'types' of epidemiology. These types are **descriptive**, **analytical**, **experimental** and **theoretical** epidemiology.

### Descriptive epidemiology

Descriptive epidemiology involves observing and recording diseases and possible causal factors. It is usually the first part of an investigation. The observations are sometimes partially subjective, but, in common with observations in other scientific disciplines, may generate hypotheses that can be tested more rigorously later. Darwin's theory of evolution, for example, was derived mainly from subjective observations, but with slight modification it has withstood rigorous testing by plant and animal scientists.

### Analytical epidemiology

Analytical epidemiology is the analysis of observations using suitable diagnostic and statistical tests.

### Experimental epidemiology

The experimental epidemiologist observes and analyses data from groups of animals from which he can select and in which he can alter the factors associated with the groups. An important component of the experimental approach is the control of the groups. Rarely, a 'natural' experiment can be conducted when the naturally occurring disease or another fortuitous circumstance approximates closely to the ideally designed experiment.

In many cases, veterinary research has proceeded directly from the descriptive to the experimental stage without much quantitative analysis of naturally occurring disease.

### Theoretical epidemiology

Theoretical epidemiology consists of the representation of disease using mathematical 'models' that attempt to simulate natural patterns of disease occurrence.

## Components of epidemiology

The components of epidemiology are summarized in *Figure 2.1*. The first stage in any investigation is the collection of relevant data. The main sources of information are outlined in Chapter 10. Methods of storing and retrieving information are discussed in Chapter 11. Investigations can be **qualitative** or **quantitative** or a combination of these two approaches.

## *Qualitative investigations*

### The natural history of disease

The ecology of diseases, including the distribution, mode of transmission and maintenance of infectious diseases, is investigated by field observation. Ecological principles are outlined in Chapter 7. Methods of transmission and maintenance are described in Chapter 6 and patterns of disease occurrence are described in Chapter 8. Field observations may also reveal information about factors that may directly or indirectly cause disease. The various factors that react to produce disease are described in Chapter 5.

### Causal hypothesis testing

If field observations suggest that certain factors may be causally associated with a disease then the association must be assessed by formulating a causal hypothesis. Causality (the relating of causes to effects) and hypothesis formulation are described in Chapter 3.

Qualitative investigations were the mainstay of epidemiologists before the Second World War. These epidemiologists were concerned largely with the identification of unknown causes of infectious disease and sources of infection. Some interesting examples of the epidemiologist acting as a medical 'detective' are described by Roueché (1967).

## *Quantitative investigations*

Quantitative investigations involve measurement (e.g. the number of cases of disease), and therefore expression and analysis of numerical values. Basic methods of expressing these values are outlined in Chapters 4 and 12. The types of measurement that are encountered in veterinary medicine are described in Chapter 9. Quantitative investigations include **surveys**, **monitoring and surveillance**, **studies**, **modelling** and the biological and economic **evaluation of disease control**.

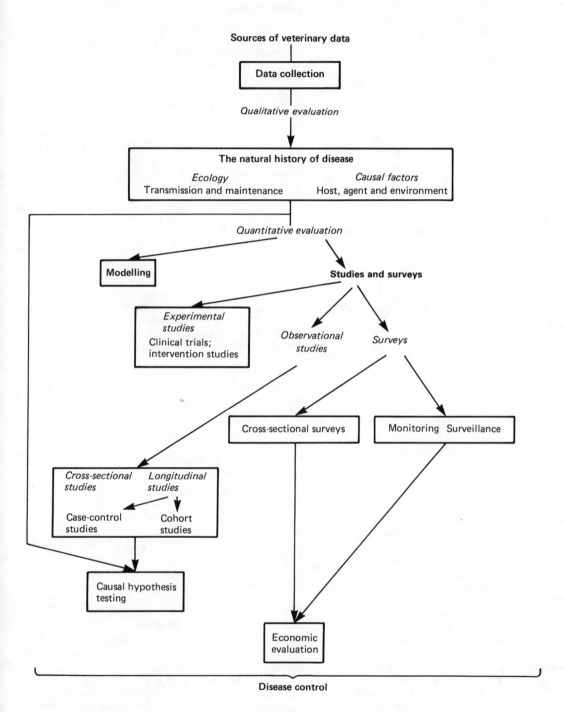

**Figure 2.1**  Components of veterinary epidemiology. (Adapted from Thrusfield, 1985a)

## Surveys

A **survey** is an examination of an aggregate of units (Kendall and Buckland, 1982). A group of animals is an example of an aggregate. The examination usually involves counting members of the aggregate and characteristics of the members. In epidemiological surveys, characteristics might include the presence of particular diseases, weight, and milk yield. Surveys can be undertaken on a **sample** of the population. Less commonly, a census, which examines the **total** animal population, can be undertaken (e.g. tuberculin testing). A **cross-sectional** survey records events occurring at a particular point in time. A **longitudinal** survey records events over a period of time. These latter events may be recorded **prospectively** from the present into the future, or may be a **retrospective** record of past events.

A particular type of diagnostic survey is **screening**. This is the identification of undiagnosed cases of disease using rapid tests or examinations. The aim is to separate individuals that probably have a disease from those that probably do not. Screening tests are not intended to be diagnostic; individuals with positive test results (i.e. classified as diseased by the screening test) require further investigation for definite diagnosis.

The design of surveys is described in Chapter 14. Serological surveys and screening are considered separately in Chapter 16.

## Monitoring and surveillance

**Monitoring** is the making of routine observations on health, productivity and environmental factors and the recording and transmission of these observations. Thus, the regular recording of milk yields is monitoring, as is the routine recording of meat inspection findings at abattoirs. The identity of individual diseased animals is not usually recorded.

**Surveillance** is a more intensive form of data recording than monitoring. Originally, surveillance was used to describe the tracing and observation of people who were in contact with cases of infectious disease. It is now used in a much wider sense (Langmuir, 1965) to include all types of disease—infectious and non-infectious—and involves the collation and interpretation of data collected during monitoring programmes, usually with the recording of the identity of diseased individuals, with a view to detecting changes in a population's health. It is normally part of control programmes for specific diseases. The recording of tuberculosis lesions at an abattoir, followed by tracing of infected animals from the abattoir back to their farms of origin, is an example of surveillance. The terms 'monitoring' and 'surveillance' have previousl, been used synonymously but the distinction between them is now generally accepted. The national and international

aspects of surveillance are reviewed by Davies (1980) and Ellis (1980) respectively.

Monitoring and surveillance can include all of the national herd. Alternatively, a few farms, abattoirs, veterinary practices or laboratories may be selected; these are then referred to as 'sentinel' units because they are designed to 'keep watch' on a disease. Similarly, stray dogs can be used as sentinels for canine parvovirus infection (Gordon and Angrick, 1985), the infection being identified serologically. Other species of animals that are also susceptible to an infectious agent can be used as 'sentinels' for infection in the main animal population. For example, wild birds can be used to monitor the activity of St Louis encephalitis virus, providing early information on the activity of the virus at a time when avian infection rates are still too low to pose an immediate threat to man (Lord *et al.*, 1974).

## Studies

'Study' is a general term that refers to any type of investigation. However, in epidemiology, a study usually involves **comparison** of groups of animals, for example a comparison of the weights of animals fed different diets. Thus, although a survey could generally be classified as a study, it is excluded from epidemiological studies because it involves only **description** rather than comparison and the analysis that the comparison requires. There are four types of epidemiological study:

(1) experimental studies;
(2) cross-sectional studies;
(3) case-control studies;
(4) cohort studies.

In an **experimental study** the investigator has the ability to allocate animals to various groups, according to factors which the investigator can randomly assign to animals (e.g. treatment regimen, preventive technique). Examples are **clinical trials** and **intervention studies**. In a clinical trial, the investigator assigns animals either to a group that is treated with one or more drugs or to an untreated control group. It is then possible to evaluate the efficacy of treatment. In an intervention study, the investigator 'intervenes' in the potential or actual development of a disease by altering possible causal factors (e.g. changing diet). Details of experimental studies may be found in standard texts such as Witts (1964) and Oldham (1968).

The other types of study—cross-sectional, case-control and cohort—are **observational**. An observational study is similar to an experimental study: animals are allocated to groups with respect to certain characteristics that they possess (trait, disease, etc.). However, in observational studies, it is not possible to assign animals to groups randomly because the investigator has little control over the factors that are being studied; the characteristics are **inherent** (e.g. sex, weight and usual diet).

A **cross-sectional** study investigates relationships between disease (or other health-related factors) and hypothesized causal factors in a specified population. Animals are categorized according to presence and absence of disease and hypothesized causal factors; inferences then can be made about associations between disease and the hypothesized causal factors, for example between heart valve incompetence (the disease) and breed (the hypothesized causal factor).

A **case-control** study compares a group of diseased animals with a group of healthy animals with respect to exposure to hypothesized causal factors. For example, a group of cats with urolithiasis (the disease) can be compared with a group of cats without urolithiasis with respect to consumption of dry cat food (the factor) to determine whether that type of food has an effect on the pathogenesis of the disease.

In a **cohort study**, a group exposed to factors is compared with a group not exposed to the factors with respect to the development of a disease. It is then possible to calculate a level of risk of developing the disease in relation to exposure to the hypothesized causal factors.

Case-control and cohort studies often have been applied in human medicine in which experimental investigations of cause are usually unethical. For example, it would not be possible to investigate the suspected toxicity of a drug by intentionally administering the drug to a group of people in order to study possible side-effects. However, if symptoms of toxicity have occurred, then a case-control study could be used to evaluate the association between the drug suspected of causing the toxicity and the symptoms. There are fewer ethical restraints on experimental investigation in veterinary medicine than in human medicine and so experimental investigation of serious conditions is more tenable. However, observational studies have a role in veterinary epidemiology, for example when investigating diseases in farm and companion animal populations. The increasing concern for animal welfare could make these techniques even more useful than previously.

Basic methods of assessing association between disease and hypothesized causal factors in observational studies are described in Chapters 13 and 15.

Observational studies form the majority of epidemiological studies. Observational and experimental science have their own strengths and weaknesses, which are discussed in detail by Trotter (1930). A major advantage of an observational investigation is that it studies the natural occurrence of disease. Experimentation may separate factors associated with disease from other factors that may have important interactions with them in natural outbreaks.

## Modelling

Disease dynamics and the effects of different control strategies can be simulated using mathematical equations. This simulation is 'modelling'. Many modern methods rely heavily on computers. Another type of modelling is biological simulation using experimental animals (frequently laboratory animals) to simulate the pathogenesis of diseases that occur naturally in animals and man. Mathematical modelling is outlined in Chapter 17.

## Disease control

The goal of epidemiology is to improve the veterinarian's knowledge so that diseases can be controlled effectively. This can be fulfilled by treatment, prevention or eradication. The economic evaluation of disease and its control is discussed in Chapter 18. Herd health schemes are described in Chapter 19. Finally, the principles of disease control are outlined in Chapter 20.

The different components of epidemiology apply the four epidemiological approaches to varying degrees. Surveys and studies, for example, consist of a descriptive and an analytical part. Modelling additionally may include a theoretical approach.

# Is epidemiology a science?

## *The interplay between epidemiology and other sciences*

During the first half of the 20th century most epidemiologists were trained initially as bacteriologists, reflecting epidemiologists' early involvement in the investigation of outbreaks of infectious disease. The epidemiological approach is now practised by veterinarians from many disciplines: the parasitologist studying the life-cycles and dynamics of helminth, arthropod and protozoan infections, the geneticist concerned with an hereditary defect in a population, and the nutritionalist investigating a deficiency or toxicity.

Today, members of a variety of other sciences also take part in epidemiological studies: statisticians analysing data from groups of animals, mathematicians modelling diseases, economists costing disease outbreaks, and ecologists studying the natural history of disease. Each of these sciences is concerned with different facets of epidemiology, ranging from the purely descriptive, qualitative approach to the quantitative analytical approach. There have been many definitions of epidemiology (Lilienfeld, 1978), which reflect these facets. These definitions vary from the ecological, relating only to infectious diseases ('the study of the ecology of infectious diseases': Cockburn, 1963), to the mathematical, referring only to human populations ('the study of the distribution and dynamics of diseases in human populations': Sartwell, 1973). However, they all have the study of populations in common, and so are encompassed by the broad definition that was given at the beginning of this chapter.

Many of the techniques used in epidemiological investigations have been developed in sciences other than epidemiology: statistical tests for assessing association and methods of sampling populations are examples. This raises the question: is epidemiology a separate science or merely a way of thinking that applies a variety of methods borrowed from other sciences? (Terris, 1962). When the bacteriologist undertakes a field survey, is he practising a distinct science called epidemiology, or is he using statistical sampling methods merely to add credence to a bacteriological hypothesis, formulated from experimental results derived in the laboratory? The difference between a science and a method is more than a semantic one: 'If epidemiology is seen merely as an adjunct to experimental research, it will be shackled with the same limitations and subject to the same narrow perspectives. It will either continue to be an amateur sport—that of making subjective observations in the field in order to raise an hypothesis that can be examined at the laboratory bench—or exist simply to add some respectability to experimental findings that on their own are unconvincing' (Davies, 1983). If epidemiology is a science then it has a separate identity and is free to develop its own methods.

The differentiation between science and method may not be easy (Himsworth, 1970). There will be those who hold the opinion that a proposed new science is merely a variation of their own, and there will be those who feel, with equal conviction, that the concepts and methods of traditional subjects are inadequate, and that an allegedly new field can be approached only on its own merits.

Trotter (1932) has suggested two considerations when judging the individuality of a science: **quality** and **distinction**. The quality of data relating to the science must be such that they can be analysed scientifically and methods of analysis must be available. The field of natural experience that is to be investigated by the science must also be distinct from those investigated by other sciences, to the extent that only the methods of the new science will extend knowledge in that field.

Over the last decade, veterinary epidemiology has fulfilled these two criteria (Davies, 1983). An example is the field investigation of foot-and-mouth disease by Smith and Hugh-Jones (1969), mentioned earlier in this chapter. They plotted the spread of the disease during the 1967/68 epidemic in the UK and concluded that virus particles could be disseminated by wind. The epidemiological data have been refined by laboratory investigation of virus excretion and, with meteorological data, have been used to formulate a model to predict dispersion of the virus that is of direct value in the planning of disease control campaigns (Gloster *et al.*, 1981). This work fulfils the two criteria of quality and distinction: the quality of the data is such that they can be analysed, and the field of natural experience—spread of disease in this case—provides distinctive knowledge. The results of these investigations and the concomitant increased understanding of disease are possible only because of the amalgamation of the techniques of the different sciences that constitutes epidemiology.

## The relationship between epidemiology and other diagnostic disciplines

The biological sciences form an hierarchy, ranging from the study of non-replicating molecules to nucleic acids, organelles, cells, tissues, organs, systems, individuals, groups and, finally, whole communities and ecosystems (Wright, 1959). The various disciplines in veterinary medicine operate at different levels in this hierarchy. The histologist and physiologist study the structure and dynamics of the individual. The clinician and pathologist are concerned with disease processes in the individual: the clinician diagnoses disease using the signs displayed by the patient; the pathologist interprets lesions to produce a diagnosis. The epidemiologist investigates populations, using the frequency and distribution of disease to produce a diagnosis. These three diagnostic disciplines, operating at different levels in the hierarchy, are complementary (Schwabe *et al.*, 1977). The epidemiologist, dealing with the higher level, must have a knowledge of those disciplines 'lower' in the hierarchy—he must be able to see both the 'wood' and the 'trees'. This means that he must adopt a broad rather than a specialist approach, avoiding the dangers of the specialist, dangers that have been described (somewhat cynically) by Konrad Lorenz (1977) in his book on the natural history of human knowledge:

'The specialist comes to know more and more about less and less, until finally he knows everything about a mere nothing. There is a serious danger that the specialist, forced to compete with his colleagues in acquiring more and more pieces of more and more specialised knowledge, will become more and more ignorant about other branches of knowledge, until he is utterly incapable of forming any judgement on the role and importance of his own sphere within the context of human knowledge as a whole'.

Thus the major attributes required to become a competent veterinary epidemiologist are a natural curiosity, a logical approach, a general interest in and knowledge of veterinary medicine, and a capability for lateral thinking. In spite of the preceding remarks on specialists, a special interest and expertise in a particular sphere of veterinary science may, however, be useful in some investigations, for example, a knowledge of economics when undertaking an evaluation of the economic effects of disease.

Epidemiology is becoming more quantitative than previously. A knowledge of statistics is therefore desirable. However, many problems can be solved without the use of complex statistical methods. Statisticians can always be consulted; the epidemiologist should know **when** to seek their advice.

The ensuing chapters describe epidemiological concepts and techniques. They also include material from other sciences, such as statistics, immunology, economics and computer science, that is relevant to the practice of contemporary veterinary epidemiology.

## Further reading

DAVIES, G. (1983) Development of veterinary epidemiology. *Veterinary Record*, **112**, 51–53

FERRIS, D.H. (1967) Epizootiology. *Advances in Veterinary Science*, **11**, 261–320

MORRIS, R.S. (1982) New techniques in veterinary epidemiology—providing workable answers to complex problems. In *Epidemiology in Animal Health*. Proceedings of a symposium held at the British Veterinary Association's Centenary Congress, Reading, 22–25 September 1982. Pp. 1–16. Society for Veterinary Epidemiology and Preventive Medicine

RIEMANN, H. (1982) Launching the new international journal 'Preventive Veterinary Medicine'. *Preventive Veterinary Medicine*, **1**, 1–4

THRUSFIELD, M.V. (1980) The scope and content of epidemiology courses in veterinary curricula. In: *Veterinary Epidemiology and Economics*. Eds Geering, W.A., Roe, R.T. and Chapman, L.A. Proceedings of the Second International Symposium, Canberra, 7–11 May, 1979. Pp. 303–314. Australian Government Publishing Service, Canberra

# 3

# Some general epidemiological concepts

Chapters 1 and 2 have outlined the development and scope of veterinary epidemiology. This chapter introduces some specific epidemiological terms and concepts that will be applied in succeeding chapters.

## Endemic, epidemic, pandemic and sporadic occurrence of disease

### Endemic occurrence

'Endemic' is used in two senses to describe:

(1) the **usual frequency of occurrence** of a disease in a population;
(2) the **constant presence** of a disease in a population.

Thus the term implies a stable state; if a disease is well understood, its endemic level is often **predictable**. The term endemic can be applied not only to overt disease but also to disease in the absence of clinical signs and to levels of circulating antibodies. Therefore, the exact context in which the term is used should always be defined. For example, laboratory mice kept under conventional systems of 'non-barrier maintenance' (i.e. with no special precautions being taken to prevent entry and spread of infection into the population) are invariably infected with the nematode *Syphacia obvelata*. Infection of 100% of the mice would be considered the usual level of occurrence, that is, the endemic level of infection. When a disease is continuously present to a high level, affecting all age-groups equally, it is **hyperendemic**. In contrast, the endemic level of actinobacillosis in a dairy herd is likely to be less than 1%.

'Endemic' is applied not only to infectious diseases but also to non-infectious ones: the veterinary meat hygienist is just as concerned with the endemic level of carcass bruising as is the veterinary practitioner with the endemic level of pneumonia in pigs.

When endemic disease is described, the affected population and its location should be specified. Thus, although bovine tuberculosis is endemic in badgers in SW England, the infection apparently is not endemic in all badger populations in the UK (Little *et al.*, 1982).

### Epidemic occurrence

'Epidemic' originally was used only to describe a sudden, usually unpredictable, increase in the number of cases of an infectious disease in a population. In modern epidemiology, an epidemic is an occurrence of an infectious or non-infectious disease to a level **in excess of the expected (i.e. endemic) level**. Thus, infection with *S. obvelata* should be absent from specific pathogen free (SPF) mice kept under strict barrier conditions where precautions are taken to prevent entry and spread of infectious agents in the colony. If an infected mouse gained entry to the colony the infection would be transmitted throughout the resident population and an epidemic of the nematode infection would occur. Such an infection in SPF mice colonies would be **unusually frequent**, that is epidemic. Similarly, if cattle grazed on rough pasture which could abrade their mouths there might be an increase in the number of cases of actinobacillosis. Although only 2% of the animals might become infected, this would be an unusually high (epidemic) level compared with the endemic level of 1% in the herd. Thus, an epidemic need not involve a large number of individuals.

When an epidemic occurs, the population must have been subjected to one or more factors that were not present previously. In the example of the SPF mouse colony that became infected with *S. obvelata*, the factor was a breakdown in barrier maintenance and the entry of an infected mouse. In the case of the herd with actinobacillosis, the new factor was an increased consumption of vegetation that could cause buccal abrasions.

The popular conception of an epidemic is an outbreak of disease that is noticed immediately. However, some epidemics may go undetected for some time after their occurrence. Thus, in London, in 1952, the deaths of 4000 people were associated with a particularly severe smog (fog intensified by smoke). The deaths occurred at the same time as the Smithfield fat stock show (HMSO, 1954). Although an epidemic of severe respiratory disease in the cattle was recognized immediately and was associated with the air pollution caused by the smog, the epidemic of human respiratory disease was not appreciated until statistics recording human deaths were published more than a year later.

In contrast, some epidemics may be exaggerated. An increased number of deaths in foxes occurred in the UK in the late 1950s. This apparent epidemic of a 'new' fatal disease received considerable publicity and every dead fox was assumed to have died from the disease. Subsequent laboratory analyses identified chlorinated hydrocarbon poisoning as the cause of the increased fox fatality, but only 40% of foxes submitted for post-mortem examination had died from the poisoning. The other 60% had died of endemic diseases that had not previously stimulated general interest (Blackmore, 1964). This example illustrates that the endemic level of disease in a population has to be known before an epidemic can be recognized.

## Pandemic occurrence

A pandemic is a widespread epidemic that usually affects a large proportion of the population. Many countries may be affected. Pandemics of rinderpest (*see Table 1.1*), foot-and-mouth disease, and African swine fever have been the cause of considerable financial loss. More recently, in 1978 and 1979, a pandemic of parvovirus infection occurred in dogs in many parts of the world (Carmichael and Binn, 1981). Serious human pandemics have included plague (the Black Death) in the Middle Ages, cholera in the 19th century and influenza soon after the First World War.

## Sporadic occurrence

A sporadic outbreak of disease is one that occurs **irregularly and haphazardly**. This implies that appropriate circumstances have occurred **locally**, producing small localized outbreaks.

Foot-and-mouth disease is not endemic in the UK. A sporadic outbreak, thought to be associated with the importation of infected meat from South America, occurred in Oswestry in October 1967 (Hugh-Jones, 1972). Unfortunately this incident resulted in an epidemic that was not eliminated until the middle of 1968 (*Figure 3.1*). However, the disease did not become endemic because of veterinary intervention. Conversely, in 1969, a single sporadic case of rabies occurred in a dog in the UK after it had completed the statutory 6-month quarantine period (Haig, 1977). No other animal was infected and so this sporadic outbreak was confined to the original case.

Thus 'sporadic' can indicate either a single case or a cluster of cases of a disease or infection (without obvious disease) that is not normally present in an area.

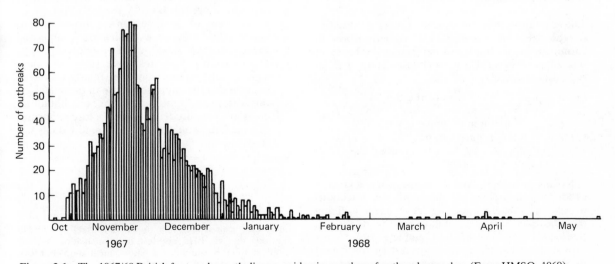

**Figure 3.1**  The 1967/68 British foot-and-mouth disease epidemic: number of outbreaks per day. (From HMSO, 1969)

Infection with *Leptospira interrogans*, serovar *pomona*, is endemic in domestic pigs in New Zealand. The bacterium is also frequently the cause of sporadic epidemics of abortion in cattle. Infected cattle excrete the bacterium in their urine only for approximately 3 months. The bacterium therefore cannot usually be maintained, and so become endemic, in the herd. If a cow becomes infected with the bacterium by direct or indirect contact with pigs, this constitutes sporadic infection. This animal may now become a short-term source of infection to other pregnant cattle in the herd, and a sporadic epidemic of abortion, of 3 or 4 months' duration, is likely to occur. Post-infection leptospiral antibodies persist for many years in cattle and sporadic infection with the bacterium is not uncommon; 18% of New Zealand cattle have detectable antibodies to this organism. Thus, although infection and the abortion that may ensue are **sporadic**, there is an **endemic** level of antibody in the bovine population (Hathaway, 1981).

## The cause of disease

The cause of events is of general relevance to all branches of science; general causal concepts are discussed by Taylor (1967). In epidemiology, studies are undertaken to identify causes of disease so that preventive measures can be developed and implemented. Chapter 1 indicated that there has been a transition from the idea that disease has a predominantly single cause to one of multiple causes. The former idea is epitomized by Koch's postulates.

### Koch's postulates

The increased understanding of microbial diseases in the late 19th century led Robert Koch to formulate his postulates to determine the cause of infectious disease. These postulates state that an organism is causal if:

(1) it is present in all cases of the disease;
(2) it does not occur in another disease as a fortuitous and non-pathogenic parasite;
(3) it is isolated in pure culture from an animal, is repeatedly passaged, and induces the same disease in other animals.

Koch's postulates brought a necessary degree of order and discipline to the study of infectious disease. Few would argue that an organism fulfilling the above criteria does not cause the disease in question; but is it the **sole** and **complete** cause? Koch provided a rigid framework for testing the causal importance of a microorganism but ignored the

influence of environmental factors that were relatively unimportant in relation to the lesions that were being studied. Microbiologists found it difficult enough to satisfy the postulates without concerning themselves with interactions between complex environmental factors. Therefore the microorganisms were assumed to be the sole causes of the diseases that the microbiologists were investigating.

Dissatisfaction became evident in two groups. Some microbiologists thought that the postulates were too difficult to satisfy because there can be obstacles to fulfilling Koch's postulates with some infectious agents that are causes of disease. Others thought that the postulates were insufficient because they did not specify the environmental conditions that turned vague associations into specific causes of disease. Furthermore, the postulates were not applicable to non-infectious diseases. A more cosmopolitan theory of cause was needed.

### Evans' postulates

Evans (1976) has produced a set of postulates that are consistent with modern concepts of causation:

(1) the proportion of individuals with the disease should be significantly higher in those exposed to the supposed cause than in those who are not;
(2) exposure to the supposed cause should be present more commonly in those with than in those without the disease, when all other risk factors are held constant;
(3) the number of new cases of disease should be significantly higher in those exposed to the supposed cause than in those not so exposed, as shown in prospective studies;
(4) temporally, the disease should follow exposure to the supposed cause with a distribution of incubation periods on a bell-shaped curve*;
(5) a spectrum of host responses, from mild to severe, should follow exposure to the supposed cause along a logical biological gradient;
(6) a measurable host response (e.g. antibody, cancer cells) should appear regularly following exposure to the supposed cause in those lacking this response before exposure, or should increase in magnitude if present before exposure; this pattern should not occur in individuals not so exposed;

---

*The bell shape is usually obtained only when the horizontal 'time' axis is mathematically transformed (Sartwell, 1950, 1966; Armenian and Lilienfeld, 1974); if a linear time scale is used then the curve is usually positively skewed, that is there are few long incubation periods relative to the number of short incubation periods. Mathematical transformation is described in Chapter 12.

(7) experimental reproduction of the disease should occur with greater frequency in animals or man appropriately exposed to the supposed cause than in those not so exposed; this exposure may be deliberate in volunteers, experimentally induced in the laboratory, or demonstrated in a controlled regulation of natural exposure;

(8) elimination (e.g. removal of a specific infectious agent) or modification (e.g. alteration of a deficient diet) of the supposed cause should decrease the frequency of occurrence of the disease;

(9) prevention or modification of the host's response (e.g. by immunization or use of specific lymphocyte transfer factor in cancer) should decrease or eliminate the disease that normally occurs on exposure to the supposed cause;

(10) all relationships and associations should be biologically and epidemiologically credible.

An important characteristic of Evans' postulates is that they require the association between an hypothesized causal factor and the disease in question to be **statistically significant**. This involves comparing **groups** of animals, rather than investigating associations in the individual.

Demonstration of a statistically significant association, however, **does not prove** that a factor is causal. The logical reduction of proof requires that the mechanism of induction of a disease by a cause needs to be explained by describing the chain of events, from cause to effect, at the molecular level. However, in the absence of experimental evidence, epidemiological identification of an association can be of considerable preventive value because it can indicate factors, the reduction or removal of which reduces the occurrence of disease. Some of the statistical techniques of demonstrating association are described in Chapter 13.

## Variables

The object of detailed statistical analysis is to identify those factors that cause disease. Disease and causal factors are examples of **variables**.

### Variable (variate)

A variable is any observable event that can vary. Examples of variables are the weight and age of an animal and the number of cases of disease.

### Study variable

A study variable is any variable that is being considered in an investigation.

### Response and explanatory variables

A response variable is one that is affected by another (explanatory) variable. For example, an animal's weight may be a response variable and food intake an explanatory variable, because weight is assumed to be affected by the amount of food consumed. In epidemiological investigations, disease is often considered as the response variable. For example, when studying the effects of dry cat food on the occurrence of urolithiasis, cat food is the explanatory variable and urolithiasis the response variable. There may also be circumstances in which disease is the explanatory variable, for example when studying the effect of disease on weight. Response variables are sometimes called 'dependent variables' and explanatory variables 'independent variables'. These terms will also be encountered in Chapters 12 and 13 and will be defined again more fully in those chapters.

## Types of association

Association is the degree of dependence or independence between two variables. There are two main types of association (*Figure 3.2*):

(1) non-statistical association;
(2) statistical association.

### Non-statistical association

A non-statistical association between a disease and an hypothesized causal factor is an association that arises by chance; that is the frequency of joint occurrence of the disease and factor is no greater than would be expected by chance.

For example, *Mycoplasma felis* has been isolated from the eyes of some cats with conjunctivitis. This represents an association between the mycoplasma and conjunctivitis in these cats. However, studies have shown that *M. felis* also can be recovered from the conjunctivae of 80% of apparently normal cats (Blackmore *et al.*, 1971). Analysis of these findings revealed that the association between conjunctivitis

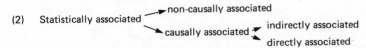

(1)   Statistically unassociated

(2)   Statistically associated — non-causally associated / causally associated — indirectly associated / directly associated

**Figure 3.2**   Types of association between disease and hypothesized causal factors.

and the presence of *M. felis* arose by chance: the mycoplasma could be present in healthy cats as well as in those with conjunctivitis. In such circumstances, where a chance non-statistical association occurs, a factor cannot be inferred to be causal.

## Statistical association

Variables are positively statistically associated when they occur together more frequently than would be expected by chance.

When attempting to establish causal relationships, even in the most carefully designed study, not all of the factors that are statistically associated with a disease are causal. This can be understood with the aid of a simple path diagram (*Figure 3.3a*). The explanatory variable, A, is the cause of a disease.

The response variables, B and C, are two manifestations of the disease. In these circumstances, there is a statistical causal association between A and B, and between A and C. There is also a statistical association between the two response variables, B and C, arising from their separate associations with A, but this is a non-causal association.

An example of these associations is given in *Figure 3.3b*. If infection of cattle with *Haemonchus contortus* were being investigated, then the following statistical associations could be found:

(1) between the presence of the parasite and abomasal mucosal hyperplasia;
(2) between the presence of the parasite and anaemia;
(3) between abomasal mucosal hyperplasia and anaemia.

The first two associations are causal and the third non-causal.

Abomasal mucosal hyperplasia and infection with *H. contortus* are **risk indicators** (**risk markers**) of anaemia, that is their presence increases the risk of anaemia. Thus risk indicators may be either causal or non-causal. Causal risk indicators are called **risk factors**. (Some authors use 'risk factor' synonymously with 'risk indicator', that is including causally and non-causally associated factors.) A knowledge of risk indicators is useful in identifying populations at which veterinary attention should be directed. Thus, high milk yield is a risk indicator of ketosis in dairy cattle. When developing preventive measures it is important to identify those risk indicators that are causal, against which control should be directed, and those that are non-causal and will not therefore affect the development of disease.

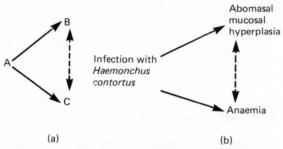

(a)    (b)

**Figure 3.3** Path diagrams indicating the paradigm (**a**) and an example (**b**) of causal and non-causal statistical associations. A = cause of disease (explanatory variable); B = manifestations of disease (response variables); ⟶ causal association; ◄---► non-causal association.

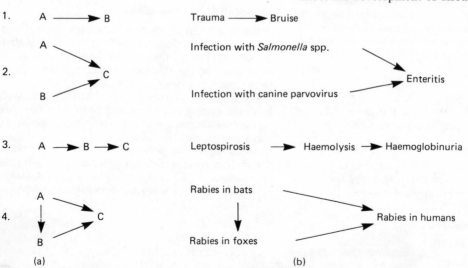

(a)    (b)

**Figure 3.4** Path diagrams indicating paradigms (**a**), and examples (**b**) of direct and indirect causal associations: 1 and 2 = direct causal associations; 3 = indirect causal association (A with C), direct causal association (B with C); 4 = direct and indirect causal association (A with C).

Explanatory and response variables can be causally associated either **directly** or **indirectly**, as shown in *Figure 3.4*. Path diagrams 1 and 2 illustrate direct causal associations. Indirect associations are characterized by an intervening variable. Path diagram 3 illustrates an indirect causal association between A and C where the effect of A is entirely through the intervening variable B, whose effect is direct. This is equivalent to saying that A and B operate at different levels, therefore either A or B can be described as the cause of C. Leptospirosis, for example, causes haemoglobinuria by haemolysing red blood cells; a clinician would say that leptospirosis causes the haemoglobinuria, whereas a pathologist might attribute it to intravascular haemolysis.

Path diagram 4 in *Figure 3.4* illustrates the situation where one explanatory variable, A, has not only a direct causal association with a response variable, C, but also an indirect effect on C by influencing another variable, B. For example, in the USA people have contracted rabies by inhalation on entering caves where rabies-infected bats roost. They can also contract rabies from foxes that have been infected by living in bat-infested caves.

## Causal models

The associations and interactions between direct and indirect causes can be viewed in two ways, producing two causal 'models'.

### Causal model 1

The relationship of causes to their effects allows the classification of causes into two types: 'sufficient' and 'necessary' (Rothman, 1976).

A cause is **sufficient** if it inevitably produces an effect (assuming that nothing happens that interrupts the development of the effect, such as death or prophylaxis). A sufficient cause virtually always comprises a range of component causes; disease therefore is **multifactorial**. Frequently, however, one component is commonly described, in general parlance, as **the** cause. For example, distemper virus is referred to as the cause of distemper, although the sufficient cause actually involves exposure to the virus, lack of immunity and, possibly, other components. It is not necessary to identify all components of a sufficient cause to prevent disease because removal of one component may render the cause insufficient. For example, an improvement in floor design can prevent foot abscesses in pigs even though the main pyogenic bacteria are not identified.

A particular disease may be produced by different sufficient causes. The different sufficient causes may have certain component causes in common, or they

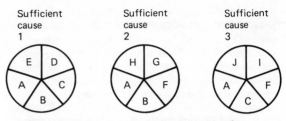

**Figure 3.5**  Conceptual scheme for the causes of an hypothetical disease (causal model 1). (From Rothman, 1976)

may not. If a cause is a component of every sufficient cause then it is **necessary**. Therefore, a necessary cause must always be present to produce an effect, for example, distemper virus is a necessary cause of distemper.

In *Figure 3.5*, A is the only necessary cause, because it is the only component appearing in all of the sufficient causes. The remaining causes (B–J) are not necessary because there are some sufficient causes without them. It is obvious that necessary causes are frequently related to the definition of a disease, for example lead is a necessary cause of lead poisoning.

A cause may be necessary, sufficient, neither, or both. It is unusual for a single component cause to be both necessary and sufficient. One example is exposure to large doses of gamma radiation and the development of radiation sickness.

An example of a cause that is necessary but not sufficient is infection with *Actinobacillus lignieresi*, which must occur before wooden tongue can develop. However, other factors that damage the buccal mucosae (e.g. sharp, abrasive vegetation) must be present before the disease occurs. In the absence of these factors the bacterium can be present without disease developing.

Therefore, factors include ones that can be classified as:

(1) **predisposing factors**, which increase the level of susceptibility in the host (e.g. age);
(2) **enabling factors**, which facilitate manifestation of a disease (e.g. housing and nutrition);
(3) **precipitating factors**, which are associated with the definitive onset of disease (e.g. many toxic and infectious agents);
(4) **reinforcing factors**, which tend to aggravate the presence of a disease (e.g. repeated exposure to an infectious agent in the absence of an immune response).

Pneumonia is an example of a disease that has sufficient causes, none of which has a necessary component. Pneumonia may have been produced in one case by heat stress where a dry, dusty environment allowed microscopic particulate matter to reach the alveoli. Cold stress could produce a clinically similar result.

Multifactorial syndromes such as pneumonia can have many sufficient causes, although none is necessary. Part of the reason is taxonomic: pneumonia is a loosely connected group of diseases whose classification (*see Chapter 9*) is based on lesions (inflammation of the lungs) rather than specific causes; the lesions can be produced by many different causes. When a disease is classified according to aetiology there is, by definition, usually only one major cause, which therefore is likely to be necessary. Examples include lead poisoning, mentioned above, and many 'simple' infectious diseases, such as tuberculosis and brucellosis.

The object of epidemiological investigations of cause is the identification of sufficient causes and their component causes. Removal of one or more components from a sufficient cause will then prevent disease produced by that sufficient cause.

### Causal model 2

Direct and indirect causes represent a chain of actions, with the indirect causes activating the direct causes (e.g. *Figure 3.4*, path diagram 3). When many such relationships occur, a number of factors can act at the same level (but not necessarily at the same intensity), and there may be several levels, producing a 'web of causation'. Again, disease is **multifactorial**. *Figure 3.6* illustrates the causal web of bovine hypomagnesaemia.

## *Confounding*

Confounding (Latin: *confundere* = to mix together) is the effect of an extraneous variable that can wholly or partly account for an apparent association between variables. Confounding can produce a spurious association between study variables, or can mask a real association. A variable that confounds is called a **confounding variable** or **confounder**.

A confounding variable is distributed non-randomly (i.e. is positively or negatively correlated with the explanatory and response variables that are being studied). A confounding variable must:

(1) be a risk indicator for the disease that is being studied;
    **and**
(2) be associated with the explanatory variable, but not be a consequence of exposure to the explanatory variable.

### Examples to illustrate the concept

An investigation of leptospirosis in dairy farmers in New Zealand (Mackintosh *et al.*, 1980) revealed that wearing an apron during milking was associated with an increased risk of contracting leptospirosis. Further work showed that the larger the herd being milked, the greater the chance of contracting leptospirosis. It was also found that farmers with large herds tended to wear aprons more frequently

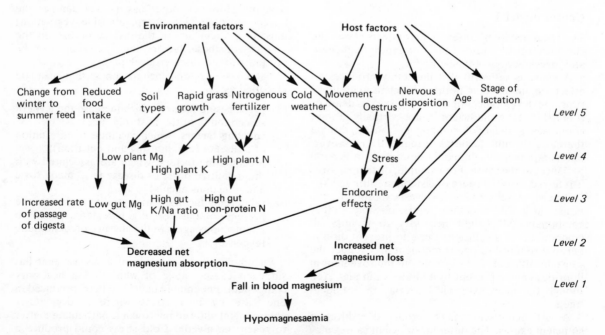

**Figure 3.6**   Causal web of bovine hypomagnesaemia (causal model 2).

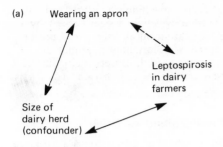

(a)      Wearing an apron

Leptospirosis
in dairy
farmers

Size of
dairy herd
(confounder)

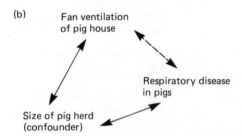

(b)      Fan ventilation
of pig house

Respiratory disease
in pigs

Size of pig herd
(confounder)

**Figure 3.7** Examples of confounding: (**a**) large dairy herds in relation to leptospirosis in dairy farmers and the wearing of milking aprons; (**b**) large pig herds in relation to respiratory disease in pigs and fan ventilation. ⟷ 'Real' association; ←- - - -→ spurious association.

for milking than farmers with small herds. The association between the wearing of aprons and leptospirosis was not causal but was produced spuriously by the confounding effect of large herd size (*Figure 3.7a*), because large herd size was associated with leptospirosis, and also with the wearing of aprons. *Figure 3.7b* illustrates a similar confounding effect in relation to respiratory disease in pigs (Willeberg, 1980b). A statistical association was demonstrated between fan ventilation and respiratory disease. This was not because fan ventilation caused respiratory disease. The association resulted from the confounding effect of herd size: large herds are more likely to develop respiratory disease than small herds, and are also more likely to have fan ventilation rather than natural ventilation.

These two examples have been selected to illustrate confounding in situations where the spurious association is obviously rather implausible. However, in many situations, confounding is less obvious but must be considered, for example in observational studies that test causal hypotheses (*see* Chapter 15).

# Formulating a causal hypothesis

The first step in any epidemiological investigation of cause is descriptive. A description of **time**, **place**, and **population** is useful initially.

## Time

Associations with year, season, month, day, or even hour in the case of food poisoning investigations should be considered. Such details may provide information on climatic influences, incubation periods and sources of infection. For example, an outbreak of salmonellosis in a group of cattle may be associated with the introduction of infected cattle feed.

## Place

The geographical distribution of a disease may indicate an association with local geological, management or ecological factors, for example nutritionally deficient soil or arthropod transmitters of infection. Epidemiological maps (*see* Chapter 4) are a valuable aid to identifying geographical associations.

## Population

The type of animal that is affected is often of considerable importance. Hereford cattle are more susceptible to squamous cell carcinoma of the eye than other breeds, suggesting that the cause may be partly genetic. In many parts of the world, meat workers are affected more often by Q fever than are other people, implying a source of infection in meat-processing plants.

When the major facts have been established, alternative causal hypotheses can be formulated. An epidemiological investigation is similar to any detective novel that unfolds a list of 'suspects' (possible causal factors), some of which may be non-statistically associated with a disease, and some statistically associated with the disease, either causally or non-causally.

There are four major methods of arriving at an hypothesis:

(1) method of difference;
(2) method of agreement;
(3) method of concomitant variation;
(4) method of analogy.

## Method of difference

If the frequency of a disease is different in two different circumstances, and a factor is present in one circumstance but is absent from the other, then the factor may be suspected of being causal. For example, Wood (1978) noted an increased occurrence of stillbirths in pigs in one of three farrowing houses. The only difference between this house and the other two was a different type of burner on its gas heaters. An hypothesis was formulated: that the different type of burner caused the stillbirths. Subsequently, the burners were shown to be defective and producing large amounts of carbon monoxide; the carbon monoxide was assumed to cause the stillbirths. The occurrence of stillbirths decreased when the faulty burners were removed, thus supporting the hypothesis.

A defect of an hypothesis based on the method of difference is that several different factors may be incriminated as possible causes. The value of an hypothesis generated by this method is reduced if many alternative hypotheses can be formulated. For example, a comparison of the different disease patterns of pigs in Africa and Denmark would involve a large number of variables, many of which could be hypothesized as causal. In contrast, the marked occurrence of mannosidosis in Angus cattle (Jolly and Townsley, 1980), compared with the absence of this disease in other breeds, strongly suggests that a genetic factor is the cause.

## Method of agreement

If a factor is common to a number of different circumstances in which a disease is present, the factor may be the cause of the disease. Thus, if a batch of meat and bone meal was associated with salmonellosis on widely different types of pig farms, and this was the only circumstance in common, then the causal hypothesis—that disease was caused by contamination of that batch—is strengthened.

A second example relates to bovine hyperkeratosis which was identified in cattle in the USA (Schwabe *et al.*, 1977). The disease was called 'X disease', because initially the cause was unknown. It occurred in different circumstances:

(1) in cattle that were fed sliced bread;
(2) in calves that had been licking lubricating oil;
(3) in cattle that were in contact with wood preservative.

The bread slicing machine was lubricated with a similar oil to that which had been licked by the calves. The lubricating oil and the wood preservative both contained chlorinated naphthalene. This chemical was common to the different circumstances and subsequently was shown to cause hyperkeratosis.

## Method of concomitant variation

This method involves a search for a factor, the frequency or strength of which varies continuously with the frequency of the disease in different situations. Thus, the distance over which cattle are transported before slaughter appears to be related to the occurrence of bruises in their carcasses (Meischke *et al.*, 1974). Similarly, there appear to be relationships between the occurrence of squamous cell carcinoma of the skin of animals and the intensity of ultraviolet radiation, between the

**Table 3.2 The relationship between number of cigarettes smoked per day and deaths by lung cancer in British doctors (1951–1961). (From Doll and Hill, 1964a)**

| Cigarettes/day in 1951 | Annual lung cancer death rate/1000 (1951–61) |
|---|---|
| None | 0.07 |
| 1–14 | 0.54 |
| 15–24 | 1.39 |
| ≥25 | 2.27 |

occurrence of bovine hypomagnesaemia and pasture levels of magnesium, and between infection of dairy personnel with leptospires and the frequency with which the personnel milk cows (*Table 3.1*). The classic medical epidemiological investigation of the association between smoking and lung cancer (Doll and Hill, 1964a,b) also illustrates this method of reasoning (*Table 3.2*): the number of deaths due to lung cancer is proportional to the number of cigarettes smoked per day.

## Method of analogy

This method of reasoning involves comparison of the pattern of the disease under study with that of a

**Table 3.1 The relationship between frequency of milking and serological evidence of exposure to leptospirosis in dairy farm personnel in the Manawatu region of New Zealand**

| Frequency of milking of cows by personnel | Serological leptospirosis | | Total number of personnel | Percentage of personnel with serological leptospirosis |
|---|---|---|---|---|
| | Present | Absent | | |
| 9 times/week | 61 | 116 | 177 | 34.5 |
| 1–8 times/week | 4 | 11 | 15 | 26.7 |
| Rarely or never | 8 | 20 | 20 | 0.0 |

disease that is already understood. The cause of a disease that is understood may be the cause of another unknown disease with a similar pattern. For example, some mammary tumours of mice are known to be caused by a virus, therefore some mammary tumours of dogs may have a viral cause. The climatic conditions associated with outbreaks of Kikuyu grass poisoning of cattle may suggest a mycotoxin as the cause because the circumstance is similar to those circumstances present in other mycotoxicoses (Bryson, 1982). Bovine petechial fever, caused by *Cytoecetes ondiri*, is present in a limited area of Kenya (Snodgrass, 1974). The mode of transmission of this infectious agent is unknown. However, other members of the genus *Cytoecetes* are known to be transmitted by arthropods, and geographic limitation is a feature of arthropod-transmitted diseases. Therefore, using the method of analogy, it has been suggested that *C. ondiri* may be transmitted by arthropods.

This method can be dangerously misleading. A classic example is the inference made by the 19th century medical epidemiologist, John Snow, that yellow fever was transmitted by sewage (Snow, 1855). He had already demonstrated that cholera was transmitted by sewage, and then observed that cholera and yellow fever were both associated with overcrowding. He then inferred that cholera and yellow fever had similar modes of transmission, whereas the latter is actually transmitted by an arthropod rather than by contaminated sewage.

When attempting to establish a causal association, five principles should be considered:

(1) the time sequence of the events;
(2) the strength of the association;
(3) biological gradient;
(4) consistency;
(5) compatibility with existing knowledge.

## Time sequence

Cause must precede effect. In a bacteriological survey, Millar and Francis (1974) found an increased occurrence of various infections in barren mares compared with others whose reproductive function was normal. However, unless the bacterial infections were present **before** the mares became infertile, it would be incorrect to infer that the bacterial infections caused infertility. The causal pathway may have been in the other direction: absence of normal reproductive cyclic activity may allow previously harmless infections to flourish.

## Strength of association

If a factor is causal, there will be a strong statistical association between the factor and the disease.

## Biological gradient

If a dose-response relationship can be found between a factor and a disease, the plausibility of a factor being causal is increased. This is the basis of reasoning by the method of concomitant variation. Examples have already been cited: frequency of milking in relation to leptospirosis (*see Table 3.1*) and smoking in relation to lung cancer (*see Table 3.2*).

## Consistency

If an association exists in a number of different circumstances, a causal relationship is probable. This is the basis of reasoning by the method of agreement. An example is bovine hyperkeratosis, mentioned above.

## Compatibility with existing knowledge

It is more reasonable to infer that a factor causes a disease if a plausible biological mechanism has been identified than if such a mechanism is not known. Thus, smoking can be suggested as a likely cause of lung cancer because other chemical and environmental pollutants are known to have a carcinogenic effect on laboratory animals. Similarly, if a mycotoxin were present in animal foodstuffs, then it might be expected to produce characteristic liver damage. On the other hand, the survey of leptospirosis of dairy farmers, mentioned earlier, showed a positive association between wearing an apron and having a leptospiral titre. This finding was not compatible with either existing knowledge or common sense and a factor that might have confounded the result was sought and found.

This chapter has discussed hypothesis formulation. The testing of hypotheses using observational studies is described in Chapter 15.

## *Further reading*

EVANS, A.S. (1976) Causation and disease. The Henle–Koch postulates revisited. *Yale Journal of Biology and Medicine*, **49**, 175–195

HILL, A.B. (1965) The environment and disease: association or causation. *Proceedings of the Royal Society of Medicine*, **58**, 295–300

LAST, A.M. (1983) *A Dictionary of Epidemiology*. Oxford University Press, London

MURPHY, E.A. (1976) *The Logic of Medicine*. Johns Hopkins University Press, Baltimore and London

SUSSER, M. (1973) *Causal Thinking in the Health Sciences. Concepts and Strategies of Epidemiology*. Oxford University Press, New York, London and Toronto

TAYLOR, R. (1967) Causation. In: *The Encyclopaedia of Philosophy*, Vol. 2. Ed. Edwards, P. Pp. 56–66. The Macmillan Company and The Free Press, New York

# 4

# Describing disease occurrence

A necessary part of the investigation of disease in a population is the counting of diseased animals so that the **amount** of disease can be described. Furthermore, it is usually desirable to describe **when** and **where** disease occurs. The amount of disease is the **morbidity** (Latin: *morbus* = disease); the number of deaths is the **mortality**. The times of occurrence of cases of a disease are its **temporal** distribution; the places of occurrence are its **spatial** distribution. The measurement and description of the size of populations and their characteristics is **demography** (Greek: *demo-* = people; *-graphia* = writing, description).

This chapter discusses the types of animal population that are encountered in veterinary medicine, and describes the methods of expressing the amount of, and temporal and spatial distribution of, disease and associated demographic data.

## The structure of animal populations

The structure of populations influences the extent to which population sizes can be assessed, as well as affecting the ways in which disease occurs and persists in animals. The organization of animal populations can usually be described as either **contiguous** or **separated**.

### Contiguous populations

A contiguous population is one in which there is much contact between individuals in the population and members of other populations. Most human populations are contiguous because there is mixing of individuals by travel. Populations of small domestic animals also are usually contiguous. Dogs and cats move freely within cities, coming into contact with other urban, suburban and rural animals of their own and different species. African nomadic tribes similarly own animals that comprise contiguous groups. Many wild animals belong to this category, too, their enumeration involving aerial and ground counts; the techniques are described by Norton-Griffiths (1978).

It is often difficult to assess the size of contiguous animal populations. Some surveys have been undertaken to establish the size of domestic small animal populations, for example, in parts of the USA (Schnurrenberger *et al.*, 1961; Dorn *et al.*, 1967; Schneider and Vaida, 1975) and in Britain (Anderson, 1983). In some developed countries, dogs must be legally registered, but this is a difficult law to enforce and so many dogs may not be recorded. There are pet registries that record and identify animals, for example, by ear or leg tattooing (Anon, 1984), but these records are voluntary and so exclude the majority of animals.

Only limited demographic data about small domestic animals are available, for example, from Kennel Club registers (Tedor and Reif, 1978; Wong and Lee, 1985). Such animals are kept in small numbers—often only one animal per household. It is therefore necessary to contact many owners to gain information about relatively few animals (i.e. the animal:owner ratio is low). This can be a difficult and costly exercise. The results may also be distorted by the lack of information on undetectable segments of the population such as strays, semi-domesticated and feral animals. Non-thoroughbred horses kept as leisure animals similarly are difficult to count.

Contiguous populations predispose to transfer and persistence of infectious diseases over large areas because of the inherent mixing and movement of animals.

## Separated populations

Separated populations occur as discrete, isolated units such as herds and flocks. They are particularly common in countries that practise intensive animal production, with many animals on one farm (e.g. many of the developed countries). *Table 4.1* illustrates the various sizes of these units in the UK; most animals of all species are kept in larger units.

A separated population can be **closed**, with no movement of animals into or out of the unit (except to slaughter). An example is a dairy herd that raises its own replacements, or is under statutory control of movement. Two of the strictest examples of closed populations are the specific pathogen free (SPF) and gnotobiotic colonies of laboratory animals.

A separated population can also be **open**, with limited movement of individuals in and out. Examples include beef herds, where animals are brought in from other farms and markets for fattening, and dairy herds that receive replacements from other farms.

It is often easier to obtain information on the size of a separated than a contiguous population. The large numbers of animals kept under conditions of intensive husbandry in a single separated unit frequently have only one owner (i.e. the animal:owner ratio is high). Many demographic data about food animals are available as a result of regular censuses and estimations. The most extensive sources are the *Animal Health Yearbook* of the *Food and Agriculture Organization of the United Nations* and *Office International des Epizooties*; animal population sizes in *Tables 1.2* and *1.4* were obtained from the first source.

Thoroughbred horses are members of separated (usually open) populations. They are concentrated in stables in major training areas and can be counted easily. Published figures, however, may not be comprehensive. Thoroughbred horses in training in the UK, for example, are recorded annually, but they make up only a small and variable age-group. Stud books provide information on stallions, mares and foals, but may be incomplete.

Separated populations, especially of the closed type, are less likely to be infected with agents from other areas than contiguous populations. However, if infection enters separated populations it may spread rapidly because the animal density frequently is high.

## Measures of disease occurrence

A major reason for determining morbidity is to assess the extent of a problem in a population. This assessment is possible only when the number of diseased animals is compared with the total number of animals in the population. A report of 10 cases of infectious enteritis in a cattery, for example, does not indicate the true extent of the problem unless the report is considered in terms of the number of cats in the cattery: there may be only 10 cats present, in which case all of the cats are affected, or there may be 100 cats, in which case only a small proportion of the cats is affected. Similarly, a knowledge of the sizes of populations and their composition (e.g. by age and sex) is necessary if disease occurrence in one population is to be compared with that in another. Thus, it is necessary to relate the number of cases of a disease to the **population at risk** of developing the disease.

## Prevalence

Prevalence, $P$, refers to the amount of disease in a known population, at a designated time, without distinction between old and new cases. Thus, annual, monthly and lifetime prevalence can be described. Prevalence is commonly expressed as **point prevalence**, that is, the amount of disease in a population at a particular point in time. Although prevalence can be defined simply as the number of affected animals, it is usually expressed in terms of the number of diseased animals in relation to the number of animals in the population at risk of developing the disease:

$$P = \frac{\text{number of individuals having a disease at a particular point in time}}{\text{number of individuals in the population at risk at that point in time}}.$$

For example, if 20 cows in a herd of 200 cows were lame on a particular day, the prevalence of lameness in the herd on that day would be 20/200, that is, 0.1. This is a **proportion** that represents the **probability** of an animal having a specified disease at a given time. Prevalence can take values between 0 and 1 and is dimensionless.

## Incidence

Incidence is an expression of the number of **new** cases that occur in a known population over a period of time. It measures the **flow** of individuals from the disease-free to the diseased state. The two essential components of an incidence value are:

(1) the number of new cases;
(2) the period of time over which the new cases occur.

Incidence, like prevalence, can be defined simply in terms of the number of affected animals, but is usually expressed in relation to the population at risk.

**Table 4.1 Holdings by size of herd or flock; UK, June 1981. (From HMSO, 1982)**

*Dairy herds*

| | 1–2 | 3–4 | 5–9 | 10–14 | 15–19 | 20–29 | 30–39 | 40–49 | 50–59 | 60–69 | 70–99 | 100–199 | 200+ | Total |
|---|---|---|---|---|---|---|---|---|---|---|---|---|---|---|
| No. of holdings | 4199 | 1253 | 2475 | 3018 | 3257 | 7140 | 6850 | 6492 | 5197 | | 12906 | 7478 | | 60265 |
| No. of cattle | 5644 | 4296 | 17481 | 36023 | 55198 | 173257 | 233666 | 286008 | 279583 | | 981249 | 1113952 | | 3186357 |

*Beef herds*

| | 1–2 | 3–4 | 5–9 | 10–14 | 15–19 | 20–29 | 30–39 | 40–49 | 50–59 | 60–69 | 70–79 | 100–199 | 200+ | Total |
|---|---|---|---|---|---|---|---|---|---|---|---|---|---|---|
| No. of holdings | 16057 | 10384 | 14658 | 9038 | 5559 | 7698 | 4578 | 2808 | 1855 | | 3288 | 1666 | | 77589 |
| No. of cattle | 23957 | 35944 | 97884 | 106034 | 93350 | 182396 | 154246 | 122587 | 99361 | | 247983 | 243340 | | 1407082 |

*Pig herds*

| | 1–2 | 3–9 | 10–19 | 20–29 | 30–49 | 50–69 | 70–99 | 100–199 | 200–399 | 400–999 | 1000–4999 | 5000+ | Total |
|---|---|---|---|---|---|---|---|---|---|---|---|---|---|
| No. of holdings | | 7155 | 3419 | | 4554 | | 3391 | 3261 | 2700 | 2973 | 1895 | | 29348 |
| No. of pigs | | 24870 | 46751 | | 145159 | | 240729 | 465395 | 768037 | 1879751 | 4209376 | | 7780068 |

*Sheep flocks*

| | 1–24 | 25–49 | 50–99 | 100–199 | 200–299 | 300–399 | 400–499 | 500–699 | 700–999 | 1000–1499 | 1500–1999 | 2000+ | Total |
|---|---|---|---|---|---|---|---|---|---|---|---|---|---|
| No. of holdings | 9572 | 7092 | 11520 | 15244 | 9454 | 10844 | | 6205 | 5120 | 5855 | | 2005 | 82911 |
| No. of sheep | 109960 | 258347 | 839352 | 2203989 | 2320670 | 4195922 | | 3656254 | 4262211 | 7995841 | | 6082867 | 31925413 |

*Laying fowls*

| | 1–25 | 26–49 | 50–99 | 100–199 | 200–499 | 500–999 | 1000–2499 | 2500–4999 | 5000–9999 | 10000–19999 | 20000–49999 | 50000+ | Total |
|---|---|---|---|---|---|---|---|---|---|---|---|---|---|
| No. of holdings | 44820 | | 4025 | 3347 | | 568 | 852 | 744 | 657 | 488 | 281 | 152 | 55934 |
| No. of fowls | 747810 | | 246791 | 635405 | | 388611 | 1382530 | 2649769 | 4534033 | 6562725 | 8481891 | 18397971 | 44027536 |

## Cumulative incidence

The cumulative incidence, *CI*, is the proportion of non-diseased individuals at the beginning of a period of study that become diseased during the period:

$$CI = \frac{\text{number of individuals that become diseased during a particular period}}{\text{number of healthy individuals in the population at the beginning of that period}}.$$

Cumulative incidence is dimensionless, and can take values between 0 and 1. Thus, if 20 animals in a cattery develop feline viral rhinotracheitis during a week, and there are 100 cats in the cattery at the beginning of the week, then, for the week:

$$CI = \frac{20}{100}$$
$$= 0.2.$$

The longer the period of observation, the greater the cumulative incidence. Thus, if 10 more cats developed the disease during a second week of observation, the cumulative incidence would be 0.3 for the 2-week period. Cumulative incidence is an indication of the average risk of developing disease during a particular period.

## Incidence rate

Incidence rate, *I*, is the usual measure of incidence:

$$I = \frac{\text{number of cases of disease that occur in a population during a particular period of time}}{\text{the sum, over all individuals, of the length of time at risk of developing disease}}.$$

The denominator is frequently measured as 'animal-years at risk'. This is the sum of the periods of observation for each animal, during which the latter is free from the disease (i.e. is at risk). For example, 6 cows, free from disease, observed for one year would constitute '6 animal-years at risk'; equally, one cow observed for 6 years would constitute '6 animal-years at risk'. An example of calculation of incidence rate is given in *Table 4.2*. This relates to enzootic bovine leucosis, in which instance diseased animals are removed from the herd when they are identified. If animals can recover from, and again become susceptible to, a disease, they contribute to the denominator for as long as they are being observed. The technique assumes that the risk of occurrence of disease is constant during the period of observation (Sheps, 1966). This assumption is generally acceptable, particularly when the risk is low, the study population is large, and the period of observation is short.

Note that incidence rate has a dimension, **time**; incidence rate is calculated **per week**, **per year**, and so on.

**Table 4.2 Example of calculation of incidence rate: enzootic bovine leucosis (EBL). (Hypothetical data)**

| Cow number | Period of observation | Time of development of EBL after beginning of observation | Contribution to animal-years at risk |
|---|---|---|---|
| 1 | 7 years | No disease | 7 years |
| 2 | 7 years | No disease | 7 years |
| 3 | 4 years | 4 years | 4 years |
| 4 | 5 years | No disease | 5 years |
| 5 | 6 years | No disease | 6 years |
| 6 | 8 years | No disease | 8 years |
| 7 | 5 years | 5 years | 5 years |
| 8 | 2 years | No disease | 2 years |
| 9 | 9 years | No disease | 9 years |
| 10 | 5 years | No disease | 5 years |
| | | *Total* = | 58 years |

*Calculation*:
Total number of cases = 2
Incidence rate     = 2 per 58 animal-years at risk
             = 3.5 per 100 animal-years at risk

This technique for calculating incidence is based on the idea that the movement to the diseased state depends on:

(1) the size of the population;
(2) the period of observation;
(3) the 'force of morbidity'.

It is the force of morbidity that is measured by the incidence rate. The measure accommodates movements into and out of the population (e.g. heifers being brought into, and cows leaving, a dairy herd).

Frequently the period of observation of individual animals cannot be recorded. Therefore, the common application of the incidence rate involves using the **average** size of the population during the period of observation, multiplied by the period of observation, as the denominator. Thus, if a herd with an average size of 70 cows was observed for one year, and seven cases of ketosis were recorded, the incidence rate would be:

$$\frac{7}{70} \text{ per year}$$

$$= 0.1/\text{year} \text{ (10 cases per 100 animals per year).}$$

Incidence is discussed in detail by Morgenstern *et al.* (1980).

## *The relationship between prevalence and incidence*

A disease with a long duration is more likely to be detected during a cross-sectional survey than is a disease of short duration. For example, chronic arthritis, lasting for several months, could be detected by a cross-sectional abattoir survey that was undertaken any time during the several months that the arthritis was present. However, clinical louping ill, lasting for a few days, could be detected by a cross-sectional survey only if the survey was conducted during the short period that the disease was apparent.

Prevalence, $P$, therefore depends on the duration, $D$, and incidence, $I$, of a disease:

$$P \propto I \times D.$$

This means that a change in prevalence can be due to:

(1) a change in incidence;
(2) a change in the average duration of the disease;
(3) a change in both incidence and duration.

A decrease in the incidence of a disease such as Johne's disease in cattle will eventually decrease the overall prevalence of the disease. Improvements in the therapy of diseases that are frequently fatal may decrease mortality, but could increase prevalence by prolonging the life of diseased animals that otherwise would have died quickly. For example, antibiotic treatment of acute bacterial pneumonia could decrease the fatality of the disease but increase the number of convalescent animals with chronic pneumonia.

The prevalence of a disease can also be decreased if the duration of the disease is reduced. Improvements in therapy, for instance, may accelerate recovery.

### Calculation of incidence from prevalence

The prevalence of a stable endemic disease **equals** the **product** of incidence and duration:

$$P = I \times D.$$

Therefore, if two components of the equation are known, the third can be calculated. For example, the annual incidence of occupationally acquired leptospirosis in New Zealand dairy farmers has been estimated (Blackmore and Schollum, 1983). Surveys had shown that 34% of farmers had serological reactions to leptospirosis (i.e. the prevalence of seropositive farmers was 0.34). Other work indicated that leptospiral titres of 1/24 or greater persist, on average, for 10 years (i.e. the duration of the infection, expressed as persistence of antibody at that titre, was 10 years). The number of notified cases of human leptospirosis had remained at approximately the same level for more than 10 years. Therefore, it could be assumed that a stable endemic level of disease existed in the human population. Thus:

prevalence (% affected) = 34,
duration (years) = 10.

Therefore:

incidence (% farmers seroconverting per year)
= 34/10
= 3.4% per year.

This estimated annual incidence compares favourably with an annual notification value of 2.1% in dairy farmers in a large dairy region of New Zealand because official notifications are generally an underestimate of the true incidence of a disease.

### Period prevalence

Prevalence and incidence values are sometimes combined as **period prevalence** ($Pp$). This is a measure of the total number of cases of a disease that have existed in a population during a defined period of study. It is the sum of the point prevalence at the beginning of the period ($P$) and the incidence ($Ip$) during the period of study:

$$Pp = P + Ip.$$

This measure is of little value because investigators usually need to distinguish between old and new cases. Whenever the term prevalence is used in this book, it refers to point prevalence, unless otherwise specified.

## *Application of prevalence and incidence values*

Epidemiological investigations of causal factors ideally require a knowledge of incidence. Causal factors operate before a disease is identified. Therefore, an incidence value, recorded as near as possible to the time of onset of a disease, can associate the disease with the action of causal factors.

Prevalence values are less useful than incidence values in investigating causal associations, because the former values are associated not only with the latter values (and therefore time of onset) but also with duration; the prevalence of a disease may be recorded a long time after the causal factors have operated. The main use of prevalence measurements is in indicating the extent of disease problems for administrative purposes and for defining research priorities and long-term disease control strategies. However, in the absence of incidence figures, changes in prevalence figures may suggest underlying changes in incidence.

When attempting to identify causal associations, disease occurrence in the presence of an hypothesized causal factor is compared with disease occurrence in the absence of the factor. This can be conducted either by:

(1) comparing the **absolute** difference between values (e.g. the absolute difference between a cumulative incidence of 0.0010 over 10 years in a group 'exposed' to a factor, and of 0.0001 in an 'unexposed' group, is 0.0009); or
(2) comparing the **relative** difference between the two groups (0.0010/0.0001 = 10, in the above example).

A relative measure obviously indicates the **magnitude** of the difference, and is usually applied in causal studies. Some of these relative measures are outlined in Chapters 13 and 15.

When prevalence is low, and the duration of disease is similar in 'exposed' and 'unexposed' groups, relative comparisons of prevalence produce similar results to relative comparisons of incidence. When prevalence increases, the ratio of prevalence in 'exposed' groups to prevalence in 'unexposed' groups approaches one, and so the association with the hypothesized causal factor is underestimated. In practice, if the prevalence is less than 0.1, underestimation is not significant.

## Ratios, proportions and rates

A ratio is a value obtained by dividing one quantity by another. For example, a male:female sex ratio might be 3:2, the upper figure being the **numerator** and the lower figure the **denominator**. A proportion is a special case of a ratio in which the numerator consists of some of (i.e. is a subset of) the individuals in the denominator. Thus, prevalence, $P$, and cumulative incidence, $CI$, are proportions.

A rate is a ratio that expresses a change in one quantity (the numerator) with respect to another quantity (the denominator). 'Time' is usually included in the denominator. Velocity (e.g. 10 feet per second) is a rate. Epidemiological rates have time as part of the denominator. Incidence rate, $I$, is the commonest epidemiological rate.

However, 'rate' has been suffixed incorrectly to epidemiological proportions in which the numerator is a subset of the denominator. Thus, 'prevalence rate' is commonly used as a synonym for prevalence, although it is not a true rate. Additionally, prevalence (often termed prevalence rate) is frequently expressed as a percentage. Thus, a prevalence of 0.1 may be seen as 'prevalence rate = 10%'. If the disease is rare, then the prevalence may be expressed as:

$$\text{prevalence (rate)} = \frac{\text{number of cases of disease}}{\text{population at risk}} \times 10^n$$

where $n$ is an integer depending on the rarity of the disease. Thus, prevalence may be expressed per 10 000 population at risk ($n = 4$) or per 1000 000 population at risk ($n = 6$).

### Case fatality rate

A case fatality rate (which, again, is a proportion rather than a true rate) is the proportion of diseased animals that die of a disease. It is therefore a measure of the probability of death in diseased animals.

### Example of calculation of prevalence, incidence, mortality and case fatality rates

Suppose a veterinarian investigates a disease that runs a clinical course ending in either recovery with permanent immunity, or death, in a herd of cattle. On 1 July 1983 the herd is investigated when the disease is already present. On 1 July 1984 the herd is re-investigated.

Total herd size on 1 July 1983: 600
Total number clinically ill on 1 July 1983: 100
Total number **becoming** clinically ill between 1 July 1983 and 1 July 1984: 200
Total number dying from the disease from 1 July 1983–1 July 1984: 120

**Prevalence** on 1 July 1983 $= \dfrac{100}{600} = 0.167$ (16.7%).

**Cumulative incidence** 1 July 1983–1 July 1984

$$= \frac{200}{500} = 0.4.$$

**Mortality rate** 1 July 1983–1 July 1984

$$= \frac{120}{600} = 20\% \text{ per year.}$$

**Case fatality rate** 1 July 1983–1 July 1984

$$= \frac{120}{300} = 40\%.$$

### Attack rate

Sometimes a population may be at risk for only a limited period of time, either because exposure to a causal agent is brief, or because the risk of developing the disease is limited to a narrow age-range such as the neonatal period. Examples of the first reason would be the feeding of a batch of food contaminated with a mycotoxin to a herd of cattle, and exposure to radiation during nuclear

**Table 4.3 Some commonly used rates and ratios (indices usually refer to a defined population of animals observed for one year\*). (Modified and expanded from Schwabe et al., 1977)**

### RATES

| Name | Definition |
|---|---|
| No-return rate at $n$ days: | $\dfrac{\text{No. animals bred that have not come back in heat in } n \text{ days after breeding}}{\text{No. animals bred}} \times 10^{a\dagger}$ |
| Pregnancy rate at $n$ days: | $\dfrac{\text{No. animals pregnant at } n \text{ days after breeding}}{\text{No. animals bred}} \times 10^{a}$ |
| Crude live birth rate: | $\dfrac{\text{No. live births occurring}}{\text{Average population}} \times 10^{a}$ |
| General fertility rate: | $\dfrac{\text{No. live births occurring}}{\text{Average no. female animals of reproductive age}} \times 10^{a}$ |
| Crude death rate: | $\dfrac{\text{No. deaths occurring}}{\text{Average population}} \times 10^{a}$ |
| Age-specific death rate: | $\dfrac{\text{No. deaths among animals in a specified age-group}}{\text{Average no. in the specified age-group}} \times 10^{a}$ |
| Calf (lamb, piglet, puppy, etc.) mortality rate: | $\dfrac{\text{No. deaths under a specified age}^{**}}{\text{No. live births}} \times 10^{a}$ |
| Neonatal (calf, lamb, etc.) mortality rate: | $\dfrac{\text{No. deaths under a specified age}^{**}}{\text{No. live births}} \times 10^{a}$ |
| Fetal death rate (also called stillbirth rate): | $\dfrac{\text{No. fetal deaths}}{\text{No. live births plus fetal deaths}} \times 10^{a}$ |
| Cause-specific death rate: | $\dfrac{\text{No. deaths from a specified cause}}{\text{Average population}} \times 10^{a}$ |
| Proportional mortality rate: | $\dfrac{\text{No. deaths from a specified cause}}{\text{Total no. deaths}} \times 10^{a}$ |
| Case fatality rate: | $\dfrac{\text{No. deaths from a specified cause}}{\text{Total no. cases of the same disease}} \times 10^{a}$ |

### RATIOS

| Name | Definition |
|---|---|
| Fetal death ratio (also called stillbirth ratio): | $\dfrac{\text{No. fetal deaths}}{\text{No. live births}} \times 10^{a}$ |
| Maternal mortality ratio: | $\dfrac{\text{No. deaths in dams from puerperal causes}}{\text{No. live births}} \times 10^{a}$ |
| Zoonosis incidence ratio (ZIR): | $\dfrac{\text{No. new cases of a zoonotic disease in an animal species in a given geographic area in a stated time period}}{\text{Average human population in the same area during the same period} \times \text{time}} \times 10^{a}$ |
| Area incidence ratio (AIR): | $\dfrac{\text{No. new cases of a disease in a given time period}}{\text{Unit geographic area in which the observations are made} \times \text{time}} \times 10^{a}$ |

\*All rates could use other specified time periods.
\*\*There is not a universal agreement on the age at which animals cease to be neonates in veterinary medicine.
†$a$ = a whole number, usually between 2 and 6; for example, if $a = 3$, then $10^{a} = 10^{3} = 1000$.

accidents. Even if observations were made on the animals for a long time, the incidence would not change. In these circumstances, when the period of risk is brief, the term **attack rate** is used to describe the proportion of animals that develop the disease.

*Table 4.3* lists some common epidemiological rates.

Proportions and rates are expressed in three main forms: **crude**, **specific** and **adjusted**.

## Crude measures

Crude prevalence and incidence values are an expression of the total amount of a disease in a population; they take no account of the structure of the population affected. For instance, the crude mortality rate of two laboratory colonies of mice could be 10/1000/day and 20/1000/day respectively. Initially this might suggest that the second colony has twice the disease problem of the first, but this difference in crude rates might be due only to a difference in age structure. Mice have a life span of about 2 years, and so if the second colony consisted of much older animals than the first, greater mortality would be expected in the second than the first colony, even without concurrent disease. Although crude rates may express the prevalence or incidence of a particular disease, they take no account of specific host characteristics such as age, sex, breed or method of husbandry, which can have a profound effect on the occurrence of a disease in a population.

## Specific measures

Specific measures of disease are those that describe disease occurrence in specific categories of the population related to certain host attributes, such as age, sex, breed and method of husbandry, and, in man, also race, occupation and socioeconomic group. Specific measures can be calculated for prevalence and incidence.

Specific measures are calculated in a similar manner to crude ones, except that the numerator and denominator apply to one or more categories of a population with specific host attributes. For instance, a whole series of different age-specific incidence rates could be calculated that would cover the entire life span of a particular population. Age-specific incidence rates of many enteric diseases, such as salmonellosis and colibacillosis, can be higher in young animals than in old animals. Sex-specific incidence rates of diabetes mellitus are higher in females than in males.

The breed-specific prevalence of intestinal carcinoma of sheep in New Zealand can reveal more information than the crude prevalence for all sheep. The specific values show that for British breeds the prevalence is 1.25%, and for fine wool breeds it is 0.24% (Simpson, 1972), suggesting a possible genetic association of the disease. The geographic distribution of different breeds of sheep in New Zealand varies considerably. In the Manawatu region, almost 70% of the population is Romney (a British breed) and 25% Perendale, other breeds accounting for the remaining 5%, while in the Christchurch area it probably would include approximately 55% Corriedale, 20% Romney and 20% half-breeds. Therefore, comparison of crude prevalence and mortality in sheep in these two areas would be of little value because no account would be taken of the different breed composition of the populations. The influence of breed in this example is apparently of greater significance to the prevalence of intestinal carcinoma than is the geographical distribution of sheep.

The breed-specific prevalence of squamous cell carcinoma of the eye in cattle reveals that Herefords have the highest prevalence: although there is a crude prevalence of 93/100 000 for all breeds of cattle, the specific prevalence for Herefords and Hereford crosses is 403/100 000. The prevalence of goitre in budgerigars is higher in pet birds than in breeders' birds (Blackmore, 1963). Similarly, the occupation-specific prevalence values of human Q fever in Australia indicate that meat workers are the highest group at risk (Scott, 1981).

The data in *Table 4.4* can be used to illustrate the superiority of specific measures over crude measures. *Table 4.4* lists the period prevalence of testicular Leydig cell tumours in Channel Island and other breeds of dairy cattle over 28 years, in two groups of bulls, calculated as the ratio of the number of recorded cases of the disease to the total of the number of animals present at any time during the period of observation. The data relating to group A

**Table 4.4 Period prevalence of Leydig cell tumours, over a 28-year period, in two groups of bulls. (Data for group A extracted from Sponenberg, 1979; data for group B are hypothetical)**

| Group | Crude period prevalence per 1000 | Period prevalence specific to breed of bull per 1000 | | Proportion of population | |
|---|---|---|---|---|---|
| | | *Channel Island* | *Other breeds* | *Channel Island* | *Other breeds* |
| A | 98 | 198 | 44 | 0.35 | 0.65 |
| B | 88 | 76 | 107 | 0.60 | 0.40 |

refer to bulls resident in an insemination centre at any time during the 28-year period. The data relating to group B are hypothetical. Although the crude period prevalence values, 98 per 1000 and 88 per 1000, are similar for both groups, the values specific to the category of bull are much lower for Channel Island breeds in group B (76/1000) than in group A (198/1000). Conversely, the values specific to other breeds are higher in group B than in group A. These differences are masked by the crude values because of the different proportions of Channel Island and other breeds in each population. The crude values are the weighted summation of the values specific to each class of bull:

Group A:
crude period prevalence (per 1000)
= (198 × 0.35) + (44 × 0.65)
= 69.3 + 28.6
= 98.

Group B:
crude period prevalence (per 1000)
= (76 × 0.60) + (107 × 0.40)
= 45.6 + 42.8
= 88.

Similarly, *Table 4.5a* illustrates that the crude incidence rate of testicular neoplasia in castrated dogs (12.67 per 1000 dog-years at risk) reveals much

**Table 4.5 Specific incidence rates of testicular neoplasia in cryptorchid dogs. (From Reif *et al.*, 1979)**

| (a) Age-specific rates | | | | |
|---|---|---|---|---|
| *Age (years)* | *No. of dogs* | *Dog-years at risk* | *No. of neoplasms* | *Age-specific rate/1000 dog-years* |
| ≤2 | 262 | 411.3 | 0 | 0.00 |
| 2–3 | 153 | 288.8 | 0 | 0.00 |
| 4–5 | 93 | 199.4 | 0 | 0.00 |
| 6–7 | 49 | 103.0 | 7 | 67.96 |
| 8–9 | 31 | 59.2 | 4 | 67.57 |
| ≥10 | 21 | 43.3 | 3 | 69.28 |
| *Total* | 609 | 1 105.0 | 14 | 12.67 |

| (b) Rates specific to location | | | | |
|---|---|---|---|---|
| *Location of testicles* | *No. of dogs* | *Dog-years at risk* | *No. of neoplasms* | *Incidence/ 1000 dog-years* |
| Bilateral scrotal (controls) | 329 | 680.0 | 0 | 0.00 |
| Abdominal-scrotal | 210 | 392.8 | 5 | 12.73 |
| Inguinal-scrotal | 188 | 372.2 | 9 | 24.18 |
| Bilateral abdominal | 54 | 96.8 | 0 | 0.00 |
| Bilateral inguinal | 27 | 52.5 | 0 | 0.00 |
| Inguinal-abdominal | 16 | 30.5 | 0 | 0.00 |
| Cryptorchid unknown | 114 | 160.2 | 0 | 0.00 |

less about the period at risk in a dog's life than the age-specific values. Likewise, the rates specific to location (*Table 4.5b*) indicate at which sites the lesion is most likely to occur.

In most circumstances specific morbidity values are the most useful type of value to calculate when investigating a disease and attempting to describe its pattern and identify possible causal associations. However, if specific values are not available, this deficiency can be solved partly by **adjustment (standardization)**.

## Adjusted (standardized) measures

If, in the example above, morbidity due to Leydig cell tumours were being compared between the two groups of bulls, **irrespective of breed of bull**, which is acting as a confounder, then the crude period prevalence would be misleading owing to difference in breed weighting, whereas the period prevalence specific to breed gives accurate information only about individual categories of the bull population. These difficulties can be partially overcome by using the technique known as **adjustment (standardization)**, by direct or indirect methods.

In **direct** adjustment, a standard population is chosen as a reference, and the prevalence or incidence in specific categories in the population under investigation is multiplied or weighted by the proportion of the similar specific category in the standard population. When these adjusted specific values are summed, the crude values in the population under study then become adjusted to the standard population. A comparison can then be made between the population under study and other populations, similarly adjusted to the standard population, without the comparison being distorted by different proportions of various categories of the population:

$$\text{direct adjusted value} = sr_1 \times \frac{S_1}{N} + sr_2 \times \frac{S_2}{N}$$

where $sr$ = specific value of study population
$S$ = number of specific category in the standard population
$N$ = total number in the standard population ($S_1 + S_2 = N$).

For example, direct adjustment may be applied to the specific period prevalence relating to the two classes of bull (Channel Island and other breeds) in *Table 4.4*, using information on bulls from breed societies as a standard in relation to the overall proportion of the Channel Island and other breeds in the total bull population. If there were 67 000 bulls in the standard population, of which 5600 were Channel Island, then:

for group A:

$$sr_1 \text{ (Channel Island)} = 198$$
$$S_1 = 5600$$
$$N = 67000$$

$$sr_2 \text{ (other breeds)} = 44$$
$$S_2 = 61400$$
$$\qquad \text{(i.e. } 67000 - 5600)$$
$$N = 67000.$$

Adjusted value for group A

$$= 198 \times \frac{5600}{67000} + 44 \times \frac{61400}{67000}$$
$$= 16.6 + 40.3$$
$$= 56.9.$$

Similarly, for group B:

$$sr_1 = 76$$
$$S_1 = 5600$$
$$N = 67000$$

$$sr_2 = 107$$
$$S_2 = 61400$$
$$N = 67000.$$

Adjusted value for group B

$$= 76 \times \frac{5600}{67000} + 107 \times \frac{61400}{67000}$$
$$= 6.4 + 98.1$$
$$= 104.5.$$

If breed of bull were the factor responsible for the differences, the two adjusted values would have been similar. However, if factors other than breed were responsible for the difference in period prevalence between the two groups of bulls, the adjusted values would be different, as in this example, where age might account for the difference. The value could be adjusted simultaneously for age by first calculating the specific value for each age-group and then again adjusting in relation to the overall standard population.

Direct adjustment requires knowledge, for each category, of the numbers of animals and the morbidity in the population for which the adjusted value is needed. If either this information is not available or the numbers in each category are so small that large fluctuations in morbidity occur through the presence or absence of a few cases, the **indirect** method of adjustment can be used.

In an indirect adjustment, a standard population is chosen and the value in each specific category in the standard population is multiplied or weighted by the proportion of the similar specific category in the study population:

$$\text{indirect adjusted value} = Sr_1 = \frac{s_1}{n} + Sr_2 = \frac{s_2}{n}$$

where $Sr$ = specific value of standard population
  $s$ = number of specific sector in study population
  $n$ = total number in the study population $(s_1 + s_2 = n)$.

The advantages, disadvantages and pitfalls associated with adjustment are discussed in detail by Fleiss (1981). In veterinary epidemiology it is often difficult to adjust values because appropriate vital statistics may not be available to aid selection of a suitable standard population. Even when statistics are available, the choice of the standard population is somewhat arbitrary.

### Epidemiological ratios

A ratio has been defined above as a value obtained by dividing one quantity by another. In epidemiology, the term ratio is usually confined to measures where the numerator is **not** drawn from the denominator. For example:

$$\textbf{fetal death ratio} = \frac{\text{number of fetal deaths}}{\text{number of live births}}.$$

In contrast, the so-called **fetal death rate** (actually, like prevalence, a proportion) is given by:

**fetal death rate**

$$= \frac{\text{number of fetal deaths}}{\text{number of fetal deaths} + \text{number of live births}}.$$

Some common veterinary ratios are given in *Table 4.3*.

## Life tables

A life table summarizes mortality in a population; the probability of dying at various ages can then be calculated. The life table can be applied to the onset of disease as well as to death, and so can be used as another means of expressing incidence in terms of the probability of developing disease at different ages.

There are two types of life table:

(1) the **current (period)** life table;
(2) the **cohort (generation)** life table.

The **current** life table summarizes the current mortality or incidence of disease over a brief period of time (1–3 years is common in human medicine). The current life table therefore represents the combined mortality experience, by age, of the population. The age-specific death or incidence rates can be used to follow an **hypothetical** group (cohort) of animals, from birth to death, and show their mortality or disease incidence rates.

The **cohort** life table is produced by following the experience of a **real** group (cohort) of animals, from birth to either development of disease or death. The probability of developing a disease, or of dying, at different ages can then be estimated.

A full description of life tables is beyond the scope of this book. Details may be found in Hill (1971). A worked example is given by Schwabe *et al.* (1977), and an example, relating to the detection of bovine leukaemia virus infection, is described by Thurmond *et al.* (1983).

Frequently life tables cannot be constructed because the composition of a population changes during the time that it is being studied. In such circumstances, risk can be measured using incidence rates with 'animal-years at risk' as the denominator.

## Displaying morbidity and mortality values and demographic data

Morbidity and mortality values and demographic data should be recorded in a way that immediately conveys their salient features such as fluctuations in values. The methods of presentation include **tables**, **bar charts**, and **time trend graphs**.

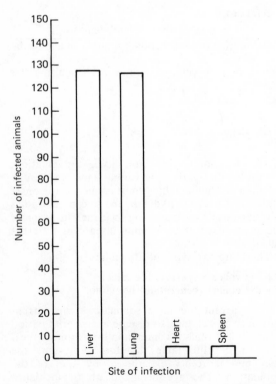

**Figure 4.1**  The distribution of hydatid cysts in organs of 765 Somalian cattle in Kuwait: an example of a bar chart. (Modified from Behbehani and Hassounah, 1976)

### Tables

Tabulation is one of the commoner techniques of displaying numerical data. It involves listing numerical values in rows and columns. An example is given in *Table 4.1*.

### Bar charts

Bar charts display variables by vertical bars that have heights proportional to the number of occurrences of the variable. The bar chart is used to display categories in which counts are **discrete**, that is, they comprise whole numbers, such as numbers of cases of disease. In the example given in *Figure 4.1* the vertical bars are separated by spaces; in some charts adjacent bars touch. (The frequency distribution of **continuous** data—defined in Chapter 9—can be displayed in a similar fashion, in which case the chart is called a **histogram**; an example is given in *Figure 12.1*.) The bar chart strikingly demonstrates differences that would not be noted as easily in tables.

### Time trend graphs

In a time trend graph the vertical position of each point represents the number of cases; the horizontal position corresponds to the midpoint of the time interval in which the cases were recorded. In *Figure 4.2*, for instance, the vertical coordinate of each point is the number of new cases of anthrax and the horizontal coordinate is the midpoint of the weekly intervals for which cases of anthrax were reported.

## Mapping

A common method of displaying the geographical (spatial) distribution of disease is by drawing maps. This is of value not only in the identification of areas where diseases exist but also in investigating the mode and direction of transmission of infectious diseases. For example, the spatial distribution of cases of foot-and-mouth disease during the British outbreak in 1967 suggested that the infection may have been disseminated by wind (Smith and Hugh-Jones, 1969). Subsequent investigations have supported this idea (Hugh-Jones and Wright, 1970; Sellers and Gloster, 1980).

Maps can also suggest possible causes of diseases of unknown aetiology. Mapping indicated that tumours (notably of the jaw) in sheep in Yorkshire clustered in areas where bracken was common (McCrea and Head, 1978). This led to the hypothesis that bracken causes tumours. Subsequently, the hypothesis was supported by experimental investigation (McCrea and Head, 1981).

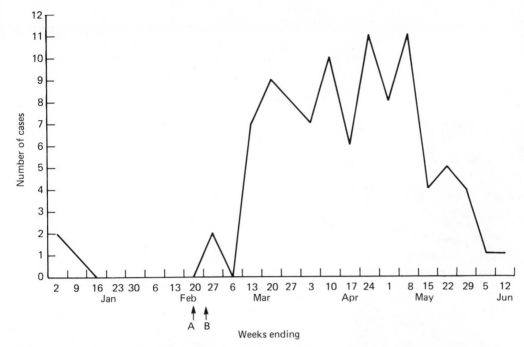

**Figure 4.2**   An anthrax outbreak in cattle in England, 1 January–12 June 1977, associated with a batch of feedstuff: an example of a time trend graph. A = feedstuff unloaded at docks; B = feedstuff arrived at mills. (Modified from MAFF, 1977)

Similarly, comparison of the maps of hypocupraemia in cattle (Leech *et al.*, 1982) with a geochemical atlas (Webb *et al.*, 1978) has indicated areas in England and Wales where bovine copper deficiency may be caused by excess dietary molybdenum.

At their simplest, maps may be qualitative, indicating location without specifying the amount of disease. They can also be quantitative, displaying the number of cases of disease (the numerator in proportions, rates and ratios), the population at risk (the denominator), and prevalence and incidence (i.e. including both numerator and denominator). Maps can be constructed according to the shape of a country or region, in which case they are often drawn to a **geographic base**. Alternatively, they can be drawn to represent the size of the population concerned. These latter, less familiar maps are drawn to a **demographic base.**

## *Geographic base maps*

*Figure 4.3* is an example of a geographic base map. It is a 'conventional' map of Great Britain, showing the shape of the country. Most atlases consist of geographic base maps. There are several types of geographic base map, each with a different purpose and displaying information in varying detail.

### Point (dot or location) maps

These maps illustrate outbreaks of disease in discrete locations, by circles, squares, dots or other symbols. An example is *Figure 4.4*, where the solid circles with adjacent names indicate the sites of outbreaks of bluetongue in Portugal. Point maps are qualitative; they do not indicate the extent of the outbreaks which could each involve any number of animals. Point maps can be refined by using arrows to indicate direction of spread of disease. A series of point maps, displaying occurrence at different times, can indicate the direction of spread of an outbreak of disease.

### Distribution maps

A distribution map is constructed to show the area over which disease occurs. An example is given in *Figure 4.5*, illustrating areas in SE Australia in which fascioliasis is continually present (endemic areas) and those that only experience the disease in wet years. Further examples, showing the world distribution of the major animal virus diseases, are presented by Odend'hal (1983).

### Choroplethic maps

It is possible to display quantitative information, such as animal density, morbidity and mortality, in

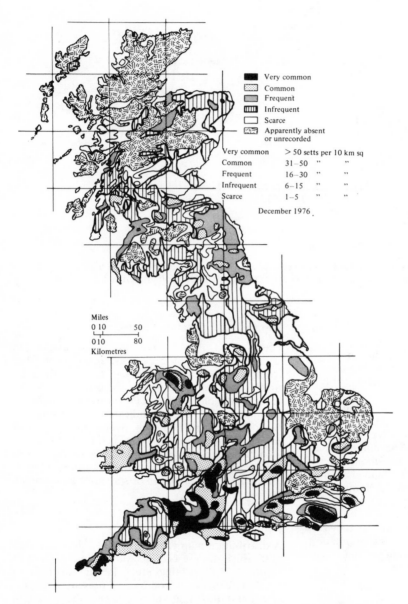

**Figure 4.3** Density of badger setts in Great Britain: an example of an isoplethic map (geographic base). (From Zuckerman, 1980)

43

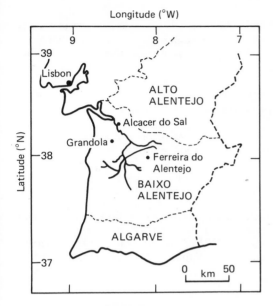

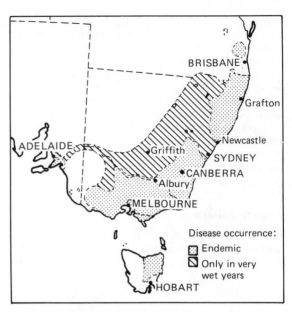

**Figure 4.4** Outbreaks of bluetongue in Portugal, July 1956: an example of a point map. (From Sellers *et al.*, 1978)

**Figure 4.5** Fascioliasis in Australia: an example of a distribution map. (Modified from Barger *et al.*, 1978)

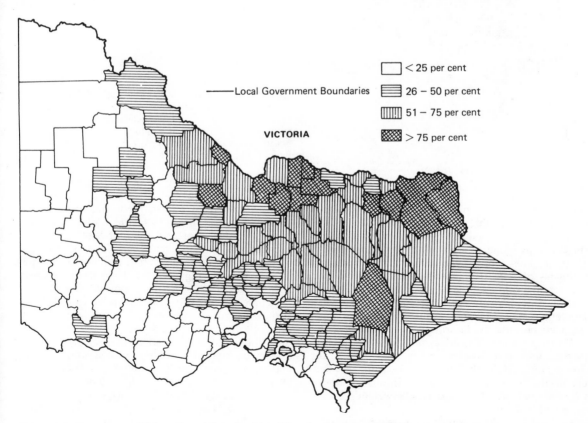

**Figure 4.6** Prevalence of fluke-affected livers by shire, Victoria, Australia, 1977–78: an example of a choroplethic map. (From Watt, 1980)

terms of discrete units of area. These units are usually administrative areas such as parishes, shires, counties or states. Maps that portray information in this way are **choroplethic** (Greek: *choros* = an area, a region; *plethos* = a throng, a crowd, the population). *Figure 4.6* is an example.

Choroplethic maps display quantitative data, but the boundaries between different recorded values are somewhat artificial. They are not the actual boundaries between, for example, high and low prevalence; they are merely the administrative boundaries of the areas for which the displayed average values are calculated.

### Isoplethic maps

True boundaries between different values can be depicted by joining all points of equal value by a line, such as joining points of equal height to

producing an apparently three-dimensional representation which, in this example, shows the occurrence of reported skunk rabies (the annual number of cases reported is proportional to the height of the peaks).

## Demographic base maps

An alternative means of presenting morbidity and mortality information is in relation to population size. Maps depicting information in this way are therefore demographically based. They have the advantage of relating morbidity and mortality to the size of the population at risk. Demographic maps require accurate information on both numerator and denominator in proportions, rates and ratios in defined areas. They are not common in veterinary medicine because this information is often missing.

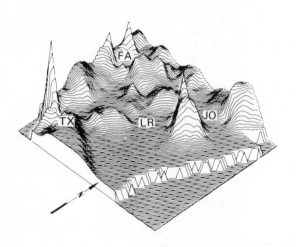

**Figure 4.7**    Occurrence of reported cases of skunk rabies in Arkansas, USA, in 1978: an example of a computer-generated map. The heights of peaks represent numbers of cases. The bases represent geographical areas. Cities: LR = Little Rock; JO = Jonesboro; TX = Texarkana; FA = Fayetteville. (From Heidt *et al.*, 1982)

produce the familiar contour map. Maps produced this way are **isoplethic** (Greek: *iso* = equal). Lines joining points of equal morbidity are **isomorbs**, and those joining points of equal mortality are **isomorts**. If these lines are to be constructed, accurate estimates of both the number of cases of disease (numerator) and the size of the population at risk (denominator) over an area must be known. Isoplethic maps are not common in veterinary medicine because this information is usually absent.

*Figure 4.3* is an isoplethic map showing badger density in Great Britain, drawn as part of an investigation into the role of badgers in the occurrence of bovine tuberculosis. In this example, the 'contours' are the boundaries between different ranges of badger density.

*Figure 4.7* is a variation of the isoplethic map. It uses modern computerized mapping techniques,

An example from human medicine, included for completeness, is shown in *Figure 4.8* which depicts average annual mortality rates of Scottish women between 45 and 54 years of age. The areas of the rectangles are proportional to the number of women in the various regions; the key in the bottom right-hand corner of the map indicates the number of people per unit area; the key in the top left-hand corner indicates mortality rates. The area of each rectangle and the mortality rate together indicate the total number of deaths for each area. These rectangles are positioned to represent their approximate geographical associations, the circled numbers locating major landmarks such as rivers.

The main application of maps in veterinary epidemiology has been to display qualitative data, commonly using point and distribution maps. However, as more animal demographic data and

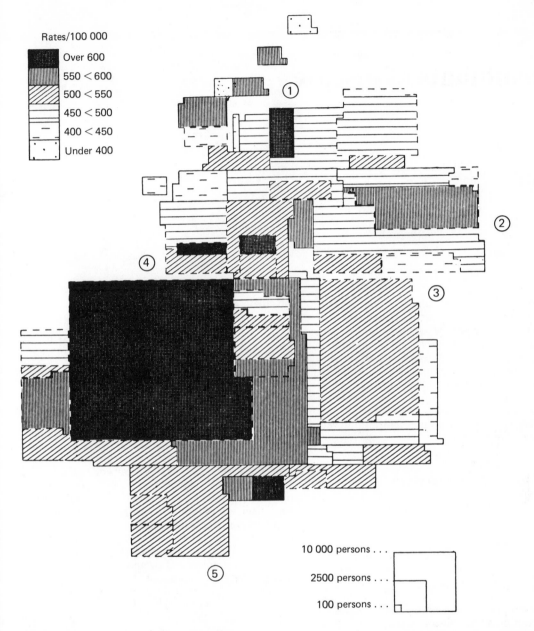

Rates/100 000

Over 600
550 < 600
500 < 550
450 < 500
400 < 450
Under 400

① ② ③ ④ ⑤

10 000 persons . . .
2500 persons . . .
100 persons . . .

**Figure 4.8** Annual average mortality of Scottish women aged 45–54 years, for the period 1959–1963: an example of a demographic base map. ① Moray Firth; ② Firth of Tay; ③ Firth of Forth; ④ Firth of Clyde; ⑤ Solway Firth. (From Forster, 1966)

information on disease morbidity become available, quantitative maps should become more common, facilitated by modern computer graphics.

## *Further reading*

AHLBOM, A. and NORELL, S. (1984) *Introduction to Modern Epidemiology*. Epidemiology Resources Inc., Chestnut Hill

HILL, A.B. (1971) *Principles of Medical Statistics*, 9th edn. *The Lancet* Limited, London

LAST, A.M. (1983) *A Dictionary of Epidemiology*. Oxford University Press, London

ROHT, L.H., SELWYN, B.J., HOLGUIN, A.H. and CHRISTENSEN, B. (1982) *Principles of Epidemiology. A Self-Teaching Guide*. Academic Press, New York

# 5

# Determinants of disease

Chapter 3 introduced the concept that disease usually is caused by multiple factors. The factors are **determinants** of disease. A determinant is any characteristic that affects the health of a population. Diet, for example, is a determinant of bovine hypomagnesaemia: reduced food intake and low levels of plant magnesium, related to rapid grass growth, are associated with an increased incidence of the disease (*see Figure 3.6*). This chapter discusses the types of determinant and the interactions that occur between them.

## Classification of determinants

Determinants can be classified in 3 ways, as:

(1) **primary** or **secondary**;
(2) **intrinsic** or **extrinsic**;
(3) associated with **host**, **agent** or **environment**.

### Primary and secondary determinants

Primary determinants are factors whose variation exerts a major effect in inducing disease. Frequently, primary determinants are necessary causes (*see* Chapter 3). Thus, exposure to distemper virus is a primary determinant of canine distemper.

Secondary determinants correspond to predisposing, enabling or reinforcing factors. For example, sex is a secondary determinant of canine heart valve incompetence: male dogs are more likely to develop incompetence than females (Buchanan, 1977; Thrusfield *et al.*, 1985). The primary determinants may include other genetically determined factors such as the rate of ageing of the valves, which may be associated with breed. Primary and secondary determinants are listed in *Table 5.1*.

### Intrinsic and extrinsic determinants

*Table 5.1* also illustrates that some determinants (both primary and secondary) are internal to the host, for example, genetic constitution including aberrant genes (which are the primary causes of genetic disorders), species, breed and sex. These determinants are **intrinsic**, also termed **endogenous** (Greek: *endon* = within). In contrast, some determinants are external to the host, for instance transportation, which may result in physical trauma, producing bruising of carcasses (Meischke *et al.*, 1974). Such determinants are **extrinsic**, also termed **exogenous** (Greek: *exo* = outside). *Table 5.2* exemplifies this classification in relation to canine pruritus (tendency to itch), a common problem in small animal practice. Internal disease, such as hepatitis or nephritis, may act as an intrinsic predisposing factor by increasing the sensitivity of the skin (Kral, 1966). Mastocytomas contain an excess of histamine and proteolytic enzymes which induce itching. Conditions that are not usually associated with pruritus, such as hypothyroidism, may become pruritic when bacterial infections are superimposed. Dietary factors, such as a high potassium:calcium ratio, also increase skin sensitivity.

### Determinants associated with host, agent and environment

Many diseases include infectious agents in their sufficient causes. Most infectious agents enter the host as challenges from the environment (the dam can be the 'environment', too, when fetal infection occurs). However, during the microbial revolution, the early emphasis on microbes as the primary causes of disease resulted in their being considered

**Table 5.1 Primary and secondary determinants**

### PRIMARY DETERMINANTS

| *Intrinsic determinants* | *Extrinsic determinants* | | | | |
|---|---|---|---|---|---|
| | *Animate* | | *Inanimate* | | |
| | *Endoparasitic* | *Ectoparasitic* | *Physical* | *Chemical* | *Allergic* |
| Genetic constitution | Viruses | Arthropods | Trauma | Excess | Allergens |
| Metabolism | Bacteria | | Climate | Deficiency | |
| Behaviour | Fungi | | Radiation | Imbalance | |
| | Protozoa | | Stressors | Poisons | |
| | Metazoa | | | Photosensitizers | |

### SECONDARY DETERMINANTS

| *Intrinsic determinants* | *Extrinsic determinants* |
|---|---|
| Genetic constitution (including sex, species and breed) | Location |
| | Climate |
| Age | Husbandry (housing, diet, general management, animal use) |
| Size and conformation | Trauma |
| Hormonal status | Concurrent disease |
| Nutritional status | Vaccination status |
| Immunological status | Stressors |
| Functional status (e.g. pregnant, lactating) | |
| Behaviour | |

**Table 5.2 Some determinants of canine pruritus. (Modified from Thoday, 1980)**

| *Intrinsic determinants* | | *Extrinsic determinants* | | | | |
|---|---|---|---|---|---|---|
| *Internal disease* | *Temperament* | *Trauma* | *Chemicals* | *Diet* | *Parasites* | *Bacteria* |
| Renal disease | Lick granuloma | Abrasion | Relative | Fat deficiency | Fleas | Causing: |
| Hepatic disease | | Aural and | primary | Carbohydrate | Lice | Juvenile impetigo |
| Diabetes mellitus | | nasal | irritants | excess | Mites: | Anal sacculitis |
| Maldigestion or | | foreign | | High potassium: | *Otodectes* spp. | Impetigo |
| malabsorption | | bodies | | calcium ratio | *Sarcoptes* spp. | Short-haired dog |
| Tumours | | | | | *Trombicula* spp. | folliculitis |
| | | | | | *Demodex* | Acute moist |
| | | | | | (pustular) | dermatitis |

separately from other environmental factors such as husbandry, trauma and toxic agents. Thus, determinants commonly are classified into those associated with the host, the agent and the environment. These three groups of factors are sometimes called the **triad** (*Figure 5.1*). Some authors (e.g. Schwabe, 1984) consider that management and husbandry are important enough in intensive animal enterprises to be classified separately from the environment, as a fourth major group.

In some diseases, an infectious agent is the main determinant, and host and environmental factors are of relatively minor importance. Such diseases are 'simple'; examples are major animal plagues like foot-and-mouth disease and tuberculosis, where a multifactorial nature is not obvious. In other diseases, termed 'complex', their multifactorial nature predominates, and an **interaction** between host, agent and environment can be identified. Thus, 'environmental' mastitis involves an interaction between *Escherichia coli* or *Streptococcus uberis* (the agent), milking machine faults, and poor

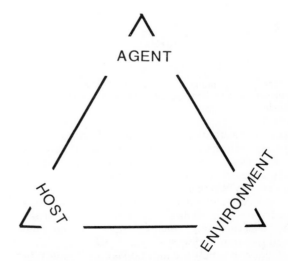

**Figure 5.1** The 'triad': three main headings under which determinants can be classified.

hygiene resulting from inadequate bedding, drainage and cleaning of passageways (the environment) (Francis *et al.*, 1979). In addition, cows (the hosts) are most susceptible in early lactation.

The complexity of a multifactorial disease depends upon the definition of disease. Most 'diseases' with which the veterinarian is initially concerned are actually clinical signs presented by animals' owners. Thus, pruritus in a dog is a clinical sign which can be caused by several different lesions each with their own sufficient causes. Further examples of signs and lesions with different causes are given in *Figures 9.1b* and *9.1c*. The causal web can become very complex when the 'disease' is defined in terms of a production shortfall in a herd or flock. Thus, 'reproductive failure' in a pig herd, reflected in unacceptably low numbers of piglets being born in a herd in a defined period of time, can be produced by decreased male or female fertility, or infection or metabolic derangement of the sow or fetus during pregnancy. *Figure 5.2* divides the causes of reproductive failure in pigs into six main areas relating to

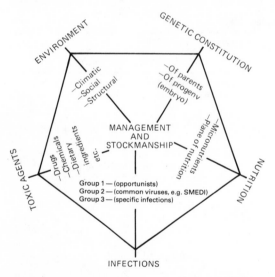

**Figure 5.2** Diagrammatic representation of causes of reproductive failure in a pig herd. (Modified from Pritchard *et al.*, 1985)

genetic constitution, nutrition, infections, toxic agents, environment and management. It therefore represents a subdivision of agent, host and environmental determinants. These six areas are discussed in detail by Wrathall (1975).

Genetic factors include genetic defects affecting the parents (e.g. abnormal genitalia or gametes) and the offspring (e.g. malformations or inherited predisposition to disease).

Failure to supply the nutritional requirements for specific micronutrients (vitamins, minor minerals and trace elements) can result in reduced litter sizes,

embryonic death and delayed puberty. The plane of nutrition can also affect performance. Restriction of diet can delay puberty. In contrast, 'flushing' (increasing the amount fed) a few days before ovulation is due can increase the number of ova released in gilts.

Infections are classified into three groups:

(1) opportunistic pathogens;
(2) common viruses;
(3) specific infectious diseases.

Group 1 pathogens are ubiquitous and frequently endogenous. They cause disease sporadically when host resistance is lowered. Examples include *Staphylococcus* and *Listeria* spp.—infections causing prenatal deaths and abortions. Notable in group 2 are the porcine parvoviruses, also termed SMEDI viruses, an acronym for stillbirth, mummification, embryonic death and infertility, which effects they produce. Group 3 infections include brucellosis, leptospirosis, toxoplasmosis and swine fever—infections caused by exogenous pathogens, which can produce low conception rates and induce abortion.

Toxic substances include those ingested in the food (e.g. mycotoxins which can induce vulvovaginitis and abnormal oestrus), and environmental pollutants such as wood preservatives which can cause abortion.

The environment affects reproduction through its climatic, social and structural components. High environmental temperatures, for example, can induce infertility in males.

Important management factors include herd age structure (young females may have a low ovulation rate and therefore small litter size), the boar:sow ratio, boar management, efficiency of heat detection and pregnancy diagnosis, breeding policy and record keeping.

The three schemes of determinant classification are not mutually exclusive. They are just three different ways of viewing the multifactorial nature of disease. Determinants are described below using the third system of classification: into those associated with host, agent or environment. This system is also followed by Schwabe *et al.* (1977) in their discussion of determinants of animal diseases, and by Reif (1983) in his consideration of determinants of diseases of dogs and cats.

## Host determinants
### *Age*

The occurrence of many diseases shows a distinct association with age. The absolute number of cases of a disease clearly is not an indication of the impact of disease in a particular age-range because the

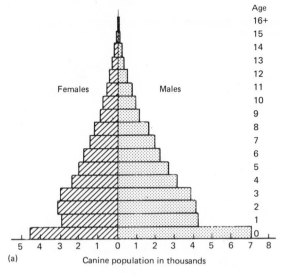

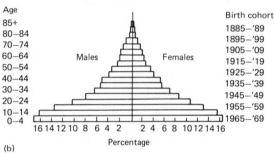

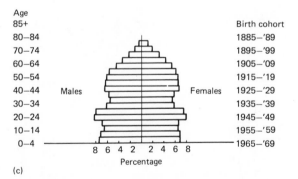

**Figure 5.3** Canine and human population pyramids. (**a**) canine: New Jersey, USA, 1957; (**b**) human: Mexico, 1970; (**c**) human: Sweden, 1970. ((**a**) From Cohen *et al.*, 1959; (**b**) and (**c**) from Ewbank and Wray, 1980)

ranges are present in different proportions in the total population. *Figure 5.3a*, which is a **population pyramid**, shows the age distribution of dogs, male and female indicated separately, in New Jersey, USA, in the late 1950s. This shape is similar to that of human populations with high fecundity and a low proportion of individuals surviving to old age, for

example 19th century European and North American populations and contemporary populations in developing countries (*Figure 5.3b*). It contrasts with the pyramid of human populations with low fecundity and a high proportion of individuals surviving to old age, for example in contemporary developed countries (*Figure 5.3c*). Thus, age-specific rates (*see* Chapter 4) provide the most valuable information about disease in particular age-groups because they relate morbidity and mortality to a uniform size of population at risk.

The life spans of animals and man differ. Therefore, it is useful to relate the ages of animals to those of man when comparing morbidity and mortality between the two groups. Lebeau (1953) has devised a method for converting canine to human age equivalents (*Figure 5.4*). A 1-year-old dog is equivalent to a 15-year-old person; a 2-year-old dog to a 24-year-old person; and, above the age of 2 years, each 1 year of a dog's life is equivalent to 4 human years. Thus, a 10-year-old dog is equivalent to a 56-year-old person (24 years, plus 4 years for each canine year from 3 years onwards). However, Reif (1983) emphasizes the problems associated with such a conversion, because large breeds of dog tend to die younger than small breeds. Applying Lebeau's conversion, *Figure 5.5* compares the age-specific incidence rates of mammary cancer in the dog and man. The rates are similar until the human menopause, when ovarian activity decreases and the human rate tends to stabilize, suggesting a hormonal determinant. This suggestion is supported by the demonstration of receptors for steroid hormones in the cytosol fractions from canine mammary carcinomas (Martin *et al.*, 1984) and the experimental reduction in the carcinomas' growth by the anti-oestrogen, tamoxifen, and by ovariectomy when the cancers are transplanted to nude mice (Pierrepoint *et al.*, 1984).

Many bacterial and virus diseases are more likely to occur, and to be fatal, in young than in old animals, either because of an absence of acquired immunity or because of a low non-immunological host resistance. Many protozoan and rickettsial infections, in contrast, induce milder responses in the young than in the old. Tumours in man and animals (e.g. *Figure 5.6*) are more common in old than in young animals, with some notable exceptions such as canine osteosarcoma and lymphosarcoma which show peak incidences between 7 and 10 years of age (Reif, 1983).

## Sex

Sexual differences in disease occurrence may be attributed to hormonal, occupational, social and ethological, and genetic determinants.

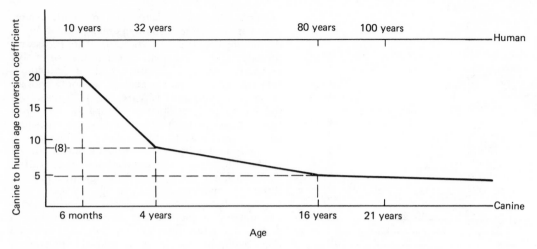

**Figure 5.4** Conversion of canine age to its human age equivalent (example: age of dog = 4 years, conversion coefficient = 8, thus human age equivalent = 4 × 8 = 32 years). (Modified from Lebeau, 1953)

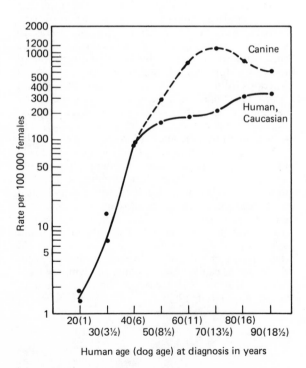

**Figure 5.5** Annual female human (Caucasian) and canine age-specific incidence rates for mammary cancer. (Modified from Schneider, 1970)

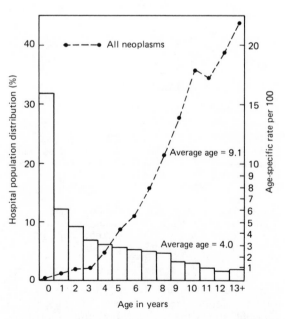

**Figure 5.6** Age distribution of a total canine hospital population (bars) and age-specific rates (graph) for canine neoplasia: University of Pennsylvania, 1952–1964. (From Reif, 1983)

## Hormonal determinants

The effects of sex hormones may predispose animals to disease. Bitches are more likely to develop diabetes mellitus than male dogs (Marmor *et al.*, 1982) and signs often develop after oestrus, possibly related to the increased insulin requirements of diabetic bitches during oestrus. Similarly, the neutering of bitches decreases the likelihood of mammary carcinoma developing (Schneider *et al.*, 1969), perhaps from the effect, outlined above, of oestrogens on this tumour.

## Occupational determinants

Sex-associated occupational hazards, although more relevant to human than animal disease, can be identified occasionally in animals, where animal use is equated with occupation. Thus, the increased risk of contracting heartworm infection by male dogs relative to bitches (Selby *et al.*, 1980) may result from increased 'occupational' exposure of male dogs during hunting to the mosquito that transmits the infection.

## Social and ethological determinants

Behavioural patterns may account for bite wound abscesses being more common in male than female cats. Social and behavioural patterns are important determinants of human disease too, for example cigarette smoking in relation to lung cancer (*see Table 3.2*) where a greater proportion of men than women smoke.

## Genetic determinants

Genetic differences in disease incidence may be inherited either by being **sex-linked**, or **sex-limited**, or **sex-influenced** (Reif, 1983). Sex-linked inheritance occurs when the DNA responsible for a disease is carried on either the X or Y sex chromosomes. Canine haemophilia A and B, for example, are associated with the X chromosome and are inherited recessively, the defects being predominant in males (Patterson and Medway, 1966). Sex-limited inheritance occurs when the DNA responsible for the disease is not in the sex chromosomes, but the disease is expressed only in one sex, for example cryptorchidism in dogs. In sex-influenced inheritance, the threshold for the overt expression of a characteristic is lower in one sex than the other, therefore there is an excess incidence in one sex over the other. Thus, canine patent ductus arteriosus is inherited through several genes (i.e. is polygeneic) but is more common in females than males, possibly because it is sex-influenced.

In many diseases, there may be excess disease occurrence in one sex over the other, but either a genetic component has not been identified clearly or the method of inheritance has not been established. Examples that are reported to occur predominantly in male dogs include epilepsy (Bielfelt *et al.*, 1971), melanoma and pharyngeal fibrosarcoma (Cohen *et al.*, 1964).

Some diseases may be apparently sex-associated, but are actually associated with other determinants that are related to gender. For instance (Schwabe *et al.*, 1977), the increased mortality rate in male dairy calves appears to be sex-associated. However, the real association is with husbandry: male dairy calves may not be given as much attention as females because they are worth less (in this instance husbandry, therefore, is a confounder).

## *Species and breed*

Species and breeds vary in their susceptibility and responses to different infectious agents. Thus, dogs do not develop heartwater. Rottweilers and Doberman pinschers react more severely to canine parvovirus enteritis than other breeds (Glickman *et al.*, 1985), and boxers appear to be more susceptible than other breeds to mycotic diseases such as coccidioidomycosis (Maddy, 1958) (distribution map of the fungus: *see Figure 7.2*).

The reasons for species susceptibility are many and not fully understood. The efficacy of the immune mechanism against an infectious agent may be important. Thus, humans are not usually susceptible to infection with *Babesia* spp. but splenectomized individuals can develop the disease. Different species have been shown to have different receptors for infectious agents on the cell surface. This is particularly important with viruses, which must enter the host cell. Monkeys are not susceptible to poliovirus because they do not have the 'right' cell receptors. Removal of the virus capsid allows the virus to divide lytically in monkey cells if it is first made to enter them. Susceptibility can vary within a species, too. Thus, only certain pigs are susceptible to the strain of *Escherichia coli* possessing the K88 antigen because susceptibility is determined by the presence of an intestinal receptor which is inherited in a simple Mendelian manner (Rutter, 1975).

Phylogenetically closely related animals are likely to be susceptible to infection by the same agent, albeit with different signs. Herpesvirus B causes labial vesicular lesions in non-human primates, and a fatal encephalitis in man. The rider to this—that phylogenetically closely related agents infect the same species of animal—is not, however, generally true. Measles, distemper and rinderpest are closely related paramyxoviruses, yet usually infect quite different species: man, dogs and cattle, respectively.

Apparently new diseases can develop when a species or breed is placed in a new ecosystem (*see* Chapter 7) which contains a pathogen that has a well-balanced relationship with local species or breeds. In such circumstances inapparent infection (discussed later in this chapter) is common in the local animals but clinical disease occurs in the exotic ones. This happened in South Africa when European breeds of sheep were exposed to bluetongue virus. The agent did not produce clinical signs in the indigenous sheep, but caused severe disease in imported Merino sheep. Malaria developed as a clinical disease in early European visitors to West Africa, whereas the local population was tolerant of the parasite. Similarly, the importation of European cattle to West Africa accentuated the problem of dermatophilosis.

There is also species and breed variation in the occurrence of non-infectious diseases. Thus, British breeds of sheep develop intestinal carcinoma more frequently than fine wool breeds, and Hereford cattle develop ocular squamous cell carcinoma more commonly than other breeds (*see* Chapter 4).

Many diseases having distinct associations with a particular familial line or breed are considered to be primarily genetic. Patterson (1980), for instance, has described over 100 such diseases in the dog. A genetic causal component is likely when disease incidence is higher in pedigree animals than in crossbreds. Examples include congenital cardiovascular defects (Patterson, 1968) and valvular heart disease (Thrusfield *et al.*, 1985) in dogs.

Diseases may be present in a range of breeds because the breeds are genetically related. Boston terriers and bull terriers show a high risk of developing mastocytoma, which may be related to their common origin (Peters, 1969). In contrast, the risk of a particular breed developing a disease may vary between countries, indicating different genetic 'pools' (or a different environment or method of management). Thus, Das and Tashjian (1965) found an increased risk of developing valvular heart disease in cocker spaniels in North America, whereas, in Scotland, Thrusfield *et al.* (1985) did not detect an increased risk in that breed.

Foley *et al.* (1979) describe in detail heritable diseases of companion animals and livestock.

## Other host determinants

### Size and conformation

Size, independent of particular breed associations, has been identified as a disease determinant. Hip dysplasia and osteosarcoma are more common in large than small breeds of dog (Tjalma, 1966). Interestingly, the latter disease is also more common in large than small children (Fraumeni, 1967). The conformation of animals may similarly increase the risk of some diseases. For instance, cows with a small pelvic outlet relative to their size (e.g. the Chianina and Belgian blue) are predisposed to dystocia.

### Coat colour

Predisposition to some diseases is associated with coat colour which is heritable and a risk indicator. For example, white cats have a high risk of developing cutaneous squamous cell carcinoma (Dorn *et al.*, 1971) related to the lack of pigment which protects the skin from the carcinogenic effects of the sun's ultraviolet radiation. In contrast, canine melanomas occur mainly in deeply pigmented animals (Brodey, 1970). White cats often have a genetic defect causing deafness (Bergsma and Brown, 1971). White hair colour is also associated with congenital deafness in Dalmatians (Anderson *et al.*, 1968).

## Agent determinants

### *Virulence and pathogenicity*

Infectious agents vary in their ability to infect and to induce disease in animals. The ability to infect is related to the inherent susceptibility of a host and whether or not the host is immune. **Virulence** is the ability of an infectious agent to cause disease, in a particular host, in terms of frequency and severity. **Pathogenicity** is sometimes used as a synonym for virulence, with virulence reserved for variations in the disease-inducing potential of different strains of the same organism. However, 'pathogenicity' refers to the quality of disease induction, and should not be used semiquantitatively to indicate the degree to which disease is induced. Thus, the protozoan parasite *Naegleria fowleri* is pathogenic to man in warm, but not in cold, water, the pathogenicity being governed in this instance by environment. More commonly, pathogenicity and virulence are intrinsic characteristics of an infectious agent and are either **phenotypically** or **genotypically** conditioned. Phenotypic changes are transient, and are lost in succeeding generations. For example, Newcastle disease virus, cultivated on the chorioallantoic membrane of hens' eggs, is more virulent to chicks than virus that is cultivated in calf kidney cells. Genotypic changes result from a change in the DNA (and RNA, in RNA viruses) of the microbial genome (the agent's total genetic complement).

Pathogenicity and virulence are determined by a variety of host and agent characteristics. The infectious agent must be able to multiply in, and resist the clearance and defence mechanisms of, the host. Multiplication and spread of bacteria are assisted by their release of toxins. An agent may achieve pathogenicity, or increase virulence, by a change in antigenic composition to a type to which the host is not genetically or immunologically resistant. However, antigenic changes are not always the cause of changes in pathogenicity and virulence. They may be simply indicators of such changes, the determinants being associated with the production of inhibitory, toxic or other substances by the agent. Genotypic changes also can alter the sensitivity of bacteria to antibiotics.

### Types of genotypic change

Genotypic changes in infectious agents can result from **mutation**, **recombination**, **conjugation**, **trans-duction** and **transformation**. Mutation is an altera-tion in the sequence of nucleic acids in the genome of a cell or virus particle. There may be either **point mutation** of one base, resulting in misreading of succeeding codon triplets, or **deletion mutation**, where whole segments of genome are removed. Deletion mutants are more likely to occur because they result in changes without redundant genetic material. Frequent mutation may produce antigenic diversity, which may induce recurrent outbreaks of disease in a population which is not immune to the new antigen. Within the same organism, mutation rates can vary for different genetic markers by a factor of 1000. Sites within the genome that frequently mutate are termed 'hot spots'. If these spots code for virulence and antigenic determinants in the infectious agent then the agent can change virulence and antigens frequently. If mutation occurs at sites that are not associated with either virulence or antigenic type, then changes in these two characteristics are rare.

Recombination is the reassortment of segments of a genome that occurs when two microbes exchange genetic material. Thus, influenza A viruses have a genome that is packaged in each virion (virus particle) as eight strands of RNA. Influenza viruses are divided into groups based on the structure of two major antigens: the haemagglu-tinin and neuraminidase (*see also Table 16.5*). Mixed infection of cells in tissue culture, and possibly of wild animals (notably birds), produces recombinants with novel haemagglutinin and neura-minidase combinations. Major changes are referred to as 'shift' and minor changes as 'drift'. The major changes are responsible for the periodic—approximately decadal—pandemics of influenza in man (Kaplan, 1982). (Note that antigenic drift also occurs in trypanosomes, but by a totally different mechanism. The superficial cell membrane is shed to reveal new antigens. The epidemiological result, though, is similar: new antigens, therefore a partially or totally susceptible population.) Recom-bination may also occur in the orbiviruses (e.g. African horse sickness and bluetongue) where the

precise mechanism is not known, and the term 'genetic reassortment' has been applied (Gorman *et al.*, 1979).

Conjugation (Finnegan, 1976) involves transmis-sion of genetic material from one bacterium to another by a conjugal mechanism (i.e. they touch) through a sex pilus. Not only can surface antigens change by this means but also drug resistance, especially to antibiotics. This is common in *E. coli*, and *Salmonella*, *Proteus*, *Shigella* and *Pasteurella* spp.

Transduction (Primrose, 1976) is the transfer of a small portion of genome from one bacterium to another by a bacterial virus (bacteriophage). Again, resistance factors, as well as surface antigens, may be transferred in this way. It occurs in *Shigella*, *Pseudomonas* and *Proteus* spp.

Transformation is transmission of naked nucleic acid between bacteria, without contact. It occurs spontaneously in *Neisseria* spp. but, to occur in other bacterial species, DNA has to be extracted in the laboratory. (This type of transformation should not be confused with the *in vitro* production of malignant cells, which is also called transformation.)

In addition to these five methods of genetic alteration, infection by more than one type of virus particle may be necessary to produce disease. Such infections do not strictly involve a change in a virus genome, rather a complementation of it, which may render a non-pathogenic virus particle pathogenic. This occurs in some plant virus infections because several plant viruses have split genomes that are packaged in separate virions. Each virion carries a portion of the total genome which is, itself, non-infectious, but which contributes to the whole infectious unit. For example, tobacco rattle virus has two virions: one containing a promoting gene, and the other containing replication and maturation genes. All three genes, and therefore both types of virion, are necessary to instigate the successful infection of a tobacco plant. In animals, Rous sarcoma virus has capsid proteins that are genetical-ly determined by a separate helper virus. Similarly, some adeno-associated viruses require an adenovir-us for infectivity. The different virions present in human hepatitis B virus fall into this double infection group too.

Conversely, infection by one virus may prevent infection by, or lessen the virulence of, a second virus. This occurs when the first virus induces the host's cells to release an inhibitory substance now known as interferon.

The ways in which virulence and pathogenicity affect the transmission and maintenance of infection are discussed in Chapter 6.

## *Gradient of infection*

'Gradient of infection' refers to the variety of responses of an animal to challenge by an infectious

Increasing severity of disease →

| Signs in animal | No signs | No signs<br><br>(Subclinical disease) | Clinical signs | | Death |
|---|---|---|---|---|---|
| | | | (Mild disease) | (Severe disease) | |
| Type of infection | No infection | Inapparent infection | Overt infection | | |
| Status of animal | Insusceptible or immune | Susceptible | | | |

**Figure 5.7** Gradient of infection: the various responses of an animal to challenge by an infectious agent.

agent (*Figure 5.7*) and therefore represents the combined effect of an agent's pathogenicity and virulence, and host characteristics such as susceptibility and pathological and clinical reactions. These responses affect the further availability of the agent to other susceptible animals, and the ability of the veterinarian to detect, and therefore to treat and control, the infection. If an animal is either insusceptible or immune then infection and significant replication and shedding of an agent do not usually occur, and the animal is not important in the transmission of infection to others.

### Inapparent (silent) infection

This is infection of a susceptible animal without clinical signs. The infection usually runs a similar course to that which produces a clinical case, with replication and shedding of agent. The inapparently infected animal poses a considerable problem to the disease controller because it is impossible to identify without auxiliary diagnostic aids such as antigen detection or serology.

**Subclinical** infection occurs without clinical signs. Some authors use this term and inapparent infection synonymously. Others ascribe a loss of productivity to subclinical infection, which is absent from inapparent infection. 'Subclinical' can also be applied to non-infectious conditions, such as hypomagnesaemia, where there may be no clinical signs.

### Clinical infection

Clinical infection produces clinical signs. Disease may be **mild**. If the disease is very mild with an illness too indefinite to permit a clinical diagnosis then it is termed an **abortive reaction**. There is a gradation to severe disease, which is called a **frank clinical reaction**, when the intensity is sufficient to allow a clinical diagnosis. The severest reaction results in death. Paradoxically, death is the logical climax of some infections because it is the only means by which the agent can be released to infect other animals. An example is infection with *Trichinella spiralis* which is transmitted exclusively by flesh eating.

Inapparent and mild clinical infections commonly indicate an adaptation of some antiquity between host and parasite; the relationship between bluetongue virus and indigenous South African sheep has already been cited.

## *Outcome of infection*

Clinical disease may result in the development of a long-standing chronic clinical infection, recovery, or death. Chronically infected cases are potential sources of an infectious agent. Death usually removes an animal as a source of infection, although there are important exceptions such as infection with *T. spiralis*, and anthrax infection where carcasses contaminate the soil. Recovery may result in **sterile immunity** following an effective host response, which removes all of the infectious agent from the body. Animals that have sterile immunity no longer constitute a threat to the susceptible population.

Two states, however, are important determinants:

(1) the carrier state;
(2) latent infection.

### The carrier state

'Carrier' is used loosely to describe several situations. In a broad sense, a carrier is any animal that sheds an infectious agent without demonstrating clinical signs. Thus, an inapparently or subclinically infected animal may be a carrier, and may shed agent, either continuously or intermittently. The periods for which animals are carriers vary, but are rarely lifelong.

**Incubatory** and **convalescent carriers** also occur. The former are animals that excrete agent during the disease's incubation period, for instance dogs shedding rabies virus in their saliva for up to 10 days before clinical signs develop. Convalescent carriers are animals that shed agent when they are recovering from a disease. In all cases, carriers are sources of infection to susceptible animals.

### Latent infection

A latent infection is one that persists in an animal without producing clinical signs. Thus, the distinction between latency, chronic infection and the carrier state is blurred. Latency may or may not be accompanied by transmission to other susceptible animals. In persistent bacterial infections (e.g. tuberculosis) a balance occurs between host and agent such that the agent replicates, but the disease may not progress for a long time. In virus and rickettsial infections, persistence is not usually associated with demonstrable replication of the agent, unless the latter is reactivated. Many examples of virus and rickettsial latency are known, but the role of latency in perpetuating infection in a population, except in a minority of infections (e.g. with bovine virus diarrhoea virus) is still unclear. The likelihood of persistence can depend not only on the particular infectious agent and host species but also on the host's age at the time of infection. For instance, all kittens transplacentally infected with feline leukaemia virus become permanently infected (Jarrett, 1985). However, from 8 weeks of age, an increasing proportion of cats resist infection; by 4–6 months of age only about 15% of naturally infected cats become permanently infected. Latently infected cats do not appear to transmit infection (except possibly female cats to their kittens, in milk).

## Microbial colonization of hosts

Infectious agents enter a host at varying times during its life. Some—the vertically transmitted ones (*see* Chapter 6)—infect the host before birth. Initial infection may or may not be followed by the immediate development of disease.

### Exogenous and endogenous pathogens

The previous description of microbes involved with reproductive failure in pigs illustrates that pathogenic infectious agents can be classified into two groups, **exogenous** and **endogenous** (Dubos, 1965).

The exogenous pathogens are not usually present in the host. They cannot normally survive for a long time in the external environment (soil, water, etc.). They do not usually form persistent relationships with the host. They are generally acquired by exposure to an infected animal, and usually produce disease with clearly identifiable clinical signs and pathological lesions. Examples include canine distemper, rinderpest, and the other traditional animal plagues.

The endogenous pathogens are often found in healthy animals, commonly in the gastrointestinal and respiratory tracts, and usually do not cause disease unless the host is stressed. An example is *E. coli*, which is commonly found in the intestinal tract of calves, and which may cause disease only when a calf is immunodeficient, for example, due to deprivation of colostrum (Isaacson *et al.*, 1978).

This twofold classification is somewhat simplistic. Some pathogens possess characteristics of both groups. For example, *Salmonella* spp. usually produce distinct clinical signs when they infect animals. However, some animals can permanently carry and intermittently excrete the agent without showing signs, as carriers. The bacterium can also be transmitted by methods other than direct contact with infected animals, for example, in contaminated food.

### Opportunistic pathogens

Some organisms cause disease only in a host whose resistance is lowered, for example by drug therapy or other diseases. Such organisms are **opportunistic**, may colonize the host at any time during life, and may be endogenous or exogenous. Examples described earlier are the group 1 pathogens that can cause prenatal deaths and abortions in pigs.

# Environmental determinants

The environment includes location, climate, and husbandry. Particular attention has been paid to environmental determinants of disease in livestock enterprises, where intensive production systems expose animals to environmental extremes (e.g. chicken battery houses), and in human medicine, where social and occupational exposure to possible causal factors (e.g. to cigarette smoke in relation to lung cancer) can occur.

## *Location*

Local geological formations, vegetation and climate affect the spatial distribution of both animals and disease. Thus, the incidence of jaw tumours in sheep, mentioned in Chapter 4, is associated with the distribution of bracken, and illustrates the value of maps in identifying causes of disease. Non-specific chronic canine pulmonary disease in middle-aged and old dogs is associated with urban residence in the USA (Reif and Cohen, 1970); urban residence being defined in relation to atmospheric pollution. This investigation has been refined by demonstrating an urban/rural gradient in the occurrence of canine pulmonary disease (Reif and Cohen, 1979): an example of the application of the method of concomitant variation (*see* Chapter 3) in inferring cause.

Noise is associated with location and may also be considered as being related to 'occupation' and husbandry. The effect of noise on animal health has not been studied in detail. Most investigations have been conducted on man and laboratory animals where, apart from the obvious induction of temporary or permanent deafness, noise has been shown to cause a general stress reaction (discussed later in this chapter) with altered secretion of adrenocortical hormones. In a review of the effects of noise on animal health, Algers *et al*. (1978) describe leucopenia (which could be associated with immunosuppression), decreased milk production in dairy cows, and oligospermia and an increased incidence of abortion in rats.

The temporal distribution of disease is also affected by location because of the seasonal effects of climate. These effects, and methods of identifying them, are discussed in Chapter 8.

## *Climate*

Two types of climate can be identified:

(1) macroclimate;
(2) microclimate.

## Macroclimate

The macroclimate comprises the normal components of weather to which animals are exposed: rainfall, temperature, solar radiation, humidity and wind, all of which affect health (Webster, 1981). Temperature may be a primary determinant, for example low temperatures in the induction of hypothermia, to which newborn animals are particularly prone. Wind and rain increase heat loss from animals. Cold stress predisposes animals to disease, for example by reducing efficiency of digestion, which may predispose to infectious enteritis. Wind also can carry infectious agents (e.g. foot-and-mouth disease virus) and arthropod vectors (e.g. *Culicoides* spp. infected with bluetongue virus) over long distances (*see* Chapter 6).

The macroclimate can also affect the stability of infectious agents, in which circumstance it is a secondary determinant. Bovine rhinotracheitis virus survives well when humidity is low, whereas rhinoviruses survive when it is high. Porcine transmissible gastroenteritis virus is sensitive to solar ultraviolet radiation, and therefore is more likely to be inactivated in summer than winter. The statistical association between respiratory disease and cool, damp weather is probably due to a build-up of pathogens, rather than a reduction in host resistance by climatic stress (Webster, 1981).

Climatic impact can be measured in several ways. A common method is to calculate the **wind-chill index**. This combines the effects of temperature and wind-speed, and is especially important at temperatures below freezing, where convective heat losses are magnified by wind. The macroclimate, in conjunction with geological features, determines vegetation and affects the spatial distribution of disease because of the resultant distribution of hosts and vectors; this is discussed in Chapter 7.

## Microclimate

A microclimate is a climate that occurs in a small defined space. This may be as small as within a few millimetres of a plant's or an animal's surface or as large as a piggery or calf house. In the former, microclimate may be **terrestrial**, for example over the surface of leaves, or **biological**, over the surface of a host's body. The terrestrial microclimate affects the development of arthropods and helminths. The biological microclimate can change during the course of a disease, assisting in its spread. For instance, sweating during the parasitaemic phase of human malaria increases the humidity of the body's surface and attracts mosquitoes to the humid skin surface at a time when the protozoon is readily available.

The microclimate in intensive animal production units is an important determinant of disease. Thus, adequate ventilation is recommended to remove stale air, microbial aerosols and dust, and to reduce humidity (Wathes *et al.*, 1983). Although the effects of high concentrations of non-pathogenic airborne bacteria on livestock are unclear, there is evidence (Pritchard *et al.*, 1981) that reduced levels of airborne bacteria are associated with a reduced incidence of clinical and subclinical respiratory disease.

## *Husbandry*

### Housing

The importance of well-designed ventilation in an animal house has already been mentioned. The structure of bedding materials and surfaces is also a determinant. Thus, claw lesions are more common and severe in pigs reared on aluminium slats than in pigs reared on steel or concrete slats, or on soil (Fritschen, 1979). Limb lesions are more common in pigs reared on concrete than on asphalt-based floors (Kovacs and Beer, 1979). Smith (1981) suggests that excessive floor slope may predispose to rectal prolapse in pigs because of the increased effect of gravity.

### Diet

Diet has obvious effects in diseases caused by energy, protein, vitamin and mineral deficiencies. Sometimes the effects are less clearly defined. There is evidence, for example, that increased dietary levels of biotin reduce the incidence of foot lesions in sows (Penny *et al.*, 1980). However, there is no evidence of an association between a deficiency of the vitamin and an increased incidence of the lesions.

Feeding regimens may be a determinant. Thus, gastric torsion in sows kept in sow stalls has been associated with once-a-day rather than twice-a-day feeding, which may indicate that the ingestion of a relatively large amount of food is a causal factor (Crossman, 1978).

### Management (including animal use)

Management determines stocking density and production policy. Increased densities increase the challenge of microbial pathogens. An internal replacement policy (i.e. maintaining a 'closed' population) is less likely to introduce pathogens into an enterprise than a policy involving buying-in animals from outside the herd.

The use to which an animal is put (its 'occupation') can affect disease occurrence. Equine limb injuries are relatively common in hunters. 'Hump-sore' occurs more frequently in draught zebus than in non-working cattle. Apparently sex-related differences in disease occurrence, that actually are related to animal use, have been described earlier.

## *Stress*

Stress is the sum of biological reactions to any adverse physical, mental and, in man, emotional stimulus that tends to disturb homeostasis. Factors that are capable of producing stress are **stressors**; examples are climatic extremes and trauma. If the biological reactions are inappropriate or inadequate then stress may lead to pathological lesions. It has been suggested (although not universally accepted) that there is a common basic reaction irrespective of cause: Selye's hypothesis (Selye, 1946). However, the reaction may be complicated by other features that are specific to a particular stressor.

The effects of stress in laboratory animals were described by Selye (1936) as a syndrome which was later termed the **general adaptation syndrome**. This is divided into three parts:

(1) general alarm reaction;
(2) phase of resistance (phase of adaptation);
(3) phase of reaction.

The general alarm reaction occurs 6–48 hours after exposure to a stressor and comprises a decrease in the size of the liver, lymph nodes, spleen and thymus, disappearance of adipose tissue, loss of muscular tone, hypothermia, the development of erosions in the digestive tract, and increased lacrimation and salivation. The phase of resistance begins after approximately 48 hours and includes adrenal enlargement associated with increased release of adrenotropic hormones, reappearance of lipoid granules, hyperplasia of the thyroid associated with increased production of thyrotropic hormones, cessation of body growth and milk secretion, and atrophy of the gonads. The various organs become almost normal, even when the stressor is still applied. The phase of reaction results in death with signs similar to those of the first part. Stress is instigated by the hypothalamus which releases hormones that lead to the release of adrenocorticotrophic hormone which acts on the adrenal gland to produce the gland's typical enlargement.

Stress and shock (which sometimes accompanies stress) should be distinguished. However, their effects are difficult to separate because both are instigated by the hypothalamus. Shock is a clinical manifestation of acute peripheral vascular collapse which results in hypotension, tachycardia, pallor and oliguria, mediated by the release of catecholamines (adrenaline and noradrenaline). Excessive release of catecholamines can result in haemorrhagic enteropathy and death. Shock can be caused by other mechanisms including hypovolaemic shock, the endotoxic forms of septic shock as found in some bacterial infections, and anaphylactic shock.

Stress is a secondary determinant of several diseases. The maintenance of stress can produce protein wastage, abnormal organ function, and suppression of the immune system and anti-inflammatory response. Thus, shipping fever (*see* Chapter 1) is associated with transportation, de-horning, castration and winter weather. The increased incidence of malignant catarrhal fever and yersiniosis in deer in winter may be due to prolonged exposure to the stressors cold and low plane of nutrition.

Stress can be a primary determinant. A notable example is when stress results from the capture of animals, where it can produce a **postcapture myopathy** syndrome. This syndrome is reported in wild animals in South Africa (Basson and Hof-meyer, 1973). It is characterized by ataxia, paresis or paralysis, the production of brown urine, and asymmetric muscular and myocardial lesions. A similar disease occurs in red deer following capture (McAllum, 1985).

Stress is also a primary determinant of the **porcine stress syndrome**. This is the inability of susceptible pigs to tolerate the usual environmental stressors (e.g. castration, vaccination, movement and high ambient temperatures) that are associated with normal management. The syndrome occurs rapid-ly—often within minutes—after exposure to a stressor. The disease, which is considered to be identical to malignant (fulminant) hyperthermia in humans, dogs, cats, horses and pigs, is characterized initially by muscle and tail tremors. Further stress can produce dyspnoea, cyanosis, increased body temperature and acidosis. The final stage is marked by total collapse, muscle rigidity, hyperthermia and death. The condition is a genetically determined error of metabolism which induces a switch of energy utilization in muscles of affected pigs from aerobic to anaerobic metabolism. It is inherited through an autosomal recessive gene with high or complete penetrance. Susceptible pigs can be detected by the rapid development of malignant hyperthermia under halothane anaesthesia, and by certain blood group linked genes (Archibald and Imlah, 1985).

## Interaction

Determinants associated with host, agent or environment do not exert their effects in isolation, but **interact** to induce disease. 'Interaction' refers to the interdependent operation of factors to produce an effect. Thus, factors that result in net decreased magnesium intake interact with those that induce increased loss to produce hypomagnesaemia (*see*

*Figure 3.6*). Bovine alimentary papillomas, caused by a papilloma virus (the agent), can transform to carcinomas in areas where bracken fern (the environment) is common, indicating a possible interaction between agent and environment (Jarrett, 1980). There is an interaction between a gene (the host) and stressors (the environment) which induces the porcine stress syndrome.

## Diseases caused by mixed agents

An important example of interaction between agents is the **mixed infection**, that is, an infection with more than one type of agent. The main infectious disease problems in intensive production systems relate to the body surfaces. Common problems are enteric and respiratory diseases and mastitis. These diseases are frequently caused by

**Table 5.3 Examples of diseases caused by mixed infections. (From Rutter, 1982)**

| Disease | Classifi-cation* | Agents |
|---|---|---|
| Enteric disease (most species) | I (?II) | Enterotoxigenic *Escherichia coli* |
| | | Rotavirus Coronavirus Calicivirus *Cryptosporidium* spp. |
| Atrophic rhinitis (pigs) | I | *Bordetella bronchiseptica* *Pasteurella multocida* |
| Foot rot (sheep) | II | *Corynebacterium pyogenes* *Fusobacterium necrophorum* *Bacteroides nodosus* Motile fusobacteria |
| Pneumonia (sheep) | II | Parainfluenza 3 *Pasteurella haemolytica* |
| Swine dysentery (pigs) | II | *Treponema hyodysenteriae* Gut anaerobes |
| 'Coli septicaemia' (chickens) | II | *Escherichia coli* Infectious bronchitis virus |
| Respiratory disease (bovine) | ?II | *Mycoplasma bovis* *Mycoplasma dispar* Parainfluenza 3 Respiratory syncytial virus Infectious bovine rhinotracheitis virus *Pasteurella* spp. Other bacteria |
| Summer mastitis (bovine) | ?II | *Corynebacterium pyogenes* *Peptococcus indolicus* *Streptococcus dysgalactiae* Micro-aerophilic cocci |

*I = Single agents can reproduce clinical signs but mixed infections frequently occur.
II = Mixed infections are essential with cooperative or synergistic interactions.
? = Insufficient evidence for definitive classification.

mixed infections. Two categories of diseases can be identified (Rutter, 1982):

(1) those diseases in which clinical signs can be produced by single agents independently, although mixed infections usually occur in animals;
(2) those diseases in which two or more microbial components are necessary to induce disease.

Some examples are listed in *Table 5.3*. Category I agents include *E. coli*, rotaviruses, caliciviruses, and *Cryptosporidium* spp., all of which can induce diarrhoea. Category II agents are exemplified by those that cause calf pneumonia, which include 5 viruses, 4 mycoplasmata and 19 bacterial species. The precise mechanism of the interaction is unclear, but investigations in mice (Jakab, 1977) suggest that pulmonary phagocytosis of bacteria may be reduced by virus inhibition of intracellular killing mechanisms in macrophages, and that bacterial adherence to virus-infected cells may increase.

Foot rot in sheep also demonstrates interaction. There are four component organisms: *Corynebacterium pyogenes*, *Fusobacterium necrophorum*, *Bacteroides nodosus* and non-pathogenic motile fusobacteria. Each of these four alone is only poorly virulent but supplies growth factors or substances that overcome the host's defence mechanisms in the complete infection (Roberts, 1969).

In addition to this general concept of interaction, two specific meanings are attached to interaction, defining **biological** and **statistical interaction**.

## Biological interaction

Biological interaction involves a dependence between two or more factors based on an underlying physical or chemical association. For instance, there is a chemical interaction between the K88 antigen of *E. coli* (the agent) and receptors in the intestine of some pigs (the hosts), described earlier in this chapter, which results in the bacteria that possess the antigen being pathogenic to pigs with the receptors. There appears to be a physical interaction, also mentioned earlier, between the presence of bacteria and poor ventilation in the induction of calf respiratory disease, associated with the density of airborne bacteria. Biological interaction similarly is demonstrated by category II mixed agents. Biological interactions therefore relate to identifiable stages in a causal pathway, and represent many of the known general qualitative interactions.

Two or more factors can also interact biologically to produce an effect that is greater than that expected of either factor alone; this is **synergism**. An example would be the potentiating effect of certain combinations of antibiotics. Similarly, there is synergism between the four component organisms of ovine root rot, described above.

'Synergism' should be reserved to describe **biological** mechanisms. In the epidemiological literature, however, synergism has also been used to describe certain types of statistical, rather than biological, interactions, and this has led to some confusion (Kleinbaum *et al.*, 1982). The use of 'synergism' in a statistical context is discussed in the following section.

## Statistical interaction

Statistical interaction is a **quantitative** effect involving two or more factors. Often disease occurrence does not depend simply on the presence or absence of a factor; there may be continuous variation in the frequency of occurrence of disease associated with both the strength of a factor (e.g. the frequency with which dairy farm personnel milk cows and infection with *Leptospira* spp.; *see Table 3.1*) and the number of factors involved. There is often a 'background' frequency of occurrence associated with none of the factors under consideration. When two or more factors are associated with disease, the frequency of disease may be proportional to the occurrence of disease resulting from the **separate** frequencies attributable to each factor (i.e. the frequency when each factor is present singly, minus the 'background' frequency). Alternatively, the frequency may be either in excess of or less than that expected from the combined effects of each factor, in which case **statistical interaction** occurs. For example, Willeberg (1976), in his study of the feline urological syndrome (FUS), showed that castration and high levels of dry cat food intake, when present simultaneously, resulted in a frequency of the FUS in excess of that expected from the combined effects of each factor, indicating positive statistical interaction between the two factors.

When several component causes are present simultaneously, their joint effect can be explained quantitatively in terms of two causal models: **additive** and **non-additive** (Kupper and Hogan, 1978). The additive model interprets disease occurrence, when two or more factors are present, as the **sum** of the amount of disease attributable to each factor. If no interaction exists, then, for example:

when X and Y are both absent, suppose 'background' disease occurrence $= \gamma$;
when cause X is present alone, disease occurrence $= 2 + \gamma$;
when cause Y is present alone, disease occurrence $= 5 + \gamma$;
when X and Y are both present, disease occurrence $= 7 + \gamma$.

If positive interaction occurs, then the level of disease occurrence, when X and Y are present, will be greater than $7 + \gamma$.

The commonest non-additive model is the multiplicative. This interprets disease occurrence, when two or more factors are present, as the **product** of the amount of disease attributable to each factor. If no interaction exists, then, for example:

> when X and Y are both absent, suppose 'background' disease occurrence $= \delta$;
> when cause X is present alone, disease occurrence $= 2\delta$;
> when cause Y is present alone, disease occurrence $= 5\delta$;
> when X and Y are both present, disease occurrence $= 10\delta$.

If positive interaction occurs, then the level of disease occurrence, when X and Y are present, will be greater than $10\delta$.

Disease occurrence can be expressed in terms of incidence or other measures of the risk of disease developing (*see* Chapter 13). The type of model depends on the means of expressing disease occurrence; for example a multiplicative model may become additive if log transformation of the measure of occurrence is conducted.

In epidemiology the additive model is the commoner of the two models. When there is evidence of positive interaction based on the additive model  the model has sometimes been described as **synergistic**. However, there are arguable differences between interaction and synergism (Blot and Day, 1979). Evidence of a positive statistical interaction does not necessarily imply a causal relationship. However, if it can be inferred that the factors are part of an aggregate of causes with a common causal pathway then synergism is said to have occurred (MacMahon, 1972). Synergism, in a statistical context, therefore may be thought of as a positive statistical interaction where a causal pathway may be inferred. Thus, castration and high levels of dry cat food intake (usually associated with overfeeding and sometimes related to insufficient water intake) are synergistically associated in the FUS: both may result in inactivity, thereby reducing blood flow to the kidneys, impairing renal function, and therefore promoting changes in the urine that are conducive to the formation of uroliths.

The value of assessing statistical interaction lies in its ability to identify the **degree** to which various determinants interact. It then may be possible to predict the extent to which disease incidence may be reduced by modification of the determinants. The quantification of statistical interaction, using the more common additive model, is described in Chapter 15.

# The cause of cancer

The cause of cancer exemplifies interaction between host, agent and environment. The abnormal, unrestricted multiplication of cells produces a tumour. Tumours may be benign, in which growth is restricted and spread to other parts of the body does not occur, or malignant, in which growth is unrestricted and spread (metastasis) may occur. Malignant tumours are commonly termed cancers, the word taking its meaning from the zodiacal sign of the crab, because malignant tumours 'put out' extensions like the limbs of a crab.

## The induction of cancer

The mass of cancerous cells that constitutes a malignant tumour originates from a single 'founder' cell which once was normal, but which has undergone a fundamental change. This change is manifested in several abnormal characteristics such as excessive dependence on anaerobic metabolism and the presence of unusual tumour antigens, in addition to the disregard for normal territorial boundaries which is a cancer's most obvious characteristic. These complex alterations in cell behaviour appear to originate from a single genetic change (Weinberg, 1983), as shown by the induction of cancer in laboratory animals by the introduction of cells that had been transformed to the cancerous state, *in vitro*, by infection with polyoma virus.

Epidemiological investigations previously had revealed that, in addition to viruses, chemical and physical agents can induce cancer. Soot was the first chemical to be incriminated. In 1775, Percival Pott, a London surgeon, recorded an increased incidence of scrotal epithelioma in chimney sweeps. Since then, a range of chemical carcinogens (cancer inducers) has been identified (Coombs, 1980), including hydrocarbons, aromatic amines (associated with bladder cancer in dyestuff workers), N-nitroso compounds (associated with liver cancer in fish, birds and mammals), steroids (e.g. oestrone, inducing mammary cancer in mice), inorganic products such as asbestos (associated with mesothelioma in man) and some natural products (e.g. the fungal aflatoxins, which are contaminants of peanut oil, and possibly implicated in human liver cancer).

Evidence suggests that tumour-inducing (oncogenic) viruses, chemical and physical carcinogens, and spontaneous mutations alter cellular DNA and, therefore, that cancer results from alterations to genetic material. Oncogenic viruses carry genes that can transform normal cells to cancerous ones. These genes (**oncogenes**) are slightly altered versions of certain normal avian and mammalian cell genes, **proto-oncogenes**, which, also if slightly altered, for example by chemical carcinogens (causing a mutation), may become oncogenes and induce tumours. Presumably such potentially dangerous proto-oncogenes are conserved because they also fulfil useful metabolic functions.

The induction of cancer occurs in two main stages (Becker, 1981):

(1) initiation;
(2) promotion.

**Initiation**, by oncogenic viruses, carcinogens or spontaneous changes in the genome, is assumed to involve an irreversible alteration in cellular DNA. There are two stages. The first is the assumed change in the cellular DNA; the second is initiation of mitosis.

Initiation alone is not sufficient to induce a cancer, but produces a cell with a high risk of becoming malignant. Malignancy results when **promotion** occurs. This step was considered to be reversible, although there is evidence that, when cells have reached a certain stage of change, they progress irreversibly to a cancerous state (e.g. Peraino *et al.*, 1977). Several chemical promotors have been identified, such as croton oil which promotes skin tumours. Many chemical carcinogens are both initiators and promotors (**complete carcinogens**).

'**Co-carcinogen**' is a general term for a factor that furthers the action of a carcinogen, such as chronic inflammation or a chemical promotor. Squamous cell carcinoma of sheep in northern Australia occurs predominantly on the ears, the prevalence increasing with decreasing latitude. Solar ultraviolet radiation has been incriminated as a physical carcinogen. An infectious agent, transmitted on ear marking instruments, may be a co-carcinogen, and would explain why the lesions are commoner on the ear than on other parts of the head (Daniels *et al.*, 1986).

Induction and promotion indicate that the progress to the cancerous state involves more than one stage. Several multistage models have been formulated (Peto, 1977), implying that several 'insults' to a cell are necessary to induce cancer. Thus, creation of an oncogene is only one of several steps that are required to produce a cancer: a particular oncogene may be a necessary, but not a sufficient, cause. The need for several distinct changes in a cell may explain why cancer is rarer in young adults than among the elderly, although there is no plausible explanation for the risk of cancer being essentially similar in old age in different species with different spans of life.

Biochemists, virologists and molecular biologists have identified inducers and promotors, using animals and tissue cultures. At the top of the biological hierarchy, epidemiologists have identified risk factors using observational studies. Two groups of factors are defined (Gopal, 1977):

(1) specific causal agents;
(2) modifying factors.

Specific physical causal agents that have been incriminated include ultraviolet and ionizing radiation (the latter experimentally inducing thyroid tumours and leukaemia in dogs), chronic irritation (associated with some horn cancers in East Indian cattle) and parasites (e.g. *Spirocerca lupi* associated with canine oesophageal osteosarcoma and fibrosarcoma). Specific chemical and biological initiators, such as viruses, have already been described. Modifying factors are not incriminated as initiators, but in some way affect the incidence of cancer, and include co-carcinogens. The genetic composition of the host is the most important modifying factor and may be related to the presence of suitable proto-oncogenes. Some cancers can be hereditary, for example, porcine lymphosarcoma (McTaggart *et al.*, 1979).

Interactions have been demonstrated in which chemical carcinogens enhance the production of tumours *in vitro* by oncogenic viruses, possibly by facilitating integration of the virus genome (Heidelberger, 1978). Some non-oncogenic viruses also are reported to interact with chemical carcinogens (Martin, 1964). Thus, chickens infected with pox viruses, and mice infected with influenza virus, are more susceptible to chemical carcinogenesis than non-infected animals.

## Investigating the cause of cancer

Doll (1977) has contended that most cancers have environmental causes either as initiators or promotors. Investigation of the cause of cancer involves cooperation between several disciplines: biochemistry, pathology, molecular biology and epidemiology. An example of this cooperation is the epidemiological identification of an age-related determinant of mammary carcinoma, probably associated with oestrogen activity, and the detection of steroid hormone receptors in fractions from the cancer, mentioned earlier in this chapter. Further progress includes the demonstration of stimulation of DNA-dependent RNA polymerase activity (an indicator of growth in the tumour) in tumours previously incubated with oestrogen, and containing receptors for oestrogen (Thomas and Pierrepoint, 1983).

Domestic animals can be useful biological models of human cancer (Pierrepoint, 1985). Dogs share environments with their owners, but ageing is more rapid than in man; thus assessment of the effects of possible carcinogens can be faster. For example, Bostock and Curtis (1984) described a difference between London and Melbourne in the proportion of canine oral tumours that are squamous cell carcinomas. This suggests that, since the life-styles of dogs in the two cities are similar, environmental factors may be responsible for inducing this carcinoma. A comparison of urban dogs with man also offers a means of removing the contribution of active smoking to a possible sufficient cause of lung cancer (Glickman *et al.*, 1983). Other tumours with similarities between the dog and man include spontaneous lymphoma (Johnson *et al.*, 1968) and osteosarcoma, described earlier, where body size appears to be a determinant.

Tumours of domestic animals and some of their causes are reviewed by Cotchin (1984).

## *Further reading*

ANDERSON, J.R. (1985) Tumours II. The aetiology of cancer. In: *Muir's Textbook of Pathology*, 12th edn. Ed. Anderson, J.R. Pp. 13.1–13.38. Edward Arnold, London

DOLL, R. and PETO, R. (1983) Epidemiology of cancer. In: *Oxford Textbook of Medicine*, Vol. 1. Ed. Weatherall, D.J., Ledingham, J.G.G. and Warrell, A. Pp. 4.51–4.79. Oxford University Press, Oxford

MacMAHON, B. (1972) Concepts of multiple factors. In: *Multiple Factors in the Causation of Environmentally Induced Disease*. Fogarty International Center Proceedings No. 12. Ed. Lee, D.H.K. and Kotin, P. Pp. 1–12. Academic Press, New York and London

MIMS, C.A. (1982) *The Pathogenesis of Infectious Diseases*, 2nd edn. Academic Press, London and New York

REIF, J.S. (1983) Ecologic factors and disease. In: *Textbook of Veterinary Internal Medicine. Vol. 1: Diseases of the Dog and Cat*, 2nd edn. Ed. Ettinger, S.J. Pp. 147–173. W.B. Saunders Company, Philadelphia

SAINSBURY, D.W.B. (1981) Health problems in intensive animal production. In: *Environmental Aspects of Housing for Animal Production*. Ed. Clark, J.A. Pp. 439–454. Butterworths, London

SCHWABE, C.W., RIEMANN, H.P. and FRANTI, C.E. (1977) *Epidemiology in Veterinary Practice*. Lea and Febiger, Philadelphia

SMITH, H., SKEHEL, J.J. and TURNER, M.J. (Eds) (1980) *The Molecular Basis of Pathogenicity*. Report of the Dahlem workshop on the molecular basis of the infective process. Berlin, 22–26 October 1979. Verlag Chemie, Weinheim

# 6

# The transmission and maintenance of infection

Infectious disease is the result of the invasion of a host by a pathogenic organism. The continued survival of infectious agents, with or without the induction of disease, depends on their successful transmission to a susceptible host, the instigation of an infection therein and replication of the agent to maintain the cycle of infection. The complete cycle of an infectious agent is its **life history (life-cycle)**. A knowledge of the life history of an infectious agent is essential when selecting the most applicable control technique (*see* Chapter 20). This involves knowledge of:

(1) the modes of transmission and maintenance of infection;
(2) the ecological conditions that favour the survival and transmission of infectious agents.

This chapter is concerned with the first topic; the second is considered in Chapter 7 with reference to basic ecology.

Transmission may be either **horizontal (lateral)** or **vertical**. Horizontally transmitted infections are those transmitted from any segment of a population to another, for example influenza virus from one horse to a stable-mate. Vertically transmitted infections are transmitted from one generation to the next by infection of the embryo or fetus while *in utero* (in mammals) or *in ovo* (in birds, reptiles, amphibians, fish and arthropods). Transmission by milk to offspring is also considered, by some, to be vertical.

## Horizontal transmission

Infections can be transmitted horizontally either **directly** or **indirectly** (*Figure 6.1*).

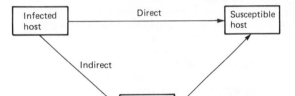

**Figure 6.1** Basic mechanisms of transmission of infectious agents.

Direct transmission occurs when a susceptible host contracts an infection, either by physical contact with an infected host or by contact with the latter's infected discharges (e.g. the transmission of canine distemper in infected urine and faeces).

Indirect transmission involves an intermediate vehicle, living or inanimate, that transmits infection between infected and susceptible hosts. This vehicle generally may be termed a **vector**, although the term is usually restricted, by common usage, to living carriers (*see below*, definition of vector). Indirect transmission can involve a vector of a different species from that of the initially infected host. The life-cycle of infectious agents may therefore be complex with several different hosts. Details of specific life-cycles are not presented in this chapter, but a basic knowledge of veterinary microbiology and parasitology is assumed. Airborne transmission of infectious agents, frequently over long distances, is also defined as indirect.

## *Types of host and vector*

A variety of terms describe the range of host/parasite relationships, and are used by the epidemiologist, protozoologist, entomologist, helminthologist and microbiologist. Each of these may use terms, specific to his discipline, that have the same general meaning, from the point of view of the life-cycle of the disease, as different words from other disciplines, for example **intermediate host** in helminthology and **biological vector** in entomology (*see below*).

### Hosts

**Host**: a plant, animal or arthropod that is capable of being infected with, and therefore giving sustenance to, an infectious agent. Replication or development of the agent usually occurs in the host.

**Definitive host**: a parasitological term describing a host in which an organism undergoes its sexual phase of reproduction (e.g. *Taenia pisiformis* in dogs; *Plasmodium* spp. in mosquitoes).

**Final host**: a term used in a more general sense (i.e. in connection with all types of infectious agent) as a synonym for **definitive host**. Both 'final' and 'definitive' imply the 'end of the line', in other words the termination of a dynamic process. They are, in most cases, therefore, improperly used.

**Primary (natural) host**: an animal that maintains an infection in the latter's endemic area (e.g. dogs infected with distemper virus). Since an infectious agent frequently depends upon a primary host for its long-term existence, the host is also called a **maintenance host.**

**Secondary host**: a species that additionally is involved in the life-cycle of an agent, especially outside typical endemic areas (e.g. cattle infected with strains of foot-and-mouth disease virus that usually cycle in buffaloes). A secondary host can sometimes act as a maintenance host.

**Paratenic host**: a host in which an agent is transferred **mechanically** by ingestion of the host, without further development (e.g. fish, containing *Diphyllobothrium* spp. larvae, which are preyed upon by larger fish). This term is exclusive to helminthology, and could be considered to have its entomological analogue in the term **mechanical vector.**

**Intermediate host**: an animal in which an infectious agent undergoes some development, frequently with **asexual reproduction** (e.g. *Cysticercus pisiformis* in rabbits and hares). This term is parasitological in origin.

**Amplifier host**: an animal which, because of temporally associated changes in population dynamics that produce a sudden increase in the host population size, may suddenly increase the amount of infectious agent. Multiplication of the agent occurs in this type of host. This term is most

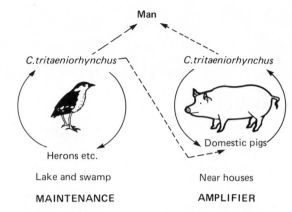

**Figure 6.2** The maintenance and amplifier hosts of Japanese encephalitis virus in Japan. The vector is the mosquito, *Culex tritaeniorhynchus*. (From Gordon Smith, 1976, based on Buescher *et al.*, 1959, and Scherer *et al.*, 1959)

commonly used in relation to virus diseases. An example is litters of baby pigs infected with Japanese encephalitis virus (*Figure 6.2*).

**Hibernating host**: an animal in which an agent is held, probably without replication, in a state of 'suspended animation' (e.g. hibernating snakes infected with either western, eastern or Japanese encephalitis virus).

**Incidental (dead-end or accidental) host**: one that does not usually transmit an infectious agent to other animals (e.g. bulls infected with *Brucella abortus*). 'Final' and 'definitive' can be applied validly to this type of host.

**Link host**: a host that forms a link between other host species (e.g. pigs linking infected herons to man in Japanese encephalitis; *Figure 6.2*).

**Reservoir**: a term commonly used as a synonym for, or prefix to, host, for instance '**reservoir**', '**reservoir host**'. A reservoir host is one in which an infectious agent normally lives and multiplies, and therefore is a common source of infection to other animals. Thus, in Kenya, buffalo and waterbuck are reservoirs of bovine ephemeral fever virus, acting as a source of infection for cattle (Davies *et al.*, 1975). Similarly, in the USA, cattle are reservoirs of bluetongue virus, and therefore can be sources of infection for sheep (Hourrigan and Klingsporn, 1975). In Sierra Leone, the multimammate mouse, *Mastomys natalensis*, is the primary host and reservoir of Lassa fever, a virus disease with a high case fatality rate in man (Monath *et al.*, 1974). The mouse is adapted to life both within houses and in fields, and comes into contact with man in rural areas, particularly during the wet season, when it may seek shelter in houses, and thus may transmit the infection to man. Reservoirs may be primary or secondary hosts.

'Reservoir' is also used to refer to any substance that is a common source of infection (e.g. soil as a source of anthrax spores).

**Vector**: an animate transmitter of infectious agents. By common usage, vectors are defined as invertebrate animals—usually arthropods—that transmit infectious agents to vertebrates. The dictionary definition of the term implies independent movement, that is, a living vehicle. Inanimate carriers of agents (e.g. feed concentrates contaminated with *Salmonella* spp.) are usually called 'fomites' (singular: fomes, from the Greek meaning 'tinder', because fomites were thought metaphorically to be the 'tinder' by which the 'fire' of an epidemic was ignited).

**Mechanical vector**: an animal (usually an arthropod) that physically carries an infectious agent to its primary or secondary host (e.g. mosquitoes and fleas transmitting myxomatosis virus between rabbits). The infectious agent neither multiplies nor develops in the mechanical vector.

**Biological vector**: a vector (usually an arthropod) in which an infectious agent undergoes either a necessary part of its life-cycle, or multiplication, before transmission to the natural or secondary host.

Three types of biological transmission occur:

(1) **developmental transmission**: with an essential phase of development occurring in the vector (e.g. *Dirofilaria immitis* in mosquitoes);
(2) **propagative transmission**: when the agent multiplies in the vector (e.g. louping ill virus in ixodid ticks);
(3) **cyclopropagative transmission**: a combination of (1) and (2) (e.g. *Babesia* spp. in ticks).

Development in the vector involves migration of the infectious agent. Thus, two types of transmission are identified in the life-cycles of members of the protozoan genus *Trypanosoma*. The African trypanosomes that parasitize the blood and tissues of infected animals are ingested by insects of the genus *Glossina*, in which they undergo a developmental cycle that involves migration from their initial focus of infection in the midgut and back to the salivary glands, from which infective forms are released; this is **salivarian** transmission. In contrast, members of the species *Trypanosoma cruzi* (the cause of Chagas' disease in man in South America, with dogs, cats and some wild animals implicated as reservoirs) are ingested by bugs of the family *Reduviidae*, from which infective forms are shed in the faeces, human infection occurring by contamination of wounds and the eyes; this is **stercorarian** transmission.

Biological vectors are frequently either definitive or intermediate hosts; for example mosquitoes are biological vectors and the definitive hosts of *Plasmodium* spp. (the cause of malaria).

## Factors associated with the spread of infection

Three factors are important in the transmission of infection (Gordon Smith, 1982):

(1) characteristics of hosts;
(2) characteristics of pathogens;
(3) effective contact.

### Characteristics of hosts

A host's **susceptibility** and **infectiousness** determine its ability to transmit infection. Susceptibility to infection may be limited to a single species or group of species. For example, only equines are naturally susceptible to equine rhinopneumonitis virus infection. Alternatively, several widely different species may be susceptible to an infection, for example, all mammals are susceptible to rabies.

Susceptibility within a species may vary markedly and may be associated with selection of genetically resistant animals following exposure to an infectious agent. For example, the mortality in rabbits, exposed experimentally to a standard dose of myxomatosis, fell from 90% to 25% over a 7-year period (Fenner and Ratcliffe, 1965).

'Infectiousness' refers to:

(1) the duration of the period when an animal is infective;
(2) the relative amount of an infectious agent that an animal can transmit.

An animal is not infectious as soon as it is infected—a period of time lapses between infection and the availability of the agent; this is the **prepatent period**. In contrast, the **incubation period** is the period of time between infection and the development of clinical signs. Thus, inapparent infections have a prepatent period, but do not have an incubation period. The **generation time** is the period between infection and maximum infectiousness. These periods, for a given agent and host species, are not the same for all animals but show natural variation. The frequency distribution of incubation periods, for example, follows a lognormal statistical distribution (*see Figure 12.4* and Sartwell, 1950, 1966).

*Figure 6.3* plots the excretion of rinderpest virus in a group of experimentally infected cattle. It illustrates that nasal excretion is the most common form of shedding of the virus, that virus is shed **before** the appearance of clinical signs, and that, **for the group**, the period of maximum infectiousness is 4 days after the onset of clinical signs (i.e. pyrexia).

Diseases with short incubation periods run a clinical course, terminating in either recovery or death relatively quickly. Thus, a relatively high host

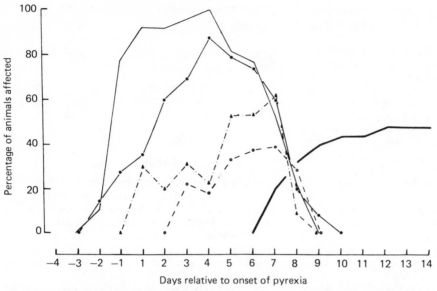

**Figure 6.3** Correlation of viraemia and virus excretion in cattle infected experimentally with virulent rinderpest virus (strain RGK/1): ——— viraemia; ●——● nasal excretion of virus; ▲–·–·–▲ urinary excretion of virus; ○ – – – ○ faecal excretion of virus; —— mortality. (From Liess and Plowright, 1964)

| | | Characteristic of host population | | |
|---|---|---|---|---|
| | | Low density | Mixed or changing densities | High density |
| **Characteristic of infectious agent** | Short incubation period | □ | ▼ | ▼▼▼▼▼ ▼▼ |
| | Mixed incubation periods | ▼▼▼ | ▼▼▼▼▼▼ | ▼▼▼▼▼▼ |
| | Long incubation | ▼▼▼▼▼ | ▼▼▼▼ | ▼▼▼▼▼ |

**Figure 6.4** The relationship between duration of incubation period of an infectious agent, density of the host, and the potential of the infectious agent to exist in a population. □: Conditions unfavourable for the existence of infectious agent. ▼: Conditions favourable for the existence of infectious agent; the number of triangles indicates the relative degree to which the conditions are favourable. (Modified from Macdonald and Bacon, 1980)

density is required to ensure that the agent's life-cycle can be perpetuated (*Figure 6.4*). An example is distemper virus infection of dogs with an incubation period of 4–5 days. This disease therefore is endemic only in urban areas where there is a high density of dogs. In contrast, infectious diseases with long incubation periods can maintain their cycles of infection in varying animal densities (*Figure 6.4*); rabies is an example.

The time between infection and availability of an infectious agent in an arthropod vector is the agent's **extrinsic incubation period**.

For transmission to occur between a vertebrate host and an arthropod vector, an infectious agent must be present to a minimum concentration in the vertebrate host's circulation. This is the **threshold level**. Some vertebrate hosts may become infected, but are unable to transmit infection to arthropods because the threshold level is not achieved. These are therefore 'dead end' hosts. For example (*Figure 6.5*), the Columbian ground squirrel is an incidental (dead end) host for Colorado tick fever. However, the golden mantled ground squirrel achieves the threshold level for the virus; therefore the vector, the tick *Dermacentor andersoni*, can ingest virus particles, and this squirrel can act as a maintenance host.

## Characteristics of pathogens

Three important characteristics of pathogens that affect transmission of infectious agents are **infectivity**, **virulence** and **stability**.

**Infectivity** relates to the amount of an organism that is required to initiate infection. The infectivity of different organisms varies considerably. For example, the **particle:infectivity ratio** (the number of virus particles required to instigate infection) of bacterial viruses (bacteriophages) in tissue culture is approximately 1:1, indicating a high degree of

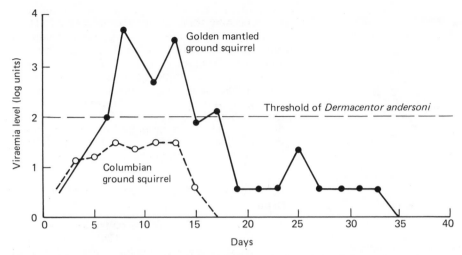

**Figure 6.5** Colorado tick fever: the relationships between viraemia levels in a maintenance host (the golden mantled ground squirrel) and an incidental host (the Columbian ground squirrel) and the threshold of infection of the arthropod maintenance host (*Dermacentor andersoni*). (From Gordon Smith, 1976, after Burgdorfer, 1960)

infectivity. Lower degrees of infectivity are demonstrated by animal viruses, with ratios of between 10:1 and 100:1. Plant viruses have an even lower infectivity, with a ratio of approximately 1000:1. Infectivity can vary between different strains of the same organism, and can depend upon the route of the infection and the age of the host.

When an agent is capable of infecting more than one species, its infectivity for different hosts is often quite different. For instance, the infective dose of strains of *Campylobacter jejuni* isolated from chickens is only 500 bacteria for chickens, whereas the infective dose of strains of the same bacterium isolated from seagulls is above $10^7$ for chickens. This example illustrates that the infectivity of an agent cannot be specified without reference to the host that it infects.

**Virulence** (*see* Chapter 5) also affects transmission and can change. Repeated passage through the same species of animal tends to increase virulence. Thus, serial passage of Ross River virus in suckling mice increases its virulence (Taylor and Marshall, 1975). However, alternate passage in mice and the mosquito *Aedes aegypti* does not alter virulence.

The length of time for which an organism can remain infective outside its host is the organism's **stability**. Some organisms survive only for short periods of time, that is they are very **labile** (e.g. *Leptospira* spp. in dry environments). Stability is frequently facilitated by protective capsules, such as those forming the outer layer of bacterial spores (e.g. *Bacillus anthracis*). The hazards presented to infectious agents by the external environment, and techniques of achieving stability, are discussed later in this chapter.

**Effective contact**

Effective contact describes the conditions under which infection is likely to occur. For a particular infection, it depends on the stability of the organism and the routes by which the organism leaves an infected host and enters a susceptible one.

Effective contact may be very short (e.g. seasonally transmitted, vector-borne diseases) or potentially of many years' duration (e.g. anthrax spores in soil). The duration of infectiousness determines the number of susceptibles that can be infected by an infected animal. Thus, upper respiratory tract infections (e.g. kennel cough in dogs) result in short periods of infectiousness of several days' duration, whereas cows infected with bovine tuberculosis may excrete the bacterium in their milk for several years.

Behaviour, which may be changed during infection, can also affect the likelihood of effective contact. Thus, feral animals that are naturally shy of man may enter houses when they contract rabies, therefore increasing the likelihood of human infection.

The pathogenesis of disease may increase the likelihood of transmission; for example, respiratory diseases may induce coughing and sneezing, thereby spreading respiratory pathogens to near neighbours.

## *Routes of infection*

The site or sites by which an infectious agent gains entry to a host, and by which it leaves the host, are the agent's routes of infection. *Figure 6.6* illustrates the main sites of infection of mammalian hosts.

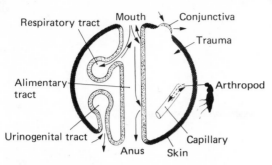

**Figure 6.6** Body surfaces as sites of horizontal infection and shedding of infectious agents. (Modified from Mims, 1982)

## The oral route

Infection via the mouth is one of the more common routes of entry, especially in relation to the enteric organisms which often 'escape' from an infected animal in the faeces. Organisms such as rotaviruses, *Salmonella* spp. and gastrointestinal parasites may contaminate water and foodstuffs, which then act as fomites. Ingested agents may be excreted in the faeces, producing the **faecal-oral** transmission cycle.

Agents that gain entry to the body orally may be disseminated from the infected animal by a variety of routes, apart from in the faeces. *Br. abortus* often infects cows orally but is excreted later in the milk and uterine discharges. Similar circumstances occur in relation to infection of ruminants with the rickettsia *Coxiella burneti*, the cause of Q fever. Such agents may then be retransmitted by both the oral and other routes. Although some organisms can be transmitted by the oral route, the low pH of gastric secretions is an effective barrier against this method of transmission for a wide variety of organisms.

## The respiratory route

The respiratory route is also a common method of transmission for many infectious agents, including those that are not restricted to the respiratory tract. Infectious agents seldom occur as individual airborne particles, but are usually associated with other organic matter in the form of droplets or dust. The nature and size of such composite particles affects their dispersal and stability. Particles of a diameter of $5\,\mu$m or greater do not reach the alveoli of the lung and therefore initially cause infection only of the upper respiratory tract.

Infections spread by the respiratory route are more likely to occur where population densities are high and ventilation is poor. Examples of such conditions are enzootic pneumonia in intensively reared pigs and occupationally acquired brucellosis in meat workers. In environmental extremes,

diseases that are rarely spread by the respiratory route become transmissible by this method. These circumstances arise in the airborne transmission of rabies from insectivorous bats to animals and man within the confines of a cave. Similarly, African swine fever virus, which is usually transmitted by *Ornithodoros* spp. ticks, spreads rapidly by the respiratory route in piggeries. In crowded and poor living conditions, pneumonic plague is transmitted directly between people, rather than by the bites of infected fleas, the latter method of transmission inducing the less severe bubonic plague.

## Infection via skin, cornea and mucous membranes

Transmission via the skin is **percutaneous** (Latin: *per* = through, across; *cut* = skin). Certain agents infect only the skin and transmission is always by direct contact with either another infected animal or a fomes; examples are 'ringworm' and ectoparasitic infestations. The incidence of such infections and infestations is particularly influenced by the population density of the susceptible hosts. Intact skin acts as an effective barrier to the majority of infectious agents, but some, particularly the immature stages of some nematodes and trematodes, can penetrate this barrier and cause infection. Examples include blood fluke (*Schistosoma* spp.) and hookworm (*Ancylostoma* spp.) infections, the latter infection also being zoonotic and the cause of cutaneous larva migrans in man.

If the skin is cut or abraded, infection by a variety of organisms can occur, resulting in localized infections of the skin (e.g. by *Staphylococcus* spp. and the cutaneous form of human anthrax). Other agents, such as leptospires, may gain entry to the body percutaneously and then develop a more generalized infection.

Another important form of percutaneous infection is from bites by both vertebrates and arthropods. Agents that are present in the saliva, such as the viruses of rabies and lymphocytic choriomeningitis, and bacteria such as *Streptobacillus moniliformis* (a common inhabitant of the oropharynx of rats), are transmitted by animal bites.

Diseases transmitted by the bites of infected arthropod vectors constitute a particular class of infections that was introduced earlier in this chapter during the description of hosts and vectors.

Infection of the cornea may remain localized, for example, bovine keratoconjunctivitis, caused by *Moraxella bovis*. Alternatively, the infection may spread to other parts of the body, for example, corneal infection of birds with Newcastle disease virus.

Although few diseases can be transmitted through intact skin, several can infect undamaged mucous membranes. An important class of such agents is those that are very labile in the external environment, and require intimate sexual contact during coitus to be transmitted to the urogenital tract, for example *Trypanosoma equiperdum* in horses.

## Methods of transmission

Six main methods of transmission, which bring infectious agents into contact with the sites of infection, can be identified:

(1) ingestion;
(2) inhalation;
(3) contact;
(4) inoculation;
(5) iatrogenic transmission;
(6) coitus.

Additionally, long-distance transfer is important in some virus infections.

### Ingestion

This may occur via a mechanical vehicle (fomes), for example, contaminated water, or by ingestion of intermediate hosts, such as cestode cysts in meat. Ingested agents are usually excreted in the faeces, producing the faecal-oral transmission cycle. Some agents are excreted only faecally because they are localized to the intestine (e.g. the Johne's disease bacillus in cattle). Other agents, if they invade the bloodstream, can be excreted by additional means, such as the urine (e.g. *Salmonella* spp.). Sometimes, agents are excreted on the breath (e.g. reoviruses).

### Inhalation

This involves airborne transmission of infectious agents via contaminated air. This mode of transfer is common with pathogens of the respiratory tract that are expired on the breath of infected animals and enter susceptible ones during inspiration.

Quasistable suspensions of liquids or solids in gases, that are capable of floating for some time, are formed only when droplet diameters do not exceed 5 $\mu$m. Expiratory droplets range in size from 15–100 $\mu$m and thus even the smallest sediment rapidly (within 3 seconds). Therefore, they cannot travel far. Direct infection from expiratory droplets is thus limited to the area directly in front of the infected individual (the 'expiratory cone'). Very localized droplet infection can occur on food bowls and by sniffing.

Other agents, which can contaminate the air, may also be airborne (e.g. foot-and-mouth disease virus shed from ruptured vesicles: *see below*, 'Long-distance transmission of infection').

### Contact

Contact transmission is transmission without transmission factors (e.g. mechanical vectors) and without participation of an external medium. This is particularly important in relation to infectious agents that are shed from the body surfaces, such as vesicular viruses, and with agents that gain entry through the body surface. Very few agents are transmitted merely by touch; some degree of trauma is necessary, albeit microscopic. Transmission may be by bites (e.g rabies and rat bite fever), or by scratches (e.g. cat scratch fever).

Diseases transmitted by contact may be described as 'contagious' (Latin: *contagio* = to touch closely) but this term is now used less commonly than previously.

### Inoculation

Inoculation (Latin: *inoculatus* = engrafted, or implanted) is the introduction into the body, by puncture of the skin or through a wound, of infectious agents.

Although classified separately here, inoculation is frequently associated with contact transmission (e.g. bites from rabid dogs). Arthropods that act as vectors may inoculate infectious agents into the blood by biting (e.g. tsetse flies infected with *Trypanosoma* spp., in which development of the parasite occurs in the salivary gland, gut and mouth parts).

### Iatrogenic transmission

**Iatrogenic** literally means 'created by a doctor'. Thus, an iatrogenically transmitted infection is one that is transferred during surgical and medical practice.

There are two main types, involving:

(1) introduction of pathogens by dirty instruments (e.g. during non-aseptic surgery and tattooing) or by contaminated body surfaces;
(2) introduction of pathogens contaminating prophylactic or therapeutic preparations (e.g. *Pseudomonas aeruginosa* in intramammary dry-cow antibiotic preparations: Nicholls *et al.*, 1981; lumpy skin disease in anaplasmosis vaccine; scrapie in louping ill vaccine; human hepatitis B virus in serum preparations) and, more rarely, by organ transplantation (e.g. rabies virus by corneal transplants).

### Coitus

Some infectious agents may be transmitted during coitus. Certain diseases are transmitted only in this way. These were called venereal diseases (Latin: *venereus* = pertaining to sexual love). In human medicine they are now referred to as sexually transmitted diseases (STDs). Sexual transmission can occur not only in vertebrates but also in arthropods. For example, African swine fever virus can be sexually transmitted from male to female ticks of the genus *Ornithodoros* (Plowright *et al.*, 1974).

The mode of transmission of agents frequently governs the epidemic picture. Thus, agents that are transmitted by the faecal-oral and airborne modes often produce sudden explosive epidemics, whereas coitally transmitted diseases spread more slowly, over a long period of time.

### Long-distance transmission of infection

Infectious diseases can be transmitted over long distances as a result of the mobility of infected animals, vectors and fomites. Previously, transportation by sea provided a period of quarantine, but the increasing use of air transport means that animals incubating infections can arrive at their destination before clinical signs of infection have appeared. The movement of horses, in connection with their sale, breeding and competition, has spread a variety of equine infections, including contagious equine metritis, equine infectious anaemia, piroplasmosis and influenza, between continents (Powell, 1985). The movement of people, for example by aeroplane, can also distribute human exotic diseases over all parts of the world (Prothro, 1977). There is concern that the screwworm fly, *Chrysomyia bezziana*, which is endemic in Papua New Guinea, may be imported into Australia as an inadvertent passenger on international flights, or by animal movement between the Torres Strait Islands (*see* the case study in Chapter 18 for further details).

Airborne transmission over long distances cannot occur with expiratory droplets because they sediment rapidly (*see above*). Transmission of respiratory and vesicular infections indirectly through the air over long distances (aerial transmission) must, therefore, be effected by other means. The evaporation of water from droplets (which can occur when droplets are airborne or on the ground) produces desiccated **droplet nuclei**, ranging in diameter from 2 $\mu$m to 10 $\mu$m. The smallest of these are quasistable and can travel over long distances, assisted by wind. The rate of formation of these nuclei depends on the temperature and relative humidity. Rain sediments the nuclei.

The distribution pattern of the nuclei can be complex. During the 1967–68 foot-and-mouth disease epidemic in England, a series of secondary outbreaks followed the primary one (*Figure 6.7a*). Initially, it was suggested that this was due to infected imported lamb, because no human or mechanical links could be established between the

secondary outbreaks and the primary outbreak at Bryn Farm. However, a complex meteorological hypothesis has been presented (Tinline, 1970, 1972) suggesting that the secondary outbreaks were caused by virus particles being pulled downwards in a current of air which is forced into vertical oscillation as it flows over a hill. This phenomenon is called a **lee wave** (*Figure 6.7b*).

Wind can also carry vectors over long distances. The outbreak of bluetongue in Portugal in 1956 (point map: *see Figure 4.4*) may have been caused by windborne transfer of the African vector *Culicoides imicola* from North Africa, although the latter is now permanently established in Portugal (Mellor *et al.*, 1985).

# Vertical transmission

## *Types and methods of vertical transmission*

There are two types of vertical transmission:

(1) hereditary;
(2) congenital.

Hereditarily transmitted diseases are carried within the genome of either parent. Thus, retroviruses, which have integrated DNA copies of the virus in the host's genome, are transferred hereditarily.

Congenitally transmitted diseases are, literally, those present at birth. According to strict etymology, hereditarily transmitted diseases are part of this group. However, by common usage, 'congenital' refers to diseases **acquired** either *in utero* or *in ovo* rather than inherited.

Transmission can occur at various stages of embryonic development. It may produce either abortion, if incompatible with life, or teratoma (literally 'monsters'). Alternatively, infection that is inapparent and continuous after birth (**innate infection**) can occur.

### Germinative transmission

This involves either infection of the superficial layers of the ovary, or infection of the ovum itself. Examples include the chicken leucosis viruses, spontaneous lymphoid leukaemias of mice (Gross, 1955), murine lymphocytic choriomeningitis and avian salmonellosis.

### Transmission to the embryo

This occurs via the placenta (transplacentally) or via the fetal circulation, through the placenta, to the fetus. For example, kittens can be transplacentally infected with feline panleucopenia virus (Csiza *et*

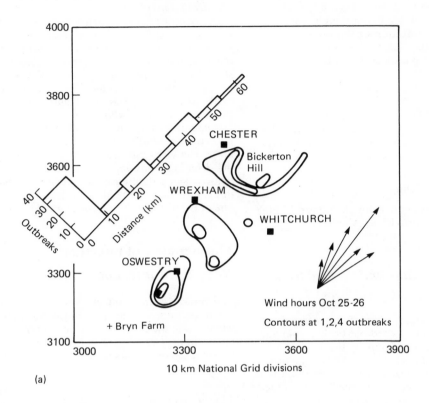

(a)

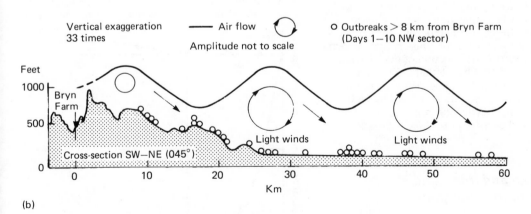

(b)

**Figure 6.7** 1967–68 English foot-and-mouth disease epidemic: (**a**) outbreaks for days 1–10; (**b**) profile through Bryn Farm illustrating the lee wave hypothesis of aerial spread of virus. (Reprinted by permission from *Nature*, Vol. 227, pp. 860–862. Copyright © 1970 Macmillan Journals Limited)

*al.*, 1971). Viruses, being small, cross the placenta with greater ease and earlier in pregnancy than larger microbes. The fetal circulation, however, can carry most microbes. Infection of the placenta does not always produce infection of the fetus. Q fever particles, for instance, may be found in large quantities in bovine placentae without infection of the developing calves.

### Ascending infection

This is infection that is transmitted from the lower genital canal to the amnion and placenta (e.g. staphylococci and streptococci).

### Infection at parturition

This is infection acquired from the lower genital canal at birth (e.g. human herpes simplex).

## *Immunological status and vertical transmission*

The immunological status of the fetus is important when agents are transmitted vertically. Immune tolerance of microbial antigens by the fetus can be detrimental in postnatal life, because 'non-self' antigens are then recognized as 'self'. The result is a lack of a protective immune response, sometimes with the development of a carrier state with the subsequent dangers to other susceptible animals, as in the case of feline panleucopenia. However, immune tolerance by the fetus can occasionally be advantageous when infections have clinical and pathological effects mediated by the immune response. The paradigm of this is lymphocytic choriomeningitis (LCM) infection of mice. In adults the disease is mediated by a lethal infiltration of the brain by responsive T lymphocytes. Prenatal infection induces a tolerance to LCM virion antigens; therefore no lymphocytic infiltration occurs in adult infections, and thus there is no clinical disease.

## *Transovarial and trans-stadial transmission in arthropods*

Some arthropods, notably ticks and mites, transmit bacteria, viruses and protozoa from one generation to another via their eggs; this is **transovarial** transmission. Examples of transovarially transmitted infections include bovine anaplasmosis (a protozoan disease causing anaemia in cattle in the tropics and subtropics, transmitted by several genera of ticks) and canine babesiosis (another protozoan disease causing anaemia in dogs, transmitted by ticks of the genera *Dermacentor* and *Haemaphysalis*).

In contrast, some arthropods only transmit infections from one developmental stage to another (e.g in ticks: larva to nymph, nymph to adult); this is **trans-stadial** transmission. An example of a transstadially transmitted disease is theileriosis, caused by protozoa of the genus *Theileria*, occurring in cattle, sheep and goats, and transmitted by ticks of the genus *Rhipicephalus*.

Some infections are spread both transovarially and trans-stadially, for example Nairobi sheep disease, a virus infection transmitted by the brown tick *Rhipicephalus appendiculatus*. Investigations of tick-transmitted diseases are revealing that many infections, once thought to be transmitted by only one of these methods, are transmitted by both.

# Maintenance of infection
## *Hazards to infectious agents*

The transmission of infection involves some stages when the infectious agent is in the host, and others when it is in the external environment or in a vector, or in both (*see Figure 6.1*). Both internal and external environments present hazards to infectious agents.

### The environment within the host

The host has its natural defence mechanisms: humoral antibodies, specific reactive cells, phagocytes and surface-active chemicals. The successful

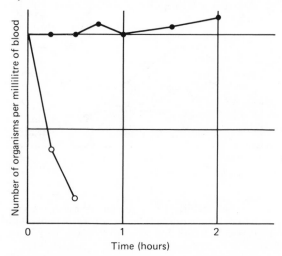

**Figure 6.8** The protective action of bacterial capsules: pneumococci, capsulated (●) and not capsulated (○), injected intravenously into mice; blood of mice then sampled every 15 minutes. (From Boycott, 1971)

parasite must be able to avoid, in part, these mechanisms, and must also avoid competition with other agents that may simultaneously infect the host in a similar niche (*see* Chapter 7). Parasites have evolved strategies to resist the host's protective mechanisms, such as acid-resistant helminth cuticles (to resist gastric acid) and an intracellular mode of life (to avoid humoral antibodies). Some bacteria possess capsules that protect them against phagocytosis, for example *Pneumococcus* spp. (*Figure 6.8*). Many parasitic nematodes have a greater fecundity than their free-living counterparts, thus ensuring that some offspring will survive the host's immune response and potentially lethal conditions in the external environment.

## The external environment

The two main hazards presented by the external environment are desiccation and ultraviolet light. Desiccation is not always lethal, but frequently inhibits multiplication. Low temperatures are not usually lethal, but can inhibit multiplication. The high temperatures attained in temperate climates are probably not lethal but those reached in tropical countries may be more effective. Many agents may be partially protected from desiccation by being discharged in moist carriers such as faeces and urine. They may also persist by being shed into favourable surroundings; leptospires, for example, persist longer in paddy fields than in semi-arid regions. Some agents (e.g. the pox viruses) are quite resistant to desiccation and can survive for long periods in dry infected scab material. Agents may also survive in inanimate material in the environment which may therefore act as fomites, for example, animal foodstuffs contaminated with *Salmonella* spp.

## *Maintenance strategies*

The ways in which infectious agents are maintained can be considered as **strategies** for maintenance. Five main strategies can be identified:

(1) avoidance of a stage in the external environment;
(2) the development of resistant forms;
(3) a 'rapidly-in, rapidly-out' strategy;
(4) persistence within the host;
(5) extension of host range.

## Avoidance of a stage in the external environment

Some agents avoid transfer via the environment. There are four main methods:

(1) by vertical transmission;

(2) by venereal transmission;
(3) by vector transmission;
(4) by transmission by sarcophaga (flesh eating), for example, the helminth *Trichinella spiralis* occurs in cysts in the muscle of pigs, rats and other animals, and is only transmitted when these animals are eaten by predators and scavengers, including man.

## Resistant forms

The harshness of the external environment can be buffered by surrounding the infectious agent with a shell that is resistant to heat and desiccation. Some bacteria form such shells (spores). Examples include members of the genera *Clostridium* and *Bacillus*, which can survive boiling water, even flames, for short periods of time, and may survive in the external environment for decades. Fungi may also produce spores. Generally these are less resistant than bacterial spores. Some helminths and protozoa form resistant shells (cysts). These can protect the agent from the host's defence mechanisms; the protozoan parasite, *Toxoplasma gondii*, for example, can survive for many years in its cystic form in the host, until the latter is eaten. Thick-shelled helminth eggs can resist the external environment and may overwinter on pasture.

## 'Rapidly-in, rapidly-out' strategy

Some agents enter the host, replicate and leave very quickly, before the host has time to mount an immune response or die. Many viruses of the upper respiratory tract can do this within 24 hours. The strategy requires a continuous supply of susceptible hosts. This may be one reason why respiratory and enteric infections, such as the common cold virus in man, are not present in primitive societies of low population density, and may not have occurred in small prehistoric societies (Brothwell and Sandison, 1967; Black, 1975).

## Persistence within the host

Agents may persist within the host, sometimes aided by a poor rejection response by the host. Examples include *Mycobacterium johnei*, tapeworm infections of the gut, and *T. gondii* and *T. spiralis* in tissues.

Persistence can be associated with a long incubation or prepatent period. A group of virus diseases, termed 'slow virus diseases' because of their long incubation period, falls into this category. Scrapie, for example, is a slow virus disease of sheep, producing neurological signs, with an incubation period of 1–5 years. Its persistence within its host facilitates vertical and possibly horizontal transmission in a flock.

**Table 6.1 Some characteristics of host/parasite relationships between fleas, acting as vectors, and infectious agents. (Simplified from Bibikova, 1977)**

| Disease and pathogen | Site of pathogen in flea | Reproduction of pathogen in flea | Duration of pathogen in flea | Pathogenic effect on flea |
|---|---|---|---|---|
| Myxomatosis *Fibromavirus myxomatosis* | Digestive tract | No | Up to 100 days | Yes |
| Tularaemia *Francisella tularensis* | Digestive tract | No | Several days | No |
| Murine typhus *Rickettsia mooseri* | Digestive tract | Yes | Lifetime | No |
| Murine trypanosomiasis *Trypanosoma lewisi* | Digestive tract | Yes | Lifetime | No |
| Salmonellosis *Salmonella enteritidis* | Digestive tract | Yes | Up to 40 days | Yes |
| Plague *Yersinia pestis* | Digestive tract | Yes | Several months to over 1 year | Yes |

Alternatively, an agent's prepatent period may be relatively short, but excretion of the agent may continue for a long time (i.e. the period of infectiousness is long). Excretion may be intermittent, for example, *Salmonella* spp. infection can be associated with intermittent clinical episodes or subclinical infection, both associated with occasional excretion of the bacterium. Infection may also result in continuous excretion. For example, infection of cattle by *Leptospira*, serovar *hardjo*, results in urinary excretion of the bacterium that can last for 12–24 months. The long period of infectiousness of hosts infected with such agents ensures that a susceptible population, resulting from regular births, is always available. Some endogenous agents (*see* Chapter 5) may persist as the bacterial flora of hosts.

Agents may persist not only within vertebrate hosts but also in arthropod vectors. *Table 6.1* lists the duration of infection of fleas by various microbial agents. Note that some agents (e.g. murine typhus) can persist in fleas for the latter's lifetime which can be very long—over 500 days in the case of unfed *Pulex irritans* (Soulsby, 1982). Additionally, agents can persist in flea excreta for long periods; murine typhus, for example, can persist for over 9 years (Smith, 1973).

## Extension of host range

Many infectious agents can infect more than one host. Indeed, their number exceeds that of one-host agents. In man, for example, over 80% of infectious agents to which he is susceptible are shared by other

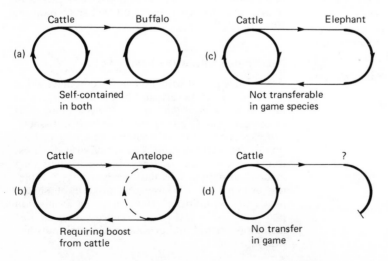

**Figure 6.9** Hypothetical interrelationship of foot-and-mouth disease in cattle and game species; see text for explanation. (From Brooksby, 1972)

species of animal. A major role of the veterinarian is to control these zoonoses (e.g. tuberculosis and canine ascarid infections).

Extension of host range is an obvious way of maintaining infection. It is facilitated by the presence of the various hosts in the same area. However, if an agent is present in two different species in the same region, it should not be assumed that transfer between these species always occurs. In Africa, for example, foot-and-mouth disease virus infections occur in both cattle and wild buffalo, but the virus rarely spreads from one species to the other (*Figure 6.9a*). Other possible relationships between cattle and game are illustrated in *Figure 6.9*. Antelope cannot maintain the infection in their own species unless it is boosted by occasional transmission to cattle (*Figure 6.9b*). Elephant can carry the virus from cattle to cattle, but cannot transmit it to members of their own species (*Figure 6.9c*). Several species of wild animals also act as dead-end hosts and are incapable of transmitting the virus to other animals (*Figure 6.9d*).

## *Further reading*

BOYCOTT, J.A. (1971) *Natural History of Infectious Disease*. Studies in Biology No. 26. Edward Arnold, London

BUSVINE, J.R. (1975) *Arthropod Vectors of Disease*. Studies in Biology No. 55. Edward Arnold, London

GORDON SMITH, C.E. (1976) *Epidemiology and Infections*. Meadowfield Press, Shildon

GORDON SMITH, C.E. (1982) Major factors in the spread of infections. In: *Animal Disease in Relation to Animal Conservation*. Symposium of the Zoological Society of London No. 50. Eds Edwards, M.A. and McDonnell, U. Pp. 207–235. Academic Press, London and New York

HERS, J.F.PH and WINKLER, K.C. (Eds) (1973) *Airborne Transmission and Airborne Infection*. Oosthoek Publishing Company, Utrecht

MATUMOTO, M. (1969) Mechanisms of perpetuation of animal viruses in nature. *Bacteriological Reviews*, **33**, 404–418

MIMS, C.A. (1982) *The Pathogenesis of Infectious Disease*, 2nd edn. Academic Press, London and New York

ROBERTSON, A. (Ed.) (1976) *Handbook on Animal Diseases in the Tropics*, 3rd edn. British Veterinary Association, London

TAYLOR, A.E.R. (Ed.) (1964) *Host-Parasite Relationships in Invertebrate Hosts*. Second Symposium of the British Society for Parasitology. Blackwell Scientific Publications, Oxford

WELLS, W.F. (1955) *Airborne Contagion and Our Hygiene: An Ecological Study of Droplet Infection*. Harvard University Press, Cambridge, Massachusetts

# The ecology of disease

The study of disease in populations requires an understanding of the relationships between organisms (hosts and agents) and their environment. These relationships govern the spatial and temporal occurrence of disease. Climate, for example, affects the survival of hosts and infectious agents and the distribution of the latter's vectors either directly or, more subtly, by regulating the occurrence of plants that support the organisms. Similarly, the type of plant can affect the availability of minerals and trace elements and therefore the occurrence of disease associated with a deficiency, an excess, or an imbalance of these chemicals. For instance, white clover (*Trifolium repens*) absorbs relatively small amounts of selenium, whereas brown top (*Agrostis tenuis*) absorbs large amounts (Davies and Watkinson, 1966). Therefore, when pasture is top-dressed with selenium salts to prevent selenium deficiency in animals, the risk of selenium toxocity is greater if the latter plant predominates.

The study of animals and plants in relation to their habits and habitation (habitat) is 'ecology' (Greek: *oikos* = house; *logo-* = discoursing). Ecology developed as a discipline relating to animals and plants, but has been extended to include microorganisms (e.g. Alexander, 1971). The scale of ecological studies therefore ranges from an investigation of leptospires in the 'environment' of the renal tubules to the distribution of sylvatic hosts of foot-and-mouth disease in the African savannahs. The study of a disease's ecology (also termed its natural history), is frequently a part of epidemiological investigations. This has two objectives:

(1) an increase in the understanding of the pathogenesis, maintenance and, for infectious agents, transmission of disease;

(2) the use of knowledge of a disease's ecology to predict when and where a disease may occur, to enable the development of suitable control techniques.

This chapter introduces basic ecological concepts and relates them to epidemiological investigations.

## Basic ecological concepts

Two major factors that determine the occurrence of disease are the distribution and size of animal populations. The former depends on the distribution of suitable food; the latter depends on availability of food, mates and the species' breeding potential.

### *The distribution of populations*

#### Vegetational zones

Botanists were among the first to note the division of the earth into different vegetational zones. In some parts of the world this division is clear, for example the border between forest and tundra in northern regions and the zoning of forests as one ascends mountains. In other areas the change is more gradual, for instance the transition from deserts to prairies. Early 18th century naturalists suggested that the world was divided into discrete **formations** of vegetation, such as tundra, savannah and desert, and they drew maps that neatly but erroneously separated formations by lines.

The first serious attempt to explain these apparent neat formations was made by de Candolle (1874), who argued that climate, particularly temperature,

**Table 7.1 Koppen's system of classification of climate based on de Candolle's plant groups. (From Colinvaux, 1973)**

| De Candolle's plant group | Postulated plant requirements | Formation | Koppen's climatic division |
|---|---|---|---|
| Megatherms (most heat) | Continuous high temperature and abundant moisture | Tropical rain forest | A (rainy with no winter) |
| Xerophiles (dry-loving) | Tolerate drought, need minimum hot season | Hot desert such as Sonoran | B (dry) |
| Mesotherms (middle heat) | Moderate temperature and moderate moisture | Temperate deciduous forest | C (rainy with mild winters) |
| Microtherms (little heat) | Less heat, less moisture, tolerate long cold winters | Boreal forest | D (rainy climates with severe winters) |
| Hekistotherms (least heat) | Tolerate polar regions 'beyond tree-line' | Tundra | E (polar climates with no warm season) |

dictated vegetation. He drew the first vegetational map based on isotherms. Rain forests were described as formations of **megatherms**, deciduous forests of **mesotherms**, and deserts of **xerophiles**. At the beginning of the 20th century Koppen used de Candolle's classification as the basis of the modern system (*Table 7.1*), which provides a good correlation between climatic and vegetational regions. Climate may dictate boundaries, but in a much more complex way than merely by ground-level temperature changes and rainfall. Recent meteorological work using satellites, and long-term studies of the thermal composition of air masses, however, suggest that the mean positions of air fronts over the earth roughly coincide with vegetational types.

## Biomes

In the 19th century, zoologists noted that the broad divisions of the earth were populated by similar animals. Even if the divisions were discontinuous (e.g. Africa and South America), some animals, especially birds, showed similar features. This assisted the evolutionists in adding credence to their theory of **convergent evolution** which states that animals of different ancestral stock evolve similar features to suit similar environments.

Zoologists attempted to classify different areas of the world according to the types of animal and plant that were present, because the distribution of animals appeared to be related to vegetation. One such person was the American Merriam (1893) who defined **life zones** in North America after studying the distribution of animals and plants at various altitudes on North American mountains.

Merriam proposed four main life zones (*Figure 7.1*):

(1) Boreal (northern), involving the Canadian, Hudsonian and Alpine Arctic;

(2) Transition, containing animals and plants from the Boreal and Sonoran;
(3) Sonoran (named after Sonora, a state in NW Mexico), comprising the Upper and Lower;
(4) Tropical.

A fifth, minor one (the Lower Californian) is also indicated in *Figure 7.1*. It is important to note that there is a gradual transition from one zone to another; the apparent boundary on the life zone map is set sharply by the cartographer. African ecological zones, based on climate, vegetation and potential for agricultural use, are described by Pratt *et al.* (1966).

Merriam, like de Candolle, thought that temperature governed the distribution of animals. He argued that, in the northern hemisphere, an animal's northern boundary was drawn by the threshold temperature below which reproduction was not possible. The animal's southern boundary was drawn by the threshold temperature above which the heat was intolerable. Although Merriam spent much time measuring mean temperatures, he was never able to match isotherms with life zones. Although reasons for the transition from one life zone to another are not available, the existence of these zones is clear. They are now commonly called **biomes**. Examples of biomes include tropical rain forest, savannah and tundra, each with its own particular range of plants and animals.

The distribution of infectious agents and their vectors, and therefore of the diseases produced by the former, may be limited by the environmental conditions of biomes. Thus, the fungus *Coccidioides immitis*, which systemically infects man, dogs, cattle and pigs, producing primary respiratory symptoms in man and dogs, appears to be endemically limited to the Lower Sonoran life zone (*Figure 7.2*: Schmelzer and Tabershaw, 1968). This zone is characterized by hot summers, mild winters, sparse

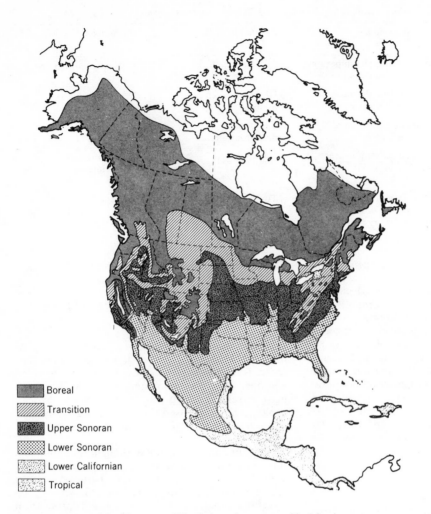

Boreal

Transition

Upper Sonoran

Lower Sonoran

Lower Californian

Tropical

**Figure 7.1** Map of the life zones of North America proposed by Merriam.

vegetation, an annual rainfall of 6–8 inches, an alkaline soil pH and wind conditions that are conducive to maintenance and dissemination of the fungus (Egeberg, 1954). The distribution of Rift valley fever (a virus disease of sheep and cattle) is associated with the wetter African ecological zones. This may be related to the abundance of mosquito vectors in these zones (Davies, 1975).

## *Regulation of population size*

### The 'balance of nature'

The early biologists were impressed by the stability of animal and plant populations. Populations grow,

reach a certain size, and then stop growing. The population becomes stable and **balanced**, with the rate of reproduction equalling the death rate.

### Control of population size by competition

Two hypotheses have been formulated to explain the balance of nature. Chapman (1928) argued that there was **environmental resistance**. Animal populations had an intrinsic rate of increase but there was some quality of the environment that resisted the increase. This theory may be good but there is no evidence to support it. The currently accepted theory is that populations are brought into balance by **competition** for the resources of the habitat, the

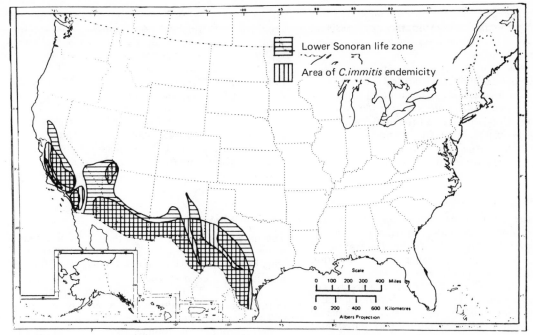

**Figure 7.2** Lower Sonoran life zone and area of endemic *Coccidioides immitis* (nosoarea) in the USA. (From Schmelzer and Tabershaw, 1968)

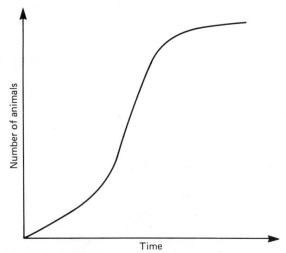

**Figure 7.3** The sigmoid growth curve for a simple population in a confined space with a limited input of energy.

most common of which is food. Competition is therefore **density-dependent**.

In order to test this hypothesis it is necessary to conduct an experiment in which food supply is controlled. Such an experiment was conducted by Gause (1934), using one species of *Paramecium* with a constant supply of food. The growth curve for this protozoon is a sigmoid (*Figure 7.3*) that approximates to a mathematical equation, called the **logistic equation**.

The logistic equation is derived thus:

If $R$ = observed rate of increase,
$r$ = intrinsic rate of increase,
$N$ = number of animals,

then, for the slope of the curve:

$R = rN.$

If $K$ = saturation number, then, with increasing competition, when $N = K$, $R = 0$.
The complete history of the sigmoid curve is:

$$R = rN \left(1 - \frac{N}{K}\right).$$

Early in growth, when growth is rapid because much food is available, $N$ is small;

therefore the quotient $N/K$ is small:

$1 - \frac{N}{K}$ approaches 1,

and $R$ approaches $rN$.

Later as growth decreases (because less food is available):

$\frac{N}{K}$ approaches $\frac{K}{K} = 1$.

Thus $1 - \frac{N}{K}$ approaches 0.

Thus $R = rN \times 0$
$= 0$.

Further laboratory studies, for example with the fruit fly *Drosophila*, supported the hypothesis of density-dependent competition for food. However, experiments with other insects, notably the flour beetle, showed that density-dependent factors other than food availability may control the size of populations, for instance the build-up of metabolic excretory products and decreased reproduction due to crowding. Thus, the competition model is a useful theoretical concept that has aided understanding of regulatory mechanisms, but in the real world other factors may also control population size.

## Dispersal

In some parts of the world, there may be dramatic seasonal variations in climate. An Australian species of grasshopper overwinters in its egg. The warmth of spring causes the eggs to hatch. The adults that develop then lay eggs as long as the weather is wet. A drought kills all of the adults. This is not density-dependent; it occurs long before competition occurs. Such insects survive only by **dispersal** over large areas to different climates so that at least some are in an area that is not wet. This phenomenon led Andrewartha and Birch (1954) to suggest that large animals too were controlled by climate, not competition for food. They emphasized the dangers of oversimplification using the logistic model.

## Predation

Predation has an obvious plausible role in controlling the size of populations, but most of the evidence suggests that this is not true for large animals because predators take only the sick and weak and young animals. Since the latter probably would not die otherwise (a small number of deaths may occur, for example by drowning during migration) predation could have some effect on population size. There is, however, contradictory evidence. In the Serengetti of Africa there are about 200 000 wildebeests, but lions will kill only 12 000–18 000 each year, an insignificant number, and mostly newborn animals that become lost.

Small predators, however, notably of insects, are efficient controllers of populations. Predators have been used to control insect pests, for example, the use of ladybirds to control cotton cushony-scale insects.

## Home range

Certain animals have a natural restriction to the area over which they roam; this is their **home range**. This may control the population and has implications for the transmission of infectious disease; infected animals may transmit infection over their home range, but no further. For example, rats are the maintenance hosts of the rickettsial disease scrub typhus. Trombiculid mites (chiggers) are the vectors; they parasitize mammals and birds. The small home range of the rats results in the mite's life-cycle being restricted to small areas, called 'mite islands' (Audy, 1961). When the mites are infected with the rickettsia, localized endemic areas of scrub typhus, associated with the mite islands, occur. Extension of the infection occurs only by dispersal of infected mites by wider-ranging incidental hosts such as birds and man in whom the infection causes serious disease.

## Territoriality

The part of an animal's home range that it defends aggressively from invaders is the animal's **territory**. This behavioural response is **territoriality**. This has an advantage, economizing movement when searching for food. Territoriality may also control the population because there is a minimum size to a territory and a finite amount of space and therefore a finite number of animals that can exist in the territory. The sizes of territories vary for the same and different species. For example, arctic birds have a larger territory when food is scarce than when it is plentiful.

## Social dominance

In the 1920s, a social hierarchy called the 'peck order' was discovered among birds. Some gregarious species, especially rodents, inhabit favourable places. When crowding occurs, the socially weaker animals are forced out. This may be a population control mechanism.

## The 'Wynne-Edwards' hypothesis

The population control consequence of territoriality, social hierarchy and behaviour may be just a side-effect. The Aberdeen zoologist, Wynne-Edwards, suggested that population control was the main purpose of **group behaviour** (Wynne-Edwards, 1962), which sometimes causes physiological stress (*see* Chapter 5). The adrenal glands are the structures that prepare the body for 'flight or fight'. The crowding of rats causes stress with associated fighting, cannibalism and reduced fecundity. Such animals have adrenals twice the size of those of unstressed animals. Sewer rats also live under stress and have hypertrophied adrenals. This is an example of the 'general adaptation syndrome' (*see* Chapter 5).

At certain times of the year animals congregate, for example, deer during the rutting season, even when equally acceptable areas are deserted. Wynne-Edwards suggested that this 'head count' of the population evoked, by feedback, the general adaptation syndrome and controlled reproduction. There are two problems with this theory: evolution tends to select individuals, not groups, and the hypothesis suggests that birth-controllers are favoured, whereas evolution usually selects the efficient producers. This theory is not fashionable today.

For whatever reason animals congregate, the increased contact can aid transmission of infectious agents, and can produce seasonal trends in disease occurrence (*see* Chapter 8). Thus, when North American leopard frogs congregate to spawn during the winter, there is seasonal transmission of Lucké's frog virus (McKinnell and Ellis, 1972).

It is difficult to produce a general theory of population control. Food availability is important, and energy availability limits the supportable biomass (*see below*, 'The distribution of energy between trophic levels'). However, different mechanisms probably operate in different circumstances.

### The implications for disease occurrence of the distribution and control of populations

The distribution, the home range of animals, and other behavioural activities of hosts of infectious agents affect the latter's transmission. An example is rabies in foxes. Rabies is maintained in Europe in foxes. The behaviour of foxes during the year alters the association between foxes. Foxes may be solitary, paired, or part of a family unit. Similarly, rabid foxes' behaviour depends on the type of rabies that they display; foxes with dumb rabies may seek a solitary existence, whereas furious rabies may cause foxes to approach other animals readily. *Figure 7.4*

| | | Grouping of foxes | | | | |
|---|---|---|---|---|---|---|
| | | Solitary | Pair | Family | Social groups | Mixed society |
| **Behaviour of rabid foxes** | Dumb | □□□□ | ▼ | ▼▼ | ▼▼▼ | ▼▼ |
| | Furious | ▼ | ▼▼ | ▼▼▼ | ▼▼▼▼ | ▼▼▼ |
| | Mixed | ▼ | ▼▼ | ▼▼▼▼▼ | ▼▼▼▼▼▼▼ | ▼▼▼▼▼ |

**Figure 7.4** Social group behaviour and behaviour of rabid foxes as determinants of rabies in foxes. □: Condition unfavourable for existence of rabies virus; number of squares indicates the relative degree to which conditions are unfavourable. ▼: Conditions favourable for the existence of rabies virus; number of triangles indicates the relative degree to which conditions are favourable. (From Macdonald and Bacon, 1980)

illustrates how these different behaviour patterns affect the survival and spread of rabies virus between animals.

Increases in home range may also increase spread of infection. Thus, during the summer months, rabies may be confined to foxes in the northern tundra and forests of Canada, but in winter, as food supplies become scarce, infected foxes may invade more southerly regions and introduce rabies to such areas.

## The niche

Gause's work with *Paramecium*, mentioned earlier in this chapter, is an example of **intraspecific** competition, that is competition between members of the same species. **Interspecific** competition can also occur when two species live together, in which case they either might both thrive, or one may be exterminated by the other.

The solving, simultaneously (in the mathematical sense) of the logistic equation for each species to find the relative size of each population produces pairs of equations that were derived independently in the USA by Lotka (1925) and in Italy by Volterra (Chapman, 1931). These equations are therefore called **Lotka–Volterra** equations. They can be derived for varying degrees of competition. The conclusion drawn from these equations is of fundamental importance in ecology. It is that **the coexistence of two strongly competing species is impossible**. Coexistence is possible only if competition is weak. This was tested again by Gause using two different species of *Paramecium* in a test-tube culture. He found that either one or the other species triumphed, depending on the composition of the environment. This led to the principle of **competitive exclusion**: that competition will exclude all but one species from a particular position defined by an animal's feeding habits, physiology, mechanical abilities and behaviour. This position is an animal's **niche** (Elton, 1927). The principle of competitive exclusion can therefore be summarized as 'one species, one niche'. (This implies that Charles Darwin's original concept of the survival of animals most suited to their environment, as a result of competition, should be modified to one of survival by the avoidance of competition.)

There are examples of competition leading to exclusion in the real world as a result of strong competition, although they are few. Probably the best-documented one is of the Abington turtles. Abington is an island in the South Atlantic that had an indigenous species of turtle. During the 19th century, sailors introduced goats to the island. The goats had exactly the same requirements as the turtles for food. Therefore there was strong competition, which led to the extinction of one of the species, in this case the turtles, according to the Lotka–Volterra prediction.

Competitive exclusion has been used as a means of disease control. The snail *Biomphalaria glabrata*, which is an intermediate host for schistosomiasis, has been replaced by the more competitive snail *Marisa cornuarietis*, which is not an intermediate host for the helminth (Lord, 1983). *M. cornuarietis* is reared and then released into streams and ponds which are the habitat of *B. glabrata*. *M. cornuarietis* dominates within a few months of its release, and *B. glabrata* virtually disappears.

However, the real world is very diverse and there are many opportunities for animals to avoid competition by finding their own niche. Sometimes the mechanism of avoidance is not obvious, for example marine zooplankton are all filter feeders but actually filter particles of different sizes and therefore do not compete.

Avoidance of competition is usual in **sympatric species**, that is, species found in the same country or area. Giraffe, Thompson's gazelles and wildebeests are sympatric species in East Africa. They avoid competition for food: the giraffe, with its long neck, feeds high up; the gazelle and wildebeests, although of similar stature, eat differently: the gazelle eats ground-hugging leaves, while the wildebeests eat side shoots.

There are two sympatric species of cormorant in England: the common cormorant and the shag. Both species look alike, occupy the same stretches of shore, are submarine feeders, nest on cliffs and are fairly abundant. They appear to occupy the same niche, but do not. The common cormorant has a mixed diet, but excludes sand eels and sprats. It fishes out to sea and nests high on cliffs on broad ledges. The shag, in contrast, eats mostly sand eels and sprats, fishes in the shallows, and nests low on cliffs or on shallow ledges.

There are many other examples of sympatric species occupying different niches, ranging from cone shells that occupy different sublittoral zones, to warblers that occupy different parts of the same tree. Short-lived animals, for example insects, can occupy the same niche and avoid competition by pursuing their activities during different seasons.

Gause noted a laboratory example of the development of a mechanism to avoid competition. During an experiment with two species of *Paramecium*, he noticed that both species survived in the same test tube because one species had changed its mode of living to inhabit only the top half of the test tube, while the other species had moved to the bottom of the tube, thus avoiding competition. This process was explained first by Darwin when he developed the concept of **divergence of character**: characters must diverge when closely related species live in the same region, be it test tube or prairie. The synonymous term **character displacement** was first used in the 1950s.

One would expect displacement to be more common than exclusion because the world offers many ways of subtly changing niches. Displacement is also a mechanism of increasing species diversity. One example illustrates this phenomenon. Two species of nuthatch occur in Greece, Turkey and other parts of Asia: *Sitta neumayer* and *S. tephronota*. The external appearance of *S. neumayer* in Greece, and *S. tephronota* in Central Asia, where the species do not overlap, is similar. However, in Iran, where the two species overlap and coexist, the external appearance of each species is different. This external divergence of characters probably reflects other changes that avoid competition.

## Some examples of niches relating to disease

### Louse infestations

Lice tend to be host species specific; pig lice do not live on man or dogs, and vice versa. By being host specific, species of lice avoid competition: they have their own niche. The human louse also demonstrates character displacement. Two types of louse live on man: the head louse and the body louse. These each parasitize the two different parts of the body, rather like Gause's two species of *Paramecium* living in the top and the bottom of the test tube.

### Intracellular parasitism

Intracellular parasites occupy a niche in cells. They include all viruses, some bacteria (e.g. *Brucella* spp., *Mycobacterium tuberculosis* and rickettsiae) and some protozoa (e.g. *Babesia* spp.). There are several advantages to this type of existence, such as

**Table 7.2 Comparison of the intracellular environment with terrestrial extreme environments. (After Moulder, 1974)**

| | Terrestrial extreme environments (e.g. deserts, salt lakes, hot springs, snowfields) | The cell |
|---|---|---|
| Diversity of inhabiting species is low | + | + |
| Dominant forms have evolved unique fitness traits | + | + |
| Dominant forms dependent on species diversity limiting factors | Factor is **abiotic**, e.g. heat, salinity, dryness | Factor is **biotic**: the cell |

safety from humoral antibodies and the avoidance of competition with extracellular agents. The intracellular environment is harsh: the agents must protect themselves from the lytic enzymes released by lysosomes. This harshness is reflected in the relatively low generation times of intracellular parasites compared with extracellular ones. The intracellular environment shares this characteristic with larger extreme environments such as snow fields and salt lakes (Moulder, 1974: *Table 7.2*).

## Epidemiological interference

Studies in India (Bang, 1975) have shown that the presence, in a human community, of one type of respiratory adenovirus prevents infection with other types, even though the latter are common in surrounding communities. This is because the first type occupies a niche (the lower respiratory tract) which therefore cannot be filled by other agents. This phenomenon is **epidemiological interference**.

Similarly, there is evidence that infection of laboratory animals and domestic livestock with one serodeme (a population demonstrating the same range of variable antigens: WHO, 1978) of *Trypanosoma congolense* delays the establishment of infection with a different serodeme in the same animals (Luckins and Gray, 1983).

Interference can affect the time of occurrence of disease. An epidemic caused by one agent may suppress epidemics caused by other similar agents. This is true of certain human respiratory infections in North America and India (Bang, 1975). Some diseases are common in the young. Interference by other agents during early life causes the diseases of the young to occur in older age cohorts, altering the age-specific incidence rates. There is evidence that this occurs with certain virus infections in man (Bang, 1975).

Interference can also affect the rate of natural immunization. If an infectious agent is present at continued high levels, and infection is followed by immunity, then there is usually a decreased incidence in older age-groups. However, if other agents interfere with the agent in the young, immunity induced by the agent is delayed, producing continued infection in older subjects. There is evidence, for example, that interference by other enteroviruses delays natural poliovirus immunization in man (Bang, 1975).

Epidemiological interference may be a general phenomenon. The delay in its discovery is probably due to the lack of long-term surveys on the incidence of infections. The phenomenon has an obvious place in the evolution of disease; it prevents massive, multiple and possibly fatal infections of the young. An example of the application of epidemiological interference to the control of enteric diseases is given in Chapter 20.

## The relationships between different types of animals and plants

A particular biome contains different types of animals and plants. Some are common, others are scarce. Some are large, others are small. Reasons for these variations have been suggested by ecological studies.

Animals tend to move about *en masse*, and so it is difficult to study them all simultaneously. Ecologists, therefore, chose to look in detail at one species of animal, in conditions that favoured easy observation. Charles Elton (1927) visited Bear Island near Spitzbergen and observed Arctic foxes, with particular reference to what they ate. Bear Island was essentially a tundra biome, thus foxes were easy to observe.

### Food chains

Elton noted what the foxes ate in the summer and the winter. In the summer, the foxes ate birds (e.g. ptarmigan and sandpiper). The birds ate berries, tundra, leaves and insects. The insects also ate leaves. Thus, Elton noted that there was a **food chain**: tundra—insects—birds—fox. In addition, the foxes ate sea birds, which in turn ate smaller marine animals, which in turn ate sea plants. Thus, there was a further food chain: marine plants—marine animals—seabird—fox.

In the winter, the birds migrated to the south, leaving only polar bear dung and the remains of carcasses of seals that had been killed by polar bears. Thus, in the winter, there was a different food chain: marine animal—seal—polar bear—fox. In animal communities, therefore, a complex system has evolved, with food chains linking animals.

### The size of animals and food webs

Elton observed that animals fed at different levels in the food chain. These levels he termed **trophic levels**. He also noted that animals occupying different trophic levels generally were of different sizes. The foxes were the largest, and the birds (one level down) were smaller. Similarly, those further down the pyramid (e.g. the insects) were even smaller. Also, moving down the food chain (e.g. from foxes to insects), the animals were **more abundant**. There were more birds than foxes, and more insects than birds. A histogram depicting animal size against number of individuals is shown in *Figure 7.5a*. If the vertical axis of the histogram is moved to the centre, and the bars are arranged symmetrically, a pyramid is produced (*Figure 7.5b*); this is the Eltonian **pyramid of numbers**. As animals become larger and rarer, they have larger home ranges and therefore, if shedding an infectious

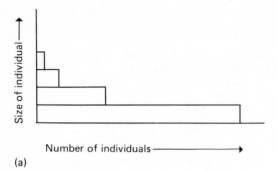

(a)

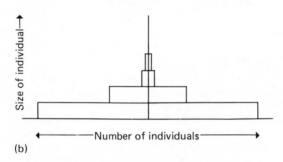

(b)

**Figure 7.5 (a)** The relationship between size of animals and size of populations; **(b)** The Eltonian 'pyramid of numbers'.

agent, transmit infections over larger areas than small animals. Thus, although hedgehogs (relatively small animals) can be infected with foot-and-mouth disease virus (McLaughlan and Henderson, 1947), they have relatively small home ranges, and so probably play only a minor role in the dissemination of the virus during epidemics.

The food chain is a simplistic view of the relationship between an animal and its food. In reality, an animal usually eats a variety of food, and so there are generally many linked food chains radiating outwards from the lower plant trophic levels to the herbivores, and then inwards towards the top carnivores, producing **food webs** (*Figure 7.6*). In addition, parasitic food webs can be identified in which the small parasites occupy a level in the food web higher than the organisms that they parasitize.

An animal's feeding habits and its place in the trophic hierarchy place restrictions on its mode of life; this led Elton to define the niche: 'an animal's place in the biotic environment; its relation to food and enemies'.

## The significance of food webs to disease transmission

The food web of an animal can determine to which orally transmitted infectious agents an animal acts as host, and from which food poisoning toxins it is at risk. Helminth diseases, for which there are definitive and intermediate hosts, are frequently transmitted via food webs. For example, the tapeworm, *Echinococcus granulosus*, includes the sheep as an intermediate host and the dog as the definitive host. The cysts in the liver and lungs of the

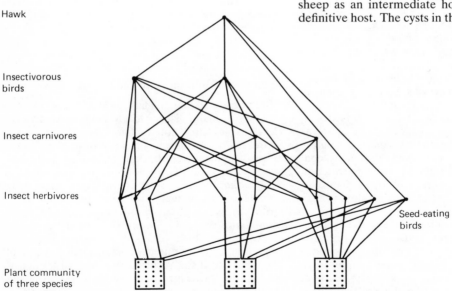

Hawk

Insectivorous birds

Insect carnivores

Insect herbivores

Seed-eating birds

Plant community of three species

**Figure 7.6** Hypothetical food web involving carnivorous, insectivorous and herbivorous birds, carnivorous and herbivorous insects, and plants.

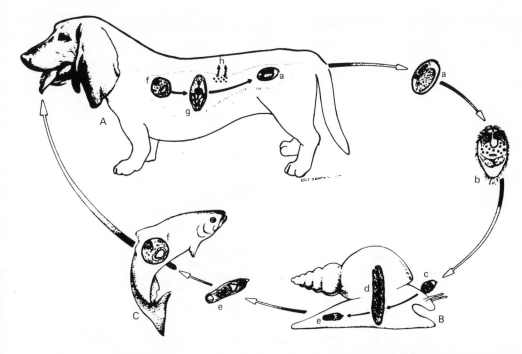

**Figure 7.7** Life-cycle of the fluke *Nanophyetus salmincola salmincola* and the microorganism *Neorickettsia helminthoeca*. A, dog (definitive host); B, *Oxytrema silicula* (first intermediate host); C, Salmonidae fish (second intermediate host); a, *Nanophyetus salmincola salmincola* egg in dog faeces; b, miracidium; c, miracidium enters snail by skin penetration; d, redia; e, cercaria; f, encysted metacercaria in salmon, ingested by the dog in raw salmon meat; g, adult fluke develops in duodenal mucosa; h, *Neorickettsia helminthoeca* leave the fluke and infect the dog systemically. (From Booth *et al.*, 1984)

intermediate host are transmitted to dogs when the latter eat sheep offal; hence the recommendations that raw sheep offal should not be fed to dogs.

*Figure 7.7* illustrates the life-cycle of *Neorickettsia helminthoeca*. This rickettsia produces a febrile disease in dogs and foxes. The disease is called 'salmon poisoning' because it is associated with the feeding of salmon to dogs. This agent's life-cycle also illustrates a parasitic food chain, in which the smallest member, the rickettsia, parasitizes a fluke which in turn parasitizes a snail for part of its life-cycle. The snail in turn releases infected miracidia which parasitize the salmon. Feeding salmon to dogs transmits the rickettsia to the latter, where the microbe produces clinical disease.

Ingestion of intermediate stages of parasites may sometimes control, rather than transmit, infection. For example, members of the genus *Utricularia* (carnivorous bladderworts) have been shown to ingest cercariae and miracidia of *Schistosoma mansoni* (Gibson and Warren, 1970). It has been suggested (Lord, 1983) that the absence of schisto-somiasis from Cuba, which has 17 species of *Utricularia*, may be related to this activity.

## The distribution of energy between trophic levels

Elton's theory explained why animals occupying different trophic levels were of different sizes but it did not explain why there were so few animals higher up the pyramid. There could be geometric restrictions: more small animals can be packed into a fixed space than larger ones. However, the sea contains few predators (e.g. sharks) at the top of the pyramid even though the sea is very large.

Lindemann (1942) explained population density at different levels of the pyramid by considering the food chain, not in terms of particulate food, but in terms of **calorific energy flow**. According to the second law of thermodynamics, the process of converting energy from one state to another is wasteful, that is, there is not 100% conversion of energy. Thus, moving up from one level to another in the Eltonian pyramid, conversion at each level wastes energy and so less protoplasm can be supported at progressively higher levels. Therefore, even if animals at different levels were of the same size, there would be fewer higher up. Since those higher up are larger, the packaging of a supportable amount of protoplasm produces even fewer animals.

It is because of the greater availability of energy at lower levels that ungulates are often bigger than their carnivorous predators. The biggest animals tend to be those that feed very low in the pyramid (e.g. filter feeders like blue whales) because much energy is available to them. When civilization dawned and man ceased to be a hunter/gatherer and began cultivating crops, he 'climbed down' the pyramid, tapping more energy. This is one reason for the increase in the world's population in the cradle of civilization in early Egypt and the associated development of horticulture and livestock farming (*see* Chapter 1).

## The analysis of predation

The association between predator and prey is a special case of interaction in a food chain. Many mathematical models have been devised to analyse predator/prey interactions. The one to be discussed here is that devised independently by Lotka and Volterra (Lotka, 1925; Chapman, 1931). They reasoned that predator/prey interactions were similar to interactions between competing species and so adapted their formulae accordingly.

The three predictions of this model are:

(1) the fluctuations of two species, one of which feeds on the other, are periodic, and the periods depend only on the coefficient of growth;
(2) the ultimate mean values of the numbers of individuals of the two species are, with fixed coefficients, independent of the initial numbers of individuals;
(3) if individuals of the two species are eliminated in proportion to their total number, then the recovery potential of the prey is greater than that of the predator; conversely, increased

protection of the prey from all risks, including the predator, allows both species to increase.

Thus, applying the first prediction, the prevalence of rabies in foxes is related to the population density of foxes (a predator) and, therefore, to the population density of mice (a prey). *Figure 7.8* illustrates this relationship, using demographic and disease prevalence data collected in Germany.

## *Ecosystems*

The relationship between animals linked by food chains defines the variety of animals in a particular area. Similarly, climate and vegetation govern the distribution of plants and therefore of the animals that live off them. These areas are characterized by the animals and plants that occupy them, and by their physical and climatic features. This unique interacting complex is called an **ecosystem** (Tansley, 1935). The components of an ecosystem can be considered separately, and ecosystems themselves can vary in size. Various terms have been devised to describe these components (Schwabe, 1984), including **biotope** and **biocenosis**.

### Biotope

A biotope is the smallest spatial unit providing uniform conditions for life. An organism's biotope therefore describes its location. This contrasts with a niche, which describes the functional position of an organism in a community. A biotope can vary in size. For example, it may be the caeca of a chicken for coccidia, or an area of poorly drained land for *Fasciola hepatica* infection of cattle.

### Biocenosis

A biocenosis is the collection of living organisms in a biotope. The organisms include plants, animals and the microorganisms in the biotope. Sometimes **biotic community** is used synonymously with biocenosis. On other occasions, 'biotic community' refers to a large biocenosis. Major biotic communities are biomes.

## *Types of ecosystem*

Three types of ecosystem can be identified, according to their origin: **autochthonous**, **anthropurgic** and **synanthropic**.

### Autochthonous ecosystems

'Autochthonous' derives from the Greek adjective *autos*, meaning 'oneself' or 'itself'; the Greek noun

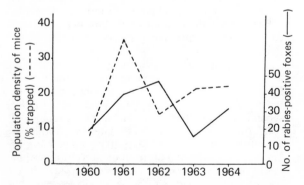

**Figure 7.8** The relationship between the population density of mice and the prevalence of fox rabies. The relationship arises from a predator/prey relationship between foxes and mice (*see* text). (From Sinnecker, 1976)

*chthon*, meaning 'the earth' or 'the land'; and the adjectival suffix -*ous*, meaning 'deriving from'. Hence an autochthonous ecosystem is one 'coming from the land itself'. Examples are to be found in biomes such as tropical rain forests and deserts.

## Anthropurgic ecosystems

'Anthropurgic' is derived from the Greek noun *anthropos*, meaning 'man'; and the Greek verb root *erg*, meaning 'to work at, to create, to produce'. Thus, an anthropurgic ecosystem is one created by man (strictly, it can also mean 'creating man'). Examples are those found in cultivated pastures and towns.

## Synanthropic ecosystems

'Synanthropic' originates from the Greek preposition *syn*, meaning 'along with, together with'; and the Greek noun *anthropos*, meaning 'man'. Thus, a synanthropic ecosystem is one that is in contact with man. An example is a rubbish tip, harbouring a variety of vermin. It follows that some synanthropic ecosystems, such as rubbish tips, are anthropurgic.

Synanthropic ecosystems facilitate the transmission of zoonotic infections from their lower animal hosts to man. For example, the brown rat, *Rattus norvegicus*, inhabits rubbish dumps and can be inapparently infected with *Leptospira*, serovar *ballum*. Humans in proximity to rubbish dumps that harbour infected rats may therefore be infected with the bacterium.

## An ecological climax

An ecological climax is said to have occurred when plants, animals and microbes have evolved to a stable, balanced relationship. Characteristically, when infections are present, they too are stable and therefore are usually endemic. Also, the balance between host and parasite usually results in inapparent infections. Such stable situations can be disrupted, frequently by man, resulting in epidemics. For example, bluetongue, a virus disease of sheep, was recognized only after the importation of European breeds of sheep to South Africa towards the end of the 19th century (Neitz, 1948). The virus, however, was present in indigenous sheep before that time, but was part of an ecological climax in which it only produced inapparent infections. The importation of exotic sheep represented a disturbance of the stable climax.

A climax involving endemic infectious agents indicates that all factors for maintenance and transmission of the agent are present. Sometimes changes in local ecology may tip the balance in favour of parasites, thus increasing disease incidence. For example, the seasonal periodicity of foot-and-mouth disease in South America may result from seasonal increases in the size of the susceptible cattle population when animals are brought into an endemic area for fattening (Rosenberg *et al.*, 1980).

## Ecological interfaces

An ecological interface is a junction of two ecosystems. Infectious diseases can be transmitted across these interfaces. An example is the transmission of yellow fever, an arbovirus disease of man. The virus is maintained in apes in Africa in an autochthonous forest ecosystem in the forest canopy (*Figure 7.9*). The canopy-dwelling mosquito, *Aedes africanus*, transmits the virus between apes. The mosquito, *A. simpsoni*, bridges the interface between the autochthonous forest ecosystem and the anthropurgic cultivated savannahs. This mosquito

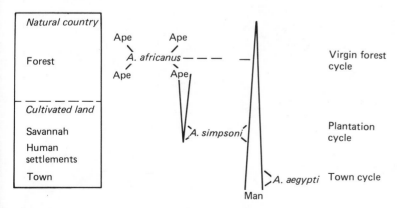

**Figure 7.9** The transmission of yellow fever between apes (primary hosts) and man (the secondary host). (From Sinnecker, 1976)

therefore maintains a plantation cycle in which man and apes may be infected. Finally, the urban mosquito, *A. aegypti*, can maintain an urban cycle in man. People who enter forests also may contract the infection from *A. africanus*.

### Ecological mosaics

An ecological mosaic is a modified patch of vegetation, created by man, within a biome that has reached a climax. Infection may spread from wild animals to man in such circumstances. For example (Schwabe, 1984), the helminth infection, loiasis, is transmitted by arthropods between man, living in small forest clearings, and canopy-dwelling monkeys. Similarly, clearing of the forest canopy encourages a close cover of weeds on the ground, creating conditions that are favourable for the incursion of field rats with mites infected with scrub typhus, which form mite islands and the resulting local areas of endemic scrub typhus (Audy, 1961).

However, transmission does not always occur in mosaics because suitable vectors may not be available. Thus, in Malaya, man lives unharmed in forests in mosaics with monkeys infected with a variety of species of *Plasmodium* (a protozoon) that are pathogenic to man. Transmission to man from monkeys does not occur because vectors that bite both types of primate are not present in the ecosystem.

## Landscape epidemiology

The study of diseases in relation to the ecosystems in which they are found is **landscape epidemiology**.

Terms conveying the same meaning are **medical ecology**, **horizontal epidemiology** (Ferris, 1967) and **medical geography**. Investigations are frequently qualitative, involving the study of the ecological factors that affect the occurrence, maintenance and, in the case of infectious agents, transmission of disease. This contrasts with the study of quantitative associations between specific diseases and hypothesized factors—sometimes termed 'vertical' epidemiology—as described in Chapters 13–15 and 17. Landscape epidemiology was developed by the Russian, Pavlovsky (1964), and later expanded by Audy (1958, 1960, 1962) and Galuzo (1975); it involves application of the ecological concepts, described above, in the study of disease.

### *Nidality*

The Russian steppe biome was the home of the great plagues such as rinderpest. Many arthropod-transmitted infections present in the steppes were also limited to distinct geographical areas. These foci were natural homes of these diseases and were called **nidi** (Latin: *nidus* = nest). The presence of a nidus depends on its limitation to particular ecosystems. An area that has ecological, social and environmental conditions that can support a disease is a **nosogenic territory** (Greek: *noso-* = sickness, disease; *gen-* = to produce, to create). A **nosoarea** is a nosogenic territory in which a particular disease is present. Thus, Britain is a nosogenic territory for rabies and foot-and-mouth disease, but is not a nosoarea for these diseases, because the microbes

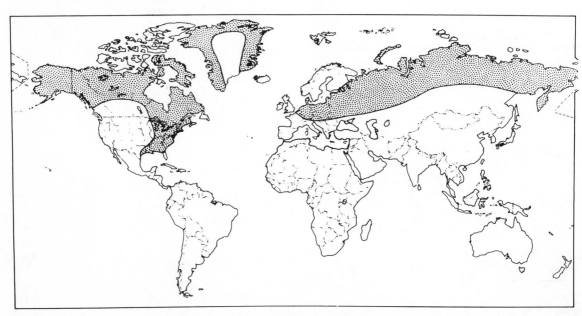

**Figure 7.10** Nosoarea (shaded) of endemic fox rabies. (From Winkler, 1975)

are prevented from entering the country by quarantine of imported animals. Diseases that show strict geographical boundaries within an ecosystem or series of ecosystems are nidal because they are confined to a specific nidus. Salmonellosis is endemic in most parts of the world because virtually all vertebrates and some invertebrates (*see Table 6.1*) can act as hosts for the various species of *Salmonella*. Rabies, when maintained in foxes, is endemic in a large zone around the northern hemisphere because this large area supports a fox population of high density (*Figure 7.10*). The nosoarea for coccidioidomycosis was described earlier in this chapter (*see Figure 7.2*).

When diseases are vector-transmitted, they are often restricted to more precise geographical boundaries than other infectious diseases. This is because the ecosystem has to satisfy the requirements of both the vertebrate host and the arthropod vector. Thus, Rocky Mountain spotted fever, a rickettsial disease of rodents transmitted by ticks, is essentially restricted to particular areas of North America, as the name of the disease suggests.

At the opposite end of the spectrum from diseases with a wide distribution are those that may be confined to relatively small areas within a town or on a farm. An isolated clump of trees that is used as a roost by starlings may be the only reservoir of infection for histoplasmosis within a large area. The faeces from these birds provide an ideal environment in which the fungal agent can survive and replicate (Di Salvo and Johnson, 1979). Even smaller nidi can be identified. For example, a focus of infestation with the tropical dog tick, *Rhipicephalus sanguineus*, has been identified in a house in London (Fox and Sykes, 1985), the warm conditions of the house providing a suitable environment for the tick. The affected dog had not been imported from abroad, but probably contracted the infestation from a quarantine kennel where it had boarded.

## Objectives of landscape epidemiology

Landscape epidemiology is founded on the concept that if the nidality of diseases is based on ecological factors then a study of ecosystems enables predictions to be made about the occurrence of disease and facilitates the development of appropriate control strategies. Three examples will illustrate this concept.

### Leptospirosis

It is known that the prevalence of *Leptospira*, serovar *ballum*, in the brown rat is density-dependent; an estimation of the number of rats inhabiting an area enables a prediction of the

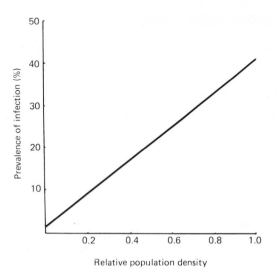

**Figure 7.11** Relationship between the relative population density and prevalence of *Leptospira*, serovar *ballum*, infection in the brown rat (*Rattus norvegicus*). (Simplified from Blackmore and Hathaway, 1980)

prevalence of serovar *ballum* infection to be made (Blackmore and Hathaway, 1980: *Figure 7.11*). The number of rat burrows in an area is a good indicator of the number of rats, and these burrows are seldom more than 100 m from the major feeding ground and are seldom more than 40 cm deep (Pisano and Storer, 1948). Thus, if inspection of the area reveals a large number of burrows and evidence of recent rat activity, it is likely that the area constitutes a reservoir of infection for serovar *ballum*. Conversely, if the rubbish dump is well managed and the area surrounding it shows evidence of regular bulldozing and few inhabited burrows, then the rat population is likely to be small and any rats present are unlikely to constitute a maintenance population for this leptospiral serovar.

### Tularaemia

In 1967 in Sweden, an epidemic of tularaemia occurred with more than 2000 human cases and a high mortality of hares (Borg and Hugoson, 1980). This epidemic was associated with the clearing of small areas of forest to create areas of grazing, which led to a sudden increase in the population density of hares and rodents. A consideration of local ecology in this instance would have suggested that the creation of these synanthropic ecosystems, in which man can be infected either by handling dead hares or through the bites of infected mosquitoes, could result in such consequences.

## Kyasanur Forest disease

Kyasanur Forest disease is caused by an arbovirus. Symptoms in man include headache, fever, back and limb pains, vomiting, diarrhoea and intestinal bleeding. Death due to dehydration can occur in untreated cases. It is apparently restricted to an area 600 miles square in the Indian state of Mysore. The virus endemically and inapparently infects some small mammals, including rats and shrews, in the local rain forest. The virus is transmitted by several species of tick (Singh *et al.*, 1964), only one of which, *Haemaphysalis spinigera*, will infest man. The usual host of the tick is the ox. Thus, when man creates ecological mosaics by cultivating areas for rice, his cattle roam into the surrounding rain forest and may become infested with virus-infected ticks. Dense populations of ticks therefore build-up around villages and, when infected, these ticks can transmit the infection to man (Hoogstraal, 1966).

## *Further reading*

BURNET, F.M. and WHITE, D.O. (1962) *Natural History of Infectious Disease*. Cambridge University Press, Cambridge

COLINVAUX, P.A. (1973) *Introduction to Ecology*. John Wiley and Sons Inc., New York

DESOWITZ, R.G. (1981) *New Guinea Tapeworms and Jewish Grandmothers. Tales of Parasites and People*. W. Norton and Company, New York and London

EDWARDS, M.A. and MCDONNELL, U. (Eds) (1982) *Animal Disease in Relation to Animal Conservation*. Symposia of the Zoological Society of London No. 50. Academic Press, London

GALUZO, I.G. (1975) Landscape epidemiology (epizootiology). *Advances in Veterinary Science and Comparative Medicine*, **19**, 73–96

LORD, R.D. (1983) Ecological strategies for the prevention and control of health problems. *Bulletin of the Pan American Health Organization*, **17**, 19–34

MAY, J.M. (Ed.) (1961) *Studies in Disease Ecology*. Hafner Publishing Company, New York

PAVLOVSKY, E.N. (1964) *Prirodnaya Ochagovost Transmissivnykh Bolezney v Svyazi s Landshoftnoy Epidemiologiey Zooantroponozov*. Translated as *Natural Nidality of Transmissible Disease with Special Reference to the Landscape Epidemiology of Zooanthroponoses*. Plous, F.K. (translator), Levine, N.D. (Ed.) (1966). University of Illinois Press, Urbana

SCHWABE, C.W. (1984) *Veterinary Medicine and Human Health*, 3rd edn. Williams and Wilkins, Baltimore

SINNECKER, H. (1976) *General Epidemiology* (translated by Walker, N.). John Wiley and Sons, London

# 8

# Patterns of disease

Methods of expressing the temporal and spatial distribution of disease were described in Chapter 4. The various patterns of disease that can be detected when disease distribution is recorded are discussed in this chapter. A considerable bulk of mathematical theory has been formulated to explain disease patterns (e.g. Bailey, 1975); this is beyond the scope of this book, although the applications of mathematics to the development of predictive models, of practical value to disease control, are described in Chapter 17.

## Basic epidemic theory

### Epidemic curves

The representation of the number of new cases of a disease by a graph, with the number of new cases on the vertical axis, and calendar time on the horizontal axis, is the most common means of expressing disease occurrence. When the time period is short, the graph describes epidemics and the graph is an **epidemic curve**. *Figure 8.1* depicts the various parts of an epidemic curve. The time between epidemics is the **interepidemic period**. An epidemic curve is given for foot-and-mouth disease in *Figure 3.1*, with the number of new outbreaks (Appendix I) approximately indicating the number of new cases. Note that the peak is shifted to the left, that is the curve is positively skewed (*see also Figures 12.3b and 17.4*).

### Factors affecting the shape of the curve

The shape of the curve and the time scale depend on:

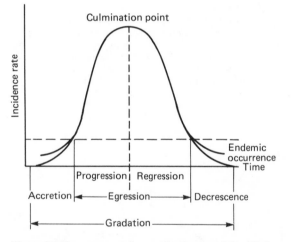

**Figure 8.1** Components of an epidemic curve (simplified to a symmetric shape for the purpose of illustration). The horizontal dotted line indicates the average number of new cases. (From Sinnecker, 1976)

(1) the incubation period of the disease;
(2) the infectivity of the agent;
(3) the proportion of susceptible animals in the population;
(4) the distance between animals (i.e. animal density).

Thus, a highly infectious agent with a short incubation period infecting a population with a large proportion of susceptible animals at high density produces a curve with a steep initial slope on a relatively small time scale, representing a rapid spread of infection among the population.

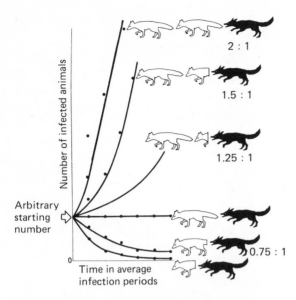

**Figure 8.2** Application of Kendall's Threshold Theorem to rabies in foxes: the theorem predicts that, if a rabid fox infects more than one other before it dies, the disease increases exponentially; if each animal infects less than one other, then the disease decreases exponentially. White animals: susceptible; black animals: infected and infectious. Numbers refer to the **contact rate**: the number of susceptible animals that are infected by an infected animal. (From Macdonald and Bacon, 1980)

A minimum density of susceptible animals is required to allow a contact-transmitted epidemic to commence. This is called the **threshold level**, and is defined mathematically by **Kendall's Threshold Theorem** (Bartlett, 1957). *Figure 8.2* illustrates application of the theorem in relation to rabies in foxes. Above a certain density of susceptible animals, one infected fox can, on average, infect more than one susceptible fox, and an epidemic can occur; the greater the density, the steeper the slope of the progressive stage of the epidemic curve. Few threshold values relating to animal diseases are known. Wierup (1983), however, has estimated that a minimum density of 12 dogs/km$^2$ is required before a canine parvovirus epidemic can occur.

Generally, 20–30% of an animal population needs to be susceptible before a contact-transmitted epidemic can **propagate** through the population (Schwabe *et al.*, 1977). As the epidemic proceeds, the proportion of susceptibles is decreased, either as a result of death of infected animals, or by increasing immunity following infection (*Figure 8.3*). Eventually, the epidemic cannot continue because there are insufficient susceptible animals available for infection. In the case of canine parvovirus, an epidemic stops when the density of susceptible dogs falls below 6/km (Wierup, 1983). A period of time is then necessary to allow replacement of susceptibles before another epidemic can commence. This explains the **cyclicity** of some epidemics.

## Common source and propagating epidemics

A **common source epidemic** is one in which all cases are infected from a source that is common to all

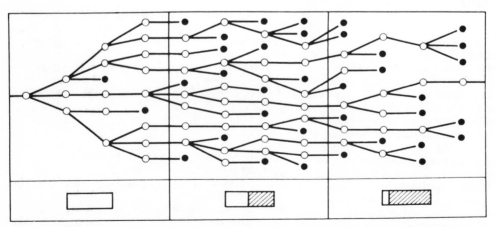

**Figure 8.3** The course of a typical epidemic caused by an infectious agent infecting a totally susceptible population. Each circle represents an infection, and the connecting lines indicate transfer from one case to the next. Black circles represent infected individuals who fail to infect others. Three periods are shown, the first when practically the whole population is susceptible, the second at the height of the epidemic, and the third at the close, when most individuals are immune. The proportions of susceptible (white) and immune (hatched) individuals are indicated in rectangles beneath the main diagram. (From Burnet and White, 1972)

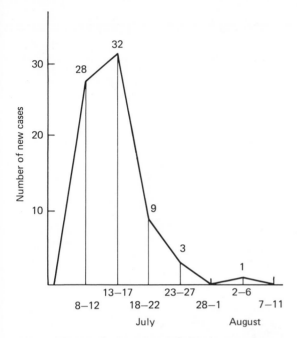

**Figure 8.4** A point source epidemic: human leptospirosis associated with contaminated water supply, Rostov-on-Don, USSR, 1955. (From Ianovich *et al.*, 1957)

individuals. If the period of exposure is brief, then a common source epidemic is a **point source** (or, more briefly, just a **point**) epidemic. A food-poisoning outbreak, in which a single batch of food is contaminated, is a typical point source epidemic. *Figure 8.4* illustrates a point source epidemic of human leptospirosis in the USSR in 1955 associated with the contamination of the water supply with the urine of infected dogs. An epidemic of leptospirosis was occurring in dogs and contaminated urine was discharged onto fields. A cloudburst occurred on 28 June during a brief period of heavy rainfall. This washed off the topsoil. Some of the soil entered a water pumping station inspection shaft which was open for repair. Thus, the water supply was contaminated, and resulted in the human epidemic.

A **propagating epidemic** is one in which initial (i.e. **primary**) cases excrete infectious agent, and thus infect, directly or indirectly, susceptible individuals which constitute **secondary** cases. Epidemics of foot-and-mouth disease in Britain (*see Figure 3.1*) typically are propagating.

The intervals between peaks of successive epidemic curves, separating the primary from subsequent secondary epidemics, reflect the incubation period of the infection. Typically, all cases of a point source epidemic occur within one incubation period of the causal agent. Thus, if the period between subsequent epidemics is less than the most common incubation period then it is difficult to

differentiate between a propagating epidemic and a series of point source epidemics. Sartwell (1950, 1966) describes a suitable technique of differentiation, based on the statistical distribution of incubation periods.

## Epidemic waves

### The primary epidemic wave

When an infectious agent enters a population that previously has not been exposed to the agent, a **primary epidemic wave** is instituted (*Figure 8.5a*). This represents a long-term interaction between host and parasite. If a balance occurs, a stable,

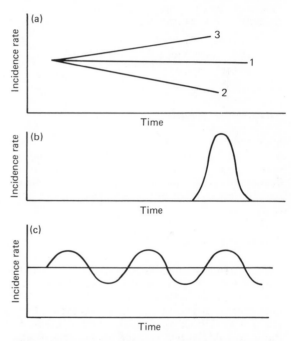

**Figure 8.5** The primary epidemic wave and the short-term disturbances of its course. (**a**) Primary epidemic wave: (1) with equilibrium between infectious agent and host; (2) host/agent interaction biased to the host; (3) host/agent interaction biased to the agent. (**b**) Secondary epidemic wave. (**c**) Tertiary epidemic wave. (From Sinnecker, 1976)

endemic level of disease is maintained (1 in *Figure 8.5a*); if the interaction is biased to the host, there is a gradual decrease in disease occurrence (2); and if the interaction is biased to the parasite, there is a gradual increase in disease occurrence (3).

### Disturbances in the primary epidemic wave

Short-term disturbances in the primary wave result from intermittent disturbances in the equilibrium between host and parasite. A classic epidemic (*Figure 8.5b*) is such a typical disturbance, resulting in a **clustering** of cases over a period of time. This may result from the action of factors related to agent, host and environment, such as the introduction of a new antigenic type (e.g. influenza A infection), or an increase in the density of the susceptible host population above the threshold level. These disturbances may be regular, in which case **cycles** of disease occur (*Figure 8.5c*).

## Trends in the temporal distribution of disease

The patterns illustrated in *Figure 8.5* can be classified into three trends:

(1) short-term (*Figure 8.5b*);
(2) cyclical (including seasonal) (*Figure 8.5c*);
(3) long term (secular) (*Figure 8.5a*).

### *Short-term trends*

Short-term trends are typical epidemics. They indicate that an event has disturbed the equilibrium between host and parasite, for example the introduction of a wild mouse infected with *Sylphacia obvelata* into a colony of SPF mice (*see* Chapter 3).

### *Cyclical trends*

Cyclical trends are associated with regular, periodic fluctuations in the level of disease occurrence. They are associated with periodic changes in susceptible host density, and density of infectious agent. Thus, the 3–4 year cycle of foot-and-mouth disease in Paraguay (*see Figure 8.11*), and the predicted 4-year periodicity of fox rabies in Britain, with a contact rate of 1.9 (*see Figure 17.3a*), are probably related to the time taken for the susceptible population to reach the threshold level. Regular, predictable cyclical fluctuations are **endemic pulsations**.

### Seasonal trends

A seasonal trend is a special case of a cyclical trend, where the periodic fluctuations in disease incidence are related to particular seasons. Fluctuations may be caused by changes in host density, management practices, survival of infectious agents, vector dynamics and other ecological factors. Thus, rinderpest occurs in Africa more commonly in the dry than the wet season because animals congregate at water holes, increasing the local density.

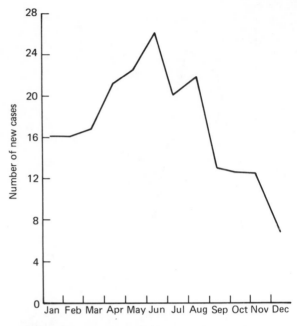

**Figure 8.6** Time trend graph depicting the seasonal occurrence of human brucellosis in the USA: average annual occurrence, 1965–1970. (Simplified from Steele *et al.*, 1972)

The prevalence of Lassa virus infection of the multimammate mouse (*see* Chapter 6) is related to density-dependent variations in mortality, competition with other rodents, and seasonal factors. The mouse may seek shelter in homes during the wet season, and this may partly explain the increased incidence of human Lassa fever during the wet season.

Human brucellosis in the USA is more common during summer than winter (*Figure 8.6*), being associated with the spring peak in calving of dairy cows and the concomitant increased risk of contracting infection from infected uterine discharges.

Rat plague demonstrates a seasonal incidence, being associated with climatically determined fluctuations in the population size of certain fleas that are vectors of the disease. Additionally, the rat population increases during the interepidemic season, thereby exacerbating the seasonal trend (Pollitzer and Meyer, 1961).

Leptospirosis is more common in the summer and early autumn than in the winter in temperate climates (*Figure 8.7*) because the warm, moist conditions during the summer predispose to survival of the pathogen (Diesch and Ellinghausen, 1975).

In contrast, transmissible gastroenteritis of pigs is more common in winter than summer (*Figure 8.8*). This may be because the survival time of the virus is very short in summer because of the stronger

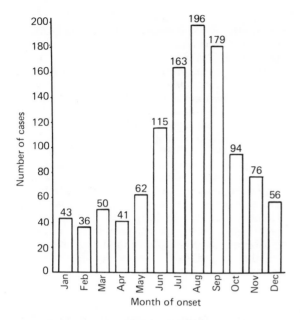

**Figure 8.7** Bar chart depicting the seasonal occurrence of human leptospirosis in the USA. (From Diesch and Ellinghausen, 1975)

ultraviolet light and higher temperatures then (Haelterman, 1963).

In the USA, feline panleucopenia shows a seasonal peak in August and September (Reif, 1976). This is associated with a peak in the number of births in the cat population in June, which increases the number of susceptible cats in the population at risk. The kittens are protected passively by maternal antibody for approximately the first 2 months of life, therefore the peak 'herd' susceptibility occurs 2 months after the birth peak. Such seasonal fluctuations are less likely in canine than in feline populations because births of puppies are distributed more evenly throughout the year than those of kittens (Tedor and Reif, 1978).

Some non-infectious diseases may show seasonal trends. Thus, bovine hypomagnesaemia is common in spring and is associated, among other factors, with low levels of magnesium in rapidly growing pastures (*see Figure 3.6*).

Sometimes seasonal determinants may be unidentified. For example, human insulin-dependent diabetes mellitus and less equivocally, canine diabetes are more common in winter than summer (Marmor *et al.*, 1982).

## Long-term (secular) trends

Secular trends occur over a long period of time. These correspond to the equilibrium in *Figure 8.5a*, being tipped either in favour of the host (2) or to the advantage of the parasite (3). *Figure 8.9* illustrates a **reported** increasing trend in the annual prevalence of rabies in wildlife in the USA, whereas the prevalence in dogs is decreasing due to adequate control. 'Reported' is emphasized to stress that accurate estimation of trends is open to errors, some of which are described below.

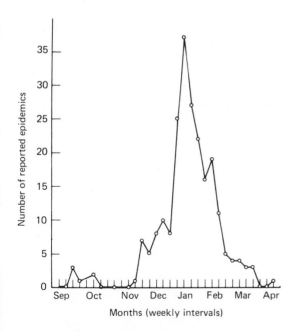

**Figure 8.8** Seasonal trend of transmissible gastroenteritis of pigs: reported epidemics in Illinois, 1968–1969. (From Ferris, 1971)

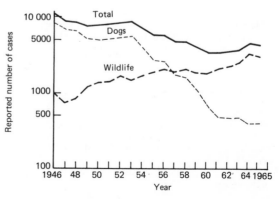

**Figure 8.9** An example of a secular trend: reported cases of rabies in the USA, 1946–1965. (From West, 1972)

Upward trends may also result from the intervention of man and changing human habits. Such trends occur with the so-called 'diseases of civilization' and 'urbanization' in man (e.g. coronary heart disease) and the diseases of intensive production in animals. Secular decreases in morbidity may be the product of prophylaxis (e.g. vaccination). Mortality may show a secular decrease due to improved therapeutic techniques.

## True and false changes in morbidity and mortality

The temporal changes that occur in recorded morbidity and mortality rates may be either true or false. The recording of mortality rates is rarer in veterinary than in human medicine because the recording of death in animals is not compulsory. Thus, details of trends in mortality in animals are usually unavailable.

The two common measures of morbidity—prevalence and incidence rate—each comprise a numerator (number of cases) and a denominator ('population at risk' for the former measure, and 'animal-years at risk', or a suitable approximation,

for the latter—Chapter 4). Changes in either numerator or denominator induce changes in prevalence and incidence rate that may be either true or false (*Table 8.1*). True changes in an incidence rate can affect the recorded incidence rate and prevalence; additionally, changes in disease duration affect prevalence (*see* Chapter 4).

A major cause of false changes is variation in the recognition and reporting of disease. Thus, the increasing secular trend in wildlife rabies in the USA between 1946 and 1965 (*Figure 8.9*) may have resulted from increased recognition and reporting of affected animals, rather than from a genuine increase in incidence. Additionally, the sampling of an animal population to record morbidity is subject to inherent **variation** in the samples (*see* Chapters 12 and 14) which may suggest changes that do not exist. Apparently changing patterns should be interpreted with due regard to the possibility that they are artificial.

## Detecting temporal trends: time series analysis

Short-term, seasonal and secular changes are temporal trends that can occur simultaneously, and may be mixed with random variation. In such circumstances, the various changes can be identified by statistical investigation. One method, originally applied in commerce, that is used in epidemiology to detect temporal trends, is **time series analysis**.

A time series is a record of events that occur over a period of time; cases of disease are typical events. The events are plotted as points on a graph, with time along the horizontal axis. *Table 8.2*, for instance, records the percentage of sheep lungs condemned monthly because of pneumonia or pleurisy at a Scottish slaughterhouse. *Figure 8.10a* plots these monthly values. There is considerable variation in the location of the points, but, by eye,

**Table 8.1 Reasons for true and false temporal changes in prevalence and incidence according to changes in the numerator (cases) and denominator (population at risk)**

*True changes*
Incidence:       change in incidence
Prevalence:      (a) change in incidence
                 (b) change in duration of disease

*False changes*
Incidence and prevalence
(1) Errors in the numerator:
     (a) changes in the recognition of disease
     (b) changes in procedures for classifying disease

(2) Errors in the denominator:
     (a) errors in enumeration of the population at risk

**Table 8.2 Percentages of sheep lungs condemned monthly because of pneumonia and/or pleurisy and average monthly and yearly percentage condemnation rates (1979–83) at a Scottish abattoir. (From Simmons and Cuthbertson, 1985)**

|  | Jan % | Feb % | Mar % | Apr % | May % | Jun % | Jul % | Aug % | Sep % | Oct % | Nov % | Dec % | Yearly % condemnation rate |
|---|---|---|---|---|---|---|---|---|---|---|---|---|---|
| 1979 | 0.33 | 0.24 | 0.46 | 0.57 | 0.65 | 0.23 | 0.27 | 0.37 | 0.14 | 0.30 | 0.24 | 0.14 | 0.33 |
| 1980 | 0.40 | 0.38 | 0.39 | 0.65 | 0.58 | 0.49 | 0.49 | 0.19 | 0.27 | 0.34 | 0.30 | 0.44 | 0.41 |
| 1981 | 0.48 | 0.58 | 0.62 | 0.75 | 0.51 | 0.44 | 0.21 | 0.17 | 0.18 | 0.21 | 0.35 | 0.27 | 0.40 |
| 1982 | 0.72 | 0.71* | 0.75* | 0.85 | 0.45 | 0.34 | 0.26 | 0.43 | 0.95 | 0.60 | 1.41 | 0.63 | 0.68 |
| 1983 | 0.71 | 0.64 | 0.48 | 0.84 | 0.38 | 0.48 | 0.69 | 0.80 | 1.09 | 0.76 | 1.25 | 0.97 | 0.76 |
| Average monthly % condemnation rate | 0.53 | 0.51 | 0.54 | 0.73 | 0.51 | 0.40 | 0.38 | 0.39 | 0.53 | 0.44 | 0.71 | 0.49 | |

*Estimated

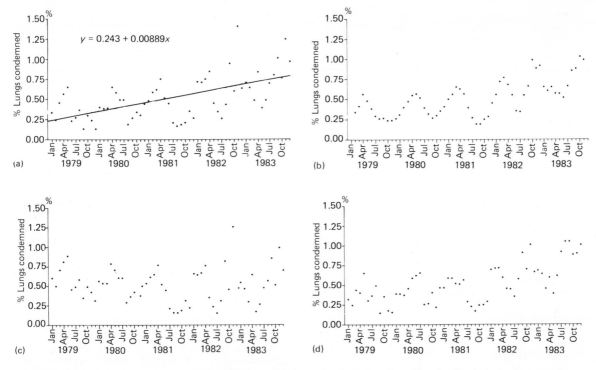

**Figure 8.10** Percentages of sheep lungs condemned monthly because of pneumonia and/or pleurisy and average monthly and yearly percentage condemnation rates (1979–1983) at a Scottish abattoir. (**a**) Percentages of lungs condemned monthly because of pneumonia and/or pleurisy (data from *Table 8.2*) with regression line. (**b**) Three-monthly rolling average percentage lung condemnation rate because of pneumonia and/or pleurisy (data from *Table 8.3*). (**c**) Percentages of lungs condemned monthly (corrected to remove secular trend) because of pneumonia and/or pleurisy. (**d**) Percentages of lungs condemned monthly (corrected to remove seasonal trend) because of pneumonia and/or pleurisy. (From Simmons and Cuthbertson, 1985)

an annual cycle is suggested, and there appears to be a slight secular trend of increased prevalence from 1979 to 1983. Trends in these data may be detected by three methods:

(1) free-hand drawing;
(2) calculation of rolling (moving) averages;
(3) regression analysis;

the object being to identify, and, if required, to remove, random variation, seasonal and secular trends.

## Free-hand drawing

The joining of points by eye is an obvious, easy method of indicating a trend. However, it is susceptible to subjective interpretation and cannot counteract random variation readily.

## Calculation of rolling (moving) averages

A rolling average is the arithmetic average of consecutive groups of measurements. Thus, to construct a rolling 3-month average of the monthly

data in *Table 8.2*, sequential sets of three adjacent values are averaged. For example, the rolling average for February 1979 is calculated by summing the monthly averages for January, February and March and dividing by 3:

$$\text{3-month rolling average} \atop \text{(February 1979)} = \frac{0.33 + 0.24 + 0.46}{3} = 0.34.$$

The 3-month rolling average for March 1979 likewise is calculated by summing the values for February, March and April 1979 and dividing by 3. *Table 8.3* presents 3-month rolling averages using the data in *Table 8.2*, and *Figure 8.10b* presents these averages graphically. This technique reduces random variation, and may therefore reveal underlying trends; a seasonal trend is clearly visible in *Figure 8.10b*.

The seasonal trend in this example cannot be readily explained. However, it is known that the prevalence of atypical pneumonia increases as the stocking density increases and as the altitude at which sheep are reared decreases (Jones and

**Table 8.3 Three-month rolling average percentage condemnation rates because of pneumonia and/or pleurisy (1979–83) at a Scottish abattoir. (Calculated from the data in *Table 8.2*)**

|      | Jan % | Feb % | Mar % | Apr % | May % | Jun % | Jul % | Aug % | Sep % | Oct % | Nov % | Dec % |
|------|-------|-------|-------|-------|-------|-------|-------|-------|-------|-------|-------|-------|
| 1979 |       | 0.34  | 0.42  | 0.56  | 0.48  | 0.38  | 0.29  | 0.26  | 0.27  | 0.23  | 0.23  | 0.26  |
| 1980 | 0.31  | 0.39  | 0.47  | 0.54  | 0.57  | 0.52  | 0.39  | 0.32  | 0.27  | 0.30  | 0.36  | 0.41  |
| 1981 | 0.50  | 0.56  | 0.65  | 0.63  | 0.57  | 0.39  | 0.27  | 0.19  | 0.19  | 0.25  | 0.28  | 0.45  |
| 1982 | 0.56  | 0.72  | 0.77  | 0.68  | 0.55  | 0.35  | 0.34  | 0.55  | 0.66  | 0.99  | 0.88  | 0.92  |
| 1983 | 0.66  | 0.61  | 0.65  | 0.57  | 0.57  | 0.52  | 0.66  | 0.86  | 0.88  | 1.03  | 0.99  |       |

Gilmour, 1983). Thus, lowland, intensively reared sheep are more likely to develop pneumonia than hill sheep. Lambs slaughtered in the spring are most frequently from the lowlands, and lambs slaughtered in the late summer and autumn are most frequently from the hill; this policy therefore could explain the seasonal trend.

Two disadvantages of rolling averages are that the first and last elements of a data set cannot be averaged (January 1979 and December 1983 in *Table 8.3*), and the averages can be affected unduly by extreme values.

## Regression analysis

Regression analysis is a statistical technique for investigating relationships between two or more variables. It requires a knowledge of statistics and so the reader who is unfamiliar with basic statistics should read Chapters 12 and 13 before proceeding further.

Regression and correlation (the latter is described in Chapter 13) are related. However, there is one major difference: a correlation coefficient may be evaluated if both or all variables exhibit random variation. Regression, however, involves the **selection** of individuals on the basis of one or more measurements (the explanatory variables) and then records the others (the response variables); therefore the explanatory variables have no random variation. Discussion here will consider only one explanatory variable and one response variable.

When observations are made at defined intervals, these **selected** intervals of time represent the explanatory variable, $x$, which is why regression, not correlation, is applied to detecting an association between events and time. The technique can be applied to the data in *Table 8.2*.

A graph showing the variation of the mean of $y$ in relation to $x$ would show the relationship between $y$ and $x$ that is observed, in practice, with random variation. If it is assumed that the true values of $y$, for each value of $x$, lie in a straight line, then this line is known as the **regression line** of the linear regression of $y$ on $x$. The slope of the line is termed the **regression coefficient** of $y$ on $x$. This may be positive, negative, or, if $x$ and $y$ are unassociated,

zero. The estimation of the regression coefficient and the intercept with the vertical axis, and the interpretation of the values of these estimates, is called **regression analysis**. If the relationship is not a linear one then a suitable transformation of $x$ or $y$ or both, such as their squares or logarithms, may transform the relationship to linearity.

Assume that the equation of the true regression line is:

$$y = \alpha + \beta x$$

where $\beta$ is the regression coefficient, and $\alpha$ is the intercept defining the point of interception of the $y$ axis by the regression line. A set of $n$ points $(x, y)$ of observations is available to estimate this line. The regression coefficient, $\beta$, is estimated by:

$$b = \frac{\Sigma(x-\bar{x})(y-\bar{y})}{\Sigma(x-\bar{x})^2}$$

$$= \frac{\Sigma(xy)-(\Sigma x)(\Sigma y)/n}{\Sigma x^2-(\Sigma x)^2/n}.$$

The intercept, $\alpha$, is estimated by:

$$a = \bar{y} - b\bar{x}.$$

Using the data in *Table 8.2*, the values of $x$ being integers from 1 to 60 (i.e. monthly intervals for 5 years) and of $y$ being the respective monthly condemnation rates:

| | |
|---|---|
| $\Sigma x = 1830.0$ | $\Sigma y = 30.820$ |
| $(\Sigma x)^2 = 3\,348\,900$ | $\Sigma x^2 = 73\,810$ |
| $\Sigma(xy) = 1\,100.0$ | $n = 60$ |
| $\bar{x} = 30.500$ | $\bar{y} = 0.51367.$ |

Thus:

$$b = \frac{1100.0 - (1830.0 \times 30.820)/60}{73810 - 3\,348\,900/60}$$

$$= 0.00889,$$

and:

$$a = 0.51367 - (0.00889 \times 30.500)$$

$$= 0.2425.$$

The regression line can now be plotted, substituting the values of $x$, from 1 to 60, in the formula for the regression line, to determine the respective values of $y$ (*Figure 8.10a*).

Thus, when $x = 1$ (January 1979)

$y = 0.2425 + 0.00889 \times 1$

$\quad = 0.2514,$

when $x = 2$ (February 1979)

$y = 0.2425 + 0.00889 \times 2$

$\quad = 0.2603,$

and so on.

Note that, in this example, the relationship between $x$ and $y$ is linear.

The effect of the secular trend can be removed by subtracting $b(x-\bar{x})$ from each value of $y$. Thus, for July 1979, $x = 7$ and:

$b(x - \bar{x}) = 0.00889(7 - 30.500)$

$\quad = 0.00889 \times -23.500$

$\quad = -0.2089,$

and the value of $y$ with the secular trend removed is:

$0.27 - (-0.2089)$

$\quad = 0.4789.$

The results for the 60-month period, with the secular trend removed, are depicted in *Figure 8.10c*.

The effect of seasonal variation can be removed by calculating a seasonal index, in this example for each month. The value of $y$ for each month of a year is taken as a proportion of the total of $y$ for that year; these proportions are averaged for a particular month over the period of study (5 years in this instance) to give a seasonal index for each month of the year. The results are 'de-seasonalized' by dividing each value of $y$ by the relevant monthly index multiplied by 12. Thus, for July 1979, the proportion of the total of $y$ contributed by July is:

$$\frac{0.27}{0.33+0.24+0.46+0.57+0.65+0.23+0.27+0.37+0.14+0.30+0.24+0.14}$$

$$= \frac{0.27}{3.95}$$

$$= 0.0684.$$

The proportions for July 1980, 1981, 1982 and 1983 are 0.0995, 0.0440, 0.0320 and 0.0759, respectively. The July seasonal index therefore is:

$$\frac{0.0684 + 0.0995 + 0.0440 + 0.0320 + 0.0759}{5}$$

$$= 0.3199/5$$

$$= 0.0640,$$

and the 'de-seasonalized' value for July 1979 is:

$$\frac{0.27}{0.0640 \times 12}$$

$$= 0.352.$$

The 'de-seasonalized' results for the period of study are shown in *Figure 8.10d*.

Note that a considerable amount of random variation remains when the secular and seasonal trends are removed (*Figures 8.10c* and *d*, respectively); this variation tends to obscure the seasonal trend in *Figure 8.10c*, and the secular trend in *Figure 8.10d*. In such circumstances, calculation of rolling averages provides a rapid means of reducing random variation. An increase in sample size should also reduce the effects of this variation. A formal significance test may be required when the effects of random variation are considerable. A description of a suitable test, and the estimation of the standard error and confidence limits of $\beta$, are given by Bailey (1981).

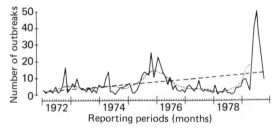

**Figure 8.11** Foot-and-mouth disease outbreaks reported by month, 12-month rolling average and trend; Paraguay, 1972–1979. ——— Raw data; ······ 12-month moving average; ------ trend. (From Peralta *et al.*, 1982)

A second example of the application of time series analysis is given by Peralta *et al.* (1982), who investigated the temporal distribution of foot-and-mouth disease in Paraguay (*Figure 8.11*). The disease shows a cycle with a periodicity of 3–4 years (peaks in 1972, 1975–76 and 1979) due to type O virus. The small peak in 1974, that was not consistent with the cycle, was caused by a sporadic outbreak due to type C virus. The reason for the cyclicity may be the changes in the proportion of the susceptible cattle population, 3–4 years being necessary to increase again the number to the threshold level. Identification of this temporal pattern can indicate times when particular attention should be paid to control.

Regression is discussed in standard introductory statistics texts such as that by Bailey (1981) and, in the context of time series analysis, in those by Sard (1979) and Wheelwright and Makridakis (1973).

## Trends in the spatial and temporal distribution of disease

### Spatial trends in disease occurrence

An epidemic represents not only the clustering of cases over a period of time, but also a clustering of cases in a defined area. An infectious disease that propagates through a population results in a **contagious** spatial pattern in contrast to sporadic outbreaks that are distributed **randomly**. These two patterns can be compared with **regular** spatial occurrence (*Figure 8.12*). 'Contagious' can also be applied, in a general sense, to the spatial clustering of disease, whether or not it is infectious (ecologists sometimes use 'over-dispersion' to refer to this type of spatial clustering in animal populations, with 'under-dispersion' referring to more regular spacing).

A variety of statistical distributions serve as models for the spatial distribution of events (Southwood, 1978). The Poisson distribution (*see* Chapter 12) has commonly been applied. The goodness of fit of a set of data to the Poisson distribution can be tested by performing a $\chi^2$-test on the observed and expected values; standard statistical texts, such as Bailey (1981), give details. If the variance is less than the mean, it implies the occurrence of a more regular distribution than is described by a Poisson series. If the variance is greater than the mean, it implies that a 'contagious' distribution is present.

Identification of spatial clustering can assist in the identification of the cause of disease. Thus, the clustering of feline leukaemia among genetically unrelated cats provided early evidence of horizontal transmission and therefore of the infectious nature of the disease (Brodey *et al.*, 1970).

The statistical methods for identifying different spatial patterns are described in detail by Cliff and Ord (1981).

### Time-space clustering

Time-space clustering is an interaction between the places of onset and the times of onset of a disease; cases that are close in space tend to be close in time. The Poisson distribution can sometimes, but not always, be applied to this type of interaction—particularly for large samples (David and Barton, 1966). Techniques for detecting time-space clustering are described by Knox (1964), David and Barton (1966), Mantel (1967), Pike and Smith (1968), and are reviewed by Williams (1984).

### Further reading

BAILEY, N.T.J. (1975) *The Mathematical Theory of Infectious Diseases*, 2nd edn. Charles Griffin and Company, London and High Wycombe

HALPIN, B. (1975) *Patterns of Animal Disease*. Baillière Tindall, London

SINNECKER, H. (1976) *General Epidemiology* (translated by Walker, N.). John Wiley and Sons, London

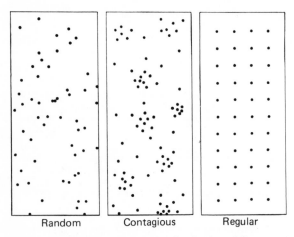

|  Random | Contagious | Regular |

**Figure 8.12** Patterns of the spatial distribution of disease. (From Southwood, 1978).

# 9

# The nature of data

The epidemiologist investigates the frequency and distribution of disease (and sometimes other characteristics, such as performance) in groups of animals. This involves the collection and analysis of **data** singular: datum): 'facts, especially numerical facts, collected together for reference or information' (*Oxford English Dictionary*, 1972). These data may relate to clinical signs, therapy, and post-mortem and laboratory examinations. If an investigation is undertaken prospectively, the epidemiologist has to decide what data should be collected. If an investigation is undertaken retrospectively, the epidemiologist may use data that have been collected by veterinary practices, abattoirs, laboratories, clinics, and other organizations. Therefore, it is necessary to know whether the types of data that are collected are suitable for a particular investigation.

Inferences about the cause of disease involve categorizing individuals into a group that has the disease and a group that does not have the disease, the object being to decide whether these two groups differ with respect to possible determinants. This is the basis of observational studies (outlined in Chapter 2 and detailed in Chapter 15). Animals are put into the diseased category because they possess certain attributes, such as clinical signs and lesions, that are used to define, and sometimes to name, the disease. A knowledge of the various features that are pertinent to the classification of disease is therefore necessary.

Some data are observations, for example, the recording of diarrhoea. Other data are interpretations of observations, for example, a diagnosis, which represents an interpretation of a set of clinical signs, lesions and laboratory results. The interpretation, and therefore the diagnosis, may be incorrect; this could result in an animal being erroneously categorized as having a particular disease. Any inferences on association between possible causal factors and disease, drawn from a study of this animal, may therefore be erroneous.

Some quantitative data are measurements, for example, body weight, milk yield, and morbidity and mortality rates. The statistical methods that are applied to analyse these data depend, to some extent, on the type of measurement.

Additionally, some data that epidemiologists use nowadays are stored in computers in unfamiliar forms, such as codes.

## Data elements

### Nomenclature and classification of disease

Data relating to disease frequently include the names of diseases. The name given to a disease is closely associated with the way in which a disease is classified. Diseases are defined at three levels (*Figure 9.1a*) in relation to:

(1) specific causes;
(2) lesions or deranged functions;
(3) presenting problems.

Diseases are generally named according to their allocation to one of these three levels, for example, parvovirus infection (specific cause), hepatitis (lesion) and ataxia (presenting problem). A fourth method of naming involves the use of eponyms, for example, Rubarth's disease and Newcastle disease.

The situation is frequently more complicated: a presenting problem may have more than one set of lesions and specific causes (*Figures 9.1b* and *9.1c*).

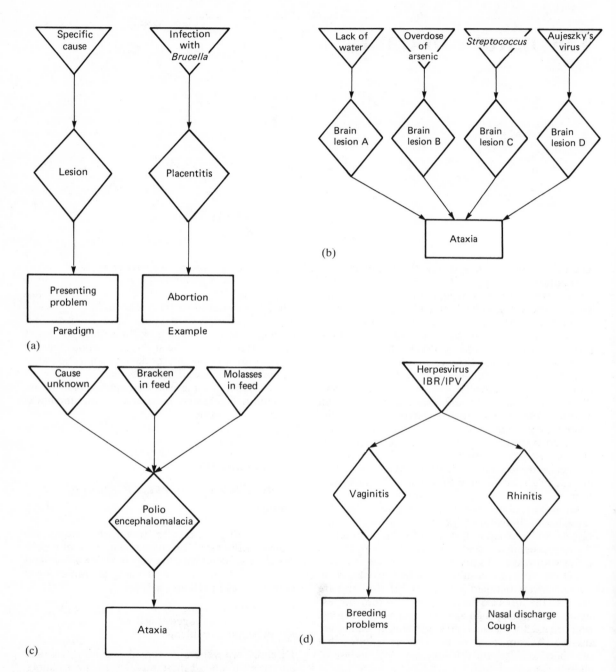

**Figure 9.1** (**a**) The three levels of disease classification. (**b**) A presenting problem common to multiple sets of lesions and specific causes. (**c**) A presenting problem and a lesion common to multiple specific causes. (**d**) A specific cause with divergent sets of lesions and presenting problems. ((**a**) Modified from Hall, 1978; (**b**), (**c**), (**d**) From Hall, 1978)

Similarly, one specific cause may produce more than one lesion and therefore more than one presenting sign (*Figure 9.1d*).

Veterinarians usually define (and therefore record) disease as a diagnosis in terms of a combination of specific cause, lesion and presenting problem. Sometimes one or more levels may be missing; the recently identified dilated pupil syndrome in cats (feline dysautonomia) is defined in terms of lesions and presenting problem, although the specific cause is still unknown (Gaskell, 1983). Initially this disease was eponymously named the Key–Gaskell syndrome.

## The significance of the nomenclature and classification of disease in epidemiological investigations

Different sectors of the veterinary profession require different types of information for their work. Pathologists have a major interest in lesions. When notifiable diseases occur, administrators act according to sets of rules that are defined by legislation; the classification of these diseases is of little consequence to the action that is taken. Similarly, epidemiologists who undertake surveys of morbidity that do not involve the testing of a causal hypothesis are concerned only with identification of a disease, irrespective of the way in which it is classified or named. However, the method of classifying disease is important in causal investigations.

The classification shown in *Figure 9.1* can be simplified to two methods:

(1) by **manifestations**, namely signs and lesions;
(2) by **cause**.

An epidemiological causal investigation attempts to detect associations between causal factors and disease. The investigation therefore is conducted because one or more component causes are not known. In such a case, the disease that is being studied is frequently named according to manifestations. For example, in *Figure 9.1b*, if the disease being studied were defined as ataxia (a presenting sign which is a manifestation), then ataxic animals would be heterogeneous with respect to cause; four separate sufficient causes, with different component causes, could be involved. This would make causal inference more difficult than if there were only a single sufficient cause that was common to all animals classified as diseased. Similarly, in *Figure 9.1c*, if disease were defined as polioencephalomalacia (a lesion, which is a manifestation), then the animals with the lesion could also be heterogeneous with respect to cause. Classification by cause in *Figure 9.1a* strengthens causal inference, because a common sufficient cause may be demonstrated in all cases of animals that are classified as diseased.

Frequently, only suboptimal data relating just to manifestations (often just signs) are available, and they must be used with due regard to their defects, or as the basis of more detailed investigations. Russell *et al.* (1982a), for example, were aware that lameness (a datum defining disease in terms of presenting signs, and frequently involving several lesions and causes) was a problem in British dairy herds, and used this as the starting point for an investigation in which they attempted to elucidate the underlying lesions and causes, by means of a questionnaire, before trying to develop suitable control strategies.

## *Diagnostic criteria*

Disease can be diagnosed using one or more of three criteria:

(1) clinical signs and symptoms*;
(2) detection of specific agents;
(3) reactions to diagnostic tests.

### Observational and interpretative data

Records relating to the three diagnostic criteria may be of either **observations** or **interpretations** (Leech, 1980). The terms overlap in that observations usually imply a comparison with the normal which itself is often a matter of judgement. For example, to observe and record that a cow is diarrhoeic implies that its faeces are less firm than its peers, and must also take into account that cows at peak yield, receiving much concentrate, usually have loose faeces.

A clinical sign may represent an observation, for example, nasal discharge. A diagnosis represents an interpretation of one or several observations. Distemper, for example, is a diagnosis that implicitly involves the interpretation of several signs, including perhaps nasal discharge, diarrhoea and coughing.

Specific agents may be observed, for instance species of *Babesia* may be identified in a blood smear. Alternatively, the presence of agents may be recorded interpretatively, for example the presence of *Escherichia coli* in the faeces of an animal with diarrhoea may be recorded as being 'not clinically significant'.

Test reactions may be observed, for example, the recording of antibody titres in serological tests. Results may also be interpreted, for example, the

---

*A sign is an abnormal feature of the patient that is observed; a symptom is a subjective abnormal feature that is described by the patient himself in human medicine.

result of an intradermal tuberculin test may be recorded as 'inconclusive'.

Interpretation involves the use of currently acceptable criteria. The recording of 'distemper', mentioned above, assumes a causal association between a particular virus and several signs. This assumption, based upon previous experimental work and many field observations, is currently acceptable. Similarly, the recording of *E. coli* as being 'not clinically significant' in some diarrhoea cases uses a criterion based upon current knowledge of commensalism.

An observational datum is easily recorded in full. However, it is difficult to record an interpretative datum fully; this would require not only the interpretation (e.g. a diagnosis) but also a record of the criteria used in the interpretation. In most cases the criteria are implicit, as in the case of distemper, and so are not recorded explicitly.

Observational and interpretative data are applied in different ways. Veterinary administrators, organizing national disease control campaigns, frequently use interpretative data to make decisions. For example, an animal's future may depend upon whether it reacts 'negatively', 'inconclusively' or 'positively' to screening tests.

Epidemiological investigations, particularly of diseases of unknown aetiology, require data such as details of diet, exposure to possible causal agents, and the various stages of a disease's pathogenesis, which are unambiguous. In this context, interpretative data may be misleading. Thus, when investigating obesity, it is better to have even an approximate estimate of an animal's body weight and food intake, than to have a subjective (interpretative) impression of its weight as 'heavy' or 'light' and its food intake as 'a little' or 'a lot' because these terms may represent different weights and amounts of food to different people.

## Sensitivity and specificity

Events may be recorded as being true when, actually, they are not. A dog, for example, may be diagnosed as having diabetes mellitus when it does not. This constitutes a **false positive** record, and renders the diagnosis inaccurate. The error in this case may have resulted from an improper inference based upon only a few clinical signs such as polyphagia and polydipsia, with no supporting biochemical evidence. Alternatively, diabetes may not be diagnosed when it actually is present. This constitutes a **false negative** record. Such errors inevitably lead to misclassification of 'diseased' and 'non-diseased' animals. These errors can occur when using clinical signs, detection of specific agents and reactions to diagnostic tests as diagnostic criteria.

**Table 9.1 Possible results of a diagnostic test**

| Test status | True status | | Totals |
| --- | --- | --- | --- |
| | *Diseased* | *Not diseased* | |
| Diseased | *a* | *b* | *a + b* |
| Not diseased | *c* | *d* | *c + d* |
| *Totals* | *a + c* | *b + d* | *a + b + c + d* |

Sensitivity = $a/(a+c)$
Specificity = $d/(b+d)$

These errors, and therefore the validity of the diagnostic techniques, can be quantified by comparing results obtained by the diagnostic method with those obtained from an independent valid criterion (*Table 9.1*). The **sensitivity** of a diagnostic method is the proportion of true positives that are detected by the method. The **specificity** of the method is the proportion of true negatives that are detected. Sensitivity and specificity can be quoted either as a probability between zero and one, or as a percentage.

The sensitivity and specificity of a diagnostic test are important in deciding the value of the test in disease control campaigns (*see* Chapter 16) and in categorizing animals in observational studies (*see* Chapter 15).

## Accuracy, refinement, precision, reliability and validity

These terms can be used in relation to qualitative data (e.g. the description of a disease) and to quantitative measures (e.g. of prevalence and weight).

### Accuracy

**Accuracy** is an indication of the extent to which an investigation or measurement conforms to the truth. Thus, if a set of scales records an animal's weight as 15 kg and this is the actual weight of the animal, then the measurement is accurate.

### Refinement

The degree of detail in a datum is its **refinement**. Thus, 13 kg and 13.781 kg may both represent the accurate weight of an animal, but the second record is more refined than the first. Similarly, 'orthopaedic surgery' is a less refined description of a surgical technique than is 'bone plating'. In *Figure 9.2*, 'otitis externa' is a less refined diagnosis than either 'otitis externa caused by bacteria' or 'otitis externa caused

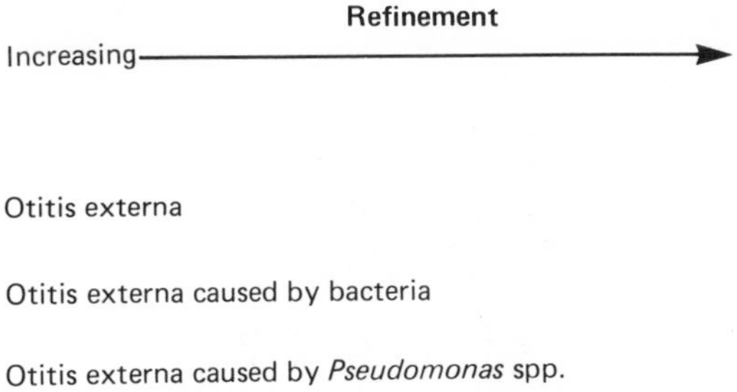

Refinement

Increasing ————————————————————➤

Otitis externa

Otitis externa caused by bacteria

Otitis externa caused by *Pseudomonas* spp.

**Figure 9.2** Example of increasing refinement of a diagnosis.

by *Pseudomonas* spp.'. The less refined definition may be described as 'coarse grained' and the more refined definitions as 'fine grained' by analogy with photographic film. Specificity is sometimes used synonymously with refinement.

Increasing the refinement of descriptive diagnostic data may improve their epidemiological value because it usually moves towards a definition of disease in terms of particular sufficient causes (*see* Chapter 3), whereas a less refined definition in terms of manifestations can include several sufficient causes (*see Figure 9.1c*).

Auxiliary tests are frequently required to increase the refinement of a diagnosis. Thus, physical examination may facilitate the diagnosis of otitis externa, but a more refined diagnosis of otitis externa involving *Pseudomonas* spp. infection would require the use of microbiological techniques. The refinement of auxiliary techniques may also vary. For example, the complement fixation test will detect types of influenza A virus, but will not detect subtypes. Identification of the latter requires more refined tests, for example haemagglutination and neuraminidase inhibition.

## Precision

**Precision** can be used in two senses. First, it can be used as a synonym for refinement. Secondly, it can be used statistically to indicate the consistency of a series of measurements. Thus, repeated sampling of a population may allow estimation of a prevalence value of, say, $40\% \pm 2\%$. Alternatively, the value may be estimated at $40\% \pm 5\%$. The first estimation is more precise than the second. Precision, in the second sense, is discussed in more detail in Chapter 14.

## Reliability

A diagnostic technique is **reliable** if it produces similar results when it is repeated. Thus **repeatability (reproducibility)** is a characteristic of a reliable technique.

## Validity

If a diagnostic technique measures what it is supposed to measure, it is **valid**. Validity is a long-term characteristic of a technique. The validity of a technique depends upon the disease that is being investigated and the method of diagnosis. A midshaft femoral fracture, for example, may be diagnosed very accurately when using only physical examination (*Figure 9.3*): the lesion is rarely misdiagnosed, thus physical examination, as a diagnostic technique, is highly valid in this instance. However, physical examination alone may not be considered sufficiently error-free, when used to diagnose diabetes mellitus. Biochemical examination, in this case urine analysis, may be used to

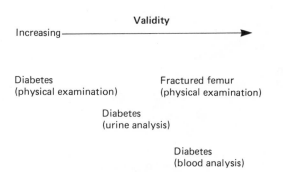

**Figure 9.3** Validity of diagnostic techniques in relation to the disease being studied.

decrease error, and fasting blood sugar estimation to decrease it further. The use of auxiliary diagnostic aids, such as biochemical, radiological and microbiological investigation, is simply a means of increasing the accuracy of a diagnosis by selecting diagnostic techniques of higher validity.

The value of a diagnostic technique is judged in terms of its **reliability** and **validity**. This can be exemplified using target shooting as an analogy (*Figure 9.4*). In target A, each shot is accurate (i.e. close to the bull's-eye, which represents the true value), therefore validity and repeatability are high. In target B, none of the shots is accurate, but the result is repeatable. In target D, none of the shots is accurate, and reliability is low because the shots are inconsistent with each other. Target C illustrates that, **on average**, it is possible to obtain high validity when the accuracy of individual shots is low. Thus, high validity corresponds to shots, on average, hitting the bull's-eye; high reliability corresponds to shots being tightly packed.

Although there has been ambiguity in the use of these five terms (Last, 1983), accuracy is best considered the property of a single diagnosis (i.e. of one shot at the bull's-eye) whereas validity should

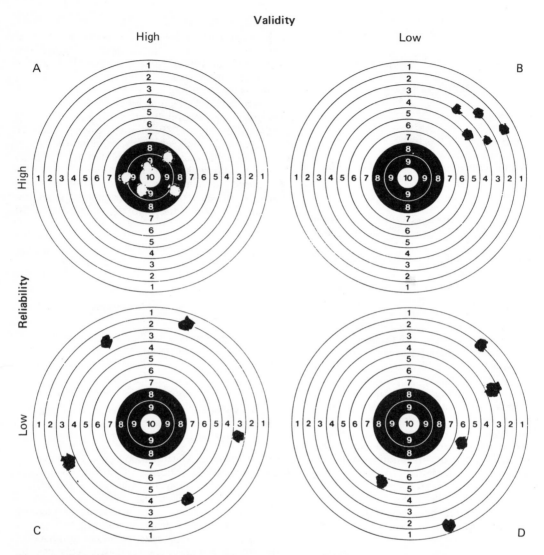

**Figure 9.4** Reliability and validity of diagnostic tests presented as analogues of target shooting.

be considered a long-term characteristic of a diagnostic technique (i.e. the average result of several shots).

## Bias

The shots fired at target B in *Figure 9.4* are not accurate, but they are repeatable. Thus, the results are reliable, but of low validity. In this example, the results may have occurred because the sights on the gun were **biased** to the right of the centre of the target. A similar bias can occur in diagnostic tests and epidemiological studies. Bias is any systematic (as opposed to random) error in the design, conduct or analysis of a study that renders results invalid.

Several types of bias can be identified (Last, 1983). Major ones are:

(1) **bias due to confounding** ( *see* Chapter 3);
(2) **interviewer bias**, where an interviewer's opinions may affect accurate reporting of data;
(3) **measurement bias**, involving inaccurate measurements or the misclassification of animals as diseased or non-diseased (e.g. when sensitivity and specificity are less than 100%);
(4) **selection bias**, where animals selected for study have systematically different characteristics from those that are not selected for study; for example, animals selected from an abattoir are unlikely to have clinical disease, whereas the general population will include some clinically diseased individuals.

Bias is a **long-run** effect. Any individual shot in target B could have been one of those in targets C or D. Only when all of the shots have been fired can the bias be detected, because it requires demonstration of reliability. Thus, an individual observation from a population cannot be biased. Similarly, if many samples produce repeatable inaccurate results then bias is present in the **population** from which the sample was drawn.

Bias can be corrected if its extent is known. Thus, the sights on the gun can be adjusted to compensate for the bias; shots will then be accurate. Similarly, biased estimates of prevalence, resulting from a test's specificity and sensitivity being less than 100%, can be corrected if the sensitivity and specificity are known (*see* Chapter 16).

# Representation of data: coding

Data are usually represented by both words and numbers. An alternative type of notation involves coding. This is a means of representing text and numerals in a standardized, usually abbreviated, form. Codes are easier and more economic to handle by a computer than plain text and so are commonly used in modern computerized recording systems (*see* Chapter 11). Representation may be by letters (**alpha codes**), numbers (**numeric codes**), a combination of each (**alphanumeric codes**) or, less frequently, by symbols.

Codes are a form of shorthand; they are briefer than their textual equivalents. Thus, it is easier and quicker to record the code numbers 274 than to write the possible textual equivalent, contagious bovine pleuropneumonia.

## *Code structure*

Data about animals divide into two groups; any system of coding must cope with both groups. The first includes categories that relate to **permanent** data such as details of species, breed, date of birth and sex. These data have been termed 'tombstone data' because they remain unchanged during the whole of an animal's life. The second group comprises data relating to events that **vary** during life, such as date of occurrence, lesions, test results, signs and diagnoses. The various categories are sometimes called **descriptors** or **specifier types**. Other data can be derived from these categories, for example the animal's age at the onset of disease.

### Components

The data that define disease can comprise a single component, called an **axis**, for example 'bronchiolitis'. Alternatively, the definition can be broken down into constituent parts. In the case of a lesion, two convenient axes are the underlying pathological process and its site (topography). Using this **biaxial** system (two axes), bronchiolitis can be recorded as 'inflammation' and 'bronchiole'. Similarly, surgical procedures can be coded biaxially, in terms of procedure and site, for example 'intramedullary pinning' and 'femur'. It is therefore possible to build up disease definitions from basic components in various axes. Codes can also be connected using suitable punctuation to produce abbreviated lines of text and numbers, termed 'text strings', which describe cases. An example is given below in the section on alphanumeric codes.

## *Numeric codes*

Numeric codes represent text by numbers, for example:

seborrhoea = 6327.

Most of the early veterinary and medical coding systems were numeric. A commonly used system, developed in North America, is the *Standard Nomenclature of Veterinary Diseases and Operations* (SNVDO: Priester, 1964, 1971). This codes diseases and operations (treatments) biaxially: diseases by topography and either aetiology or lesion, and operations by topography and procedure. Examples are:

diagnosis : 3530    3900.0 = bronchiolitis due to allergy,

treatment : 723    52 = ureteric anastomosis.

In these examples, the diagnosis includes a topographical part (3530 = bronchiole) and an aetiological part (3900.0 = allergy). Similarly, treatment is defined in terms of topography (723) and procedure (52).

Multiaxial systems have also been developed that allow the summarizing of recorded data under several axes, for example topography, aetiology, function and disease (Cordes *et al.*, 1981). An example is given below in the section on alphanumeric codes.

### Consecutive and hierarchic codes

A **consecutive** code is one in which consecutive numbers are drawn up to represent data, for example:

001 = distemper,
002 = infectious hepatitis,
003 = acute cystitis.

It is also possible to draw up a list of codes with a **hierarchic** structure, that is with initial digits

**Table 9.2 An example of hierarchic numeric codes**

|  | Code | Meaning |
|---|---|---|
| Treatment | 100 | General medical therapy |
|  | 110 | Antibiotic |
|  | 112 | Oxytetracycline |
|  | 120 | Parasiticide |
|  | 122 | Thiabendazole |
| Species and breed | 100 | Horse |
|  | 110 | Pony |
|  | 111 | Welsh mountain pony |
|  | 120 | Warm blooded |
|  | 121 | English thoroughbred |
|  | 200 | Dog |
|  | 300 | Cat |
|  | 400 | Cattle |
|  | 410 | Friesian |

**Table 9.3 An example of numeric coding of quantitative data: frequency codes for numbers of eggs per gram of faeces (epg) for use on a parasitology data report form (From Slocombe, 1975)**

| Code | epg | Code | epg |
|---|---|---|---|
| 004 | 1– 500 | 014 | 5001– 5500 |
| 005 | 501–1000 | 015 | 5501– 6000 |
| 006 | 1001–1500 | 016 | 6001– 6500 |
| 007 | 1501–2000 | 017 | 6501– 7000 |
| 008 | 2001–2500 | 018 | 7001– 7500 |
| 009 | 2501–3000 | 019 | 7501– 8000 |
| 010 | 3001–3500 | 020 | 8001– 8500 |
| 011 | 3501–4000 | 021 | 8501– 9000 |
| 012 | 4001–4500 | 022 | 9001– 9500 |
| 013 | 4501–5000 | 023 | 9501–10000 |

representing broad categories, and succeeding digits indicating more refined categories; the more digits used, the more refined the definition. An example is given in *Table 9.2*, and its hierarchic structure, resembling the roots of a tree, is illustrated in *Figure 9.5*. The use of initial digits alone produces 'coarse grain' definitions; the use of additional succeeding digits produces 'fine grain' (i.e. more detailed) definitions. There are two main advantages to hierarchic codes. First, if accurate auxiliary diagnostic techniques are not available and therefore refined diagnoses are not definable, then a coarse grain code may be used without succumbing to the temptation of offering a more refined diagnosis than can be substantiated. Secondly, the individual interests of data collectors can be accommodated. For example, someone with a specialist interest in chemotherapy may be able to record the use of a particular antibiotic, whereas those who are content with recording just that an antibiotic has been used may record in the coarser grain.

Even when the type of code is acceptable (e.g. a biaxial hierarchic format) the code may be unacceptable because the amount of detail that it contains may be unsuitable for a particular purpose. The SNVDO, for example, was considered to be insufficiently refined in relation to parasitological diagnostic techniques by Canadian parasitologists, and so they devised a more detailed code for that field (Slocombe, 1975).

In addition to recording qualitative data, it is possible to use code to record quantitative data such as test results. There is some loss of refinement compared with the use of the results themselves because coding often involves the grouping of individual values into ranges of values (blocks). *Table 9.3*, for example, illustrates the numeric codes for ranges of numbers of helminth eggs isolated from faeces. Some test results are already blocked, although the blocking is often concealed by the mode of expression. Thus, a serological test quoted as positive at a dilution of 1:1024 implies that it was

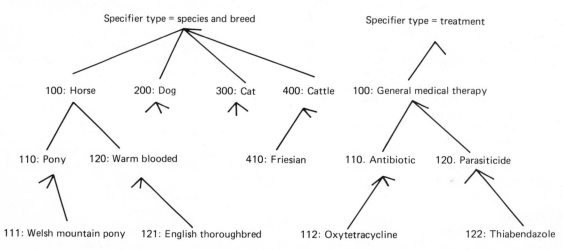

**Figure 9.5** Diagrammatic representation of a hierarchic code (code listed in *Table 9.2*).

negative at 1:1025, whereas the next dilution tested that yielded a negative result was probably 1:2048.

It is usually advantageous to use code numbers that are mathematically related to the upper limits of the intervals used to categorize the variable. In the previous example (*Table 9.3*) the code number is:

$$\frac{\text{epg upper limit}}{500} + 3$$

where epg = number of eggs per gram of faeces.

## Alpha codes

Alpha codes represent plain text by alphabetical abbreviations or acronyms, for example:

FN = female neuter,
M  = male.

Codes that are totally alpha are not common.

## Alphanumeric codes

Alphanumeric codes have evolved more recently than numeric codes. An example is given in *Table 9.4*, where the disease is located in three axes: the disease's name, its topography and its aetiology. The first axis classifies the disease according to its name. In the first example in the table, the first (alpha) part of the first axis relates to the broad disease category (abomasitis) and the second (numeric) component produces a 'finer grain' description (mycotic abomasitis); this is therefore a simple hierarchy. The second axis classifies the disease according to the anatomical system that it affects (UDIG=upper digestive system). The third axis classifies the disease according to cause (MYCO=mycosis).

Signs may also be coded alphanumerically. *Table 9.5* illustrates a hierarchic alphanumeric code of signs. Codes can virtually replace full text if suitable punctuation marks are used in the text string. The

**Table 9.5 An example of hierarchic alphanumeric codes for signs. (From White and Vellake, 1980)**

*Acoustic sense signs*
A00 Deafness

        A01 Complete deafness
        A02 Partial deafness

A10 Discharge from ear

        A11 Bloody discharge from ear
        A12 Purulent discharge from ear

A20 Excess wax/cerumen in ear

A30 Abnormal ear size

A40 Other signs referrable to the ear

        A41 Mite infestation of ear, parasite, dirt
        A42 Odour bad ear
        A43 Cold ears

*Digestive system signs*

D00 Abnormal appetite

        D01 Decreased appetite
        D02 Polyphagia—excessive appetite
        D03 Anorexia—loss of appetite
        D04 Pica—Depraved appetite

D10 Difficulty in prehension, cannot get food in mouth

D20 Chewing difficulty

D30 Signs of the jaw

        D31 Weakness of jaw
        D32 Inability to close jaw
        D33 Inability to open jaw
        D34 Malformation of jaw

D40 Odour from mouth

D50 Signs referrable to the oral mucosa

        D51 Bleeding oral mucosa
        D52 Ecchymosis oral mucosa
        D53 Petechia oral mucosa
        D54 Dryness oral mucosa
        D55 Cold oral mucosa

**Table 9.4 An example of alphanumeric diagnostic codes (3 axes). (From Stephen, 1980)**

| Code | Axis 1<br>Name of disease | Axis 2<br>Anatomical system involved | Axis 3<br>Aetiological agent or other indicated cause |
|---|---|---|---|
| ABO 10 | Abomasitis, mycotic | UDIG (upper digestive) | MYCO (mycotic) |
| BRA 10 | Brachygnathia | BOJOS (bones, joints, etc.) | CONGEN (congenital) |
| ENC 45 | Encephalomyelitis, equine, Western | NERVO (nervous) | VIRO (virus) |
| EPI 10 | Epidermitis, porcine, exudative | SKAP (skin and appendages) | BACTE (bacterial) |
| TOX 64 | Seneciosis (including pyrrolizidine poisoning) | LIVBIP (liver and biliary) | TOXO (toxicosis) |

COSREEL* code (Russell *et al.*, 1982b), for example, allows diagnoses, surgical and medical treatments, vaccinations, antiserum treatment, tests, local and general signs, and case progress to be described.

Thus: ?(DME)KED(GUT)INI(EMG,34)CL means ketosis due to dietary reasons, metritis due to infection, and clots in the milk from both left quarters, because the codes are:

| | | |
|---|---|---|
| ? | = | diagnosis |
| DME | = | Disease: MEtabolic |
| KE | = | KEtosis |
| D | = | owing to Diet |
| GUT | = | Genital system: UTerus |
| IN | = | INflammation |
| I | = | due to Infection |
| EMG | = | Epidermal system: Mammary Gland |
| 34 | = | quarters 3 and 4 (the two left) |
| CL | = | CLots. |

## Symbols

Symbols can be used as codes. Thus ↑ and ↓ are frequently used to represent elevated and lowered body temperature respectively. Symbols may be combined with letters such as D+ and D− to indicate the presence and absence, respectively, of diarrhoea. *Table 9.6* lists some examples of symbolic codes used in an international veterinary disease reporting system. These may appear to represent very vague descriptions. However, they reflect the level of knowledge of morbidity in many countries,

**Table 9.6 An example of symbolic codes. (From FAO-WHO-OIE, 1984)**

| Code | Disease occurrence |
|---|---|
| − | Not recorded; obviously not present |
| (−) | Not recorded; probably not present |
| | Year last occurrence: below symbol |
| | 0000: never |
| ? | Suspected but not confirmed |
| (+) | Exceptional occurrence |
| + | Low sporadic incidence |
| ++ | Moderate incidence |
| +++ | High incidence |
| ... | No information available |
| +\ | Disease much reduced, but still exists |
| +ø | Confined to certain regions |
| +← | Mostly in imported animals |
| +! | Disease only recently recognized in country |
| +~ | Seasonal occurrence |
| +.. | Disease exists; distribution and incidence entirely unknown |

*COSREEL is an acronym for COmputer System for Recording Events affecting Economically-important Livestock.

where reliable, accurate, quantitative data are unavailable. The value of such general terms was noted in the last century by a notable medical epidemiologist William Farr: 'The refusal to recognize terms that express imperfect knowledge has an obvious tendency to encourage reckless conjecture'.

## Choosing a code

The choice of a code is partly subjective. Some people find numbers easier to handle; others are more content with letters. There are, however, several definable advantages and disadvantages to numeric and alpha codes.

If acronymic alpha codes are used (e.g. ABO for abomasum) they may be easier to relate to the plain text data and, possibly, to remember, than numeric codes. However, users of numeric codes frequently report that they soon 'learn the numbers'.

In some cases, alpha codes, in order to be acronymic, may require more characters than their numeric counterparts, even though 26 alternatives are available for each alpha character, and 36 for alphanumeric, compared with only 10 for numeric systems. This may be an important space consideration in computerized systems which, in any case, can pack numeric data more tightly than either alpha or alphanumeric strings.

Numeric codes can be entered into computers more quickly than alpha codes. Most computer keyboards have a nine-digit numeric keypad which can be depressed more quickly than the alphabetic typewriter-style keyboard, especially if the user cannot type.

If a consecutive numeric code is used, care should be taken to ensure that it is long enough to accommodate all definitions of a specifier type. A four-digit code (e.g. 0000–9999) can accommodate 10 000 definitions (1000 if the last digit is a 'check digit'—*see below*), and would then be 'full'. If more than 10 000 definitions were required, a five-digit code would have to be used.

If there is a requirement for a variable 'grain' in the definition, a hierarchic code is the most suitable. Alpha codes can be used, although numeric codes are more common. Numeric codes can have 10 categories (0–9) at each level of the hierarchy. Alpha codes, based on the Roman alphabet, can have 26 categories (A–Z) at each level of the hierarchy.

Numeric codes are not subject to language differences. Alpha codes, however, if acronymic, may need to vary according to the language of the user.

When all of these merits are considered, subjective assessment is still a major factor. This is a reason for the considerable range of codes that are available and for the lack of a universally acceptable one.

# Error detection

Provision must be made for verifying data during the process of combining them with an existing collection of data. In general, as many checks as possible should be made on each datum and the criteria used for checking should remain a permanent characteristic of the data that have satisfied the criteria. This is important when combining data from different sources and when combining data that have satisfied different, perhaps incompatible, sets of criteria.

## Consistency

Initially, checks should be made that the codes are recognizable, and then that they are internally consistent. Thus, it is illogical to record an elevated body temperature and a lowered body temperature at the same time. Placing the event in the context of what else is known about the animal's life history may reveal other inappropriate data. For instance, the recording of 'dystocia' becomes unacceptable when the animal's existing record shows it to be either male, or juvenile, or to have undergone an ovariohysterectomy some time ago. All of these inconsistencies would suggest that the animal may have been misidentified.

The initial check that the code is recognizable is simple if consecutive codes are employed: the check is that the code that is offered is neither less than the lowest nor greater than the highest code in use. Alphanumeric codes may need to be checked against a list held within the computer containing all permissible codes. Some codes (e.g. *Table 9.4* and COSREEL) use combinations of code elements taken from different lists, for example representing organs, pathological processes and causes. Each element must be identified and checked against the appropriate list; further checks are required to ensure that any particular combination of organ, pathological process and cause is feasible.

## 'Finger trouble'

Data that are entered via keyboards (a common form of data entry in computerized systems—*see* Chapter 11) are subject to four types of error, collectively and colloquially termed 'finger trouble'. These errors are:

(1) **insertion**, where extra characters are erroneously added;
(2) **deletion**, where characters are omitted;
(3) **substitution**, where the wrong character is typed;
(4) **transposition**, where the correct characters are typed in the wrong order.

The danger is that the incorrect version may be an allowable code that means something totally different from the intended code. If the codes have the same number of characters then insertion and deletion are easily detected because the incorrectly entered code is the wrong length. The likelihood of entry of an incorrect code can be reduced by increasing the 'redundancy' of the code, that is by adding more characters to the code. For example, many transpositions and substitutions would be needed to change 'mastitis' into another plausible word. Unfortunately, highly redundant codes with many characters require many keystrokes which itself increases the chance of error. A balance must be found between these conflicting requirements.

Data that are transmitted electronically, for example, from one computer to another via telephone links (*see* Chapter 11), can be corrupted during transit by the 'noise' of the transmission medium. There are several ways of protecting data from this degradation, including the use of 'parity bits' and 'check bytes' (bits and bytes are defined in Chapter 11) to signal corruption of each character. Alternatively or additionally a 'check digit' may be incorporated in numeric codes to perform the same function while also increasing the codes' length and redundancy.

## Check digits

These are mathematical functions of the preceding digits of the code, for example:

5029 = anaemia.

The first three digits (502) are a consecutively ordered code which relates to anaemia, and the fourth digit (9) is a check digit which is a function of the code numbers. The check digit, in this case, may have been generated using the formula:

$$(\text{1st digit} \times 2) + \text{second digit} - \frac{\text{third digit}}{2}$$
$$= \text{check digit,}$$

that is $(5 \times 2) + 0 - \frac{2}{2} = 9$.

The computer will not accept 5028 or 5020 since it recognizes that the last digit is not the correct function of 502. Similarly, it will not accept 5019 or 5039 which represent two totally different diagnoses. This is therefore a useful validation check against corruption to incorrect codes. (Of course, in this example, 4229 and 4109 would be consistent with the formula used to produce the check digit, but these are so unlike 5029 that it is very improbable that they would be entered.)

# Measurements

The numeric codes mentioned above are examples of the use of numbers to describe one property of an animal: its membership of a group or class. The code 671, perhaps representing diabetes, may indicate that all animals with that code attached to them belong to a unique class: diabetics. More commonly, in veterinary medicine, numbers are used to measure **amounts** rather than just to indicate classes. Prevalence and incidence, body weight, milk yield, temperature and antibody titre are examples of amounts that are commonly measured. The measurements are often used as a basis for analysis, which frequently involves statistics. Not all measurements are amenable to the same type of statistical analysis, and an improper appreciation of the nature of measurements often leads to the use of inappropriate statistical tests. An understanding of measurement is therefore desirable.

There are two types of measurement: **discrete** and **continuous**. A discrete measurement has only one of a specified set of values, such as whole numbers (1,2,7,9, etc.), for example the number of teats on a sow. Discrete data, by their nature, can be divided into categories and therefore are **categorical** data. A continuous measurement may have any value within a defined range (though the range can be infinite). Examples are the girth of a cow and its body weight. Discrete measurements are often **nominal** or **ordinal**, and also can be **interval** or **ratio**. Continuous measurements may be either **interval** or **ratio**.

## *Discrete measurements*

### The nominal (classificatory) scale

This scale involves the use of numbers (or other symbols) to classify objects. The numeric and alpha codes described above are examples. A non-veterinary example would be the use of numbers or letters on aircraft to indicate their origin. The property of a nominal scale is **equivalence**: members in a class must possess the same property. Expressed technically, the equivalence relation is:

reflexive ($x = x$ for all values of $x$),
symmetrical (if $x = y$, then $y = x$),
transitive (if $x = y$, and $y = z$, then $x = z$).

The only legitimate operation that can be performed on a nominal scale is transformation of the symbols. For example, the code 671 for diabetes could be transformed or changed to 932 for **all** diabetics. This scale is a 'weak' form of measurement.

### The ordinal (ranking) scale

The ordinal scale allows groups to be related to other groups. Most commonly, the relation can be expressed in terms of equal to, greater than ($>$) or less than ($<$). An example is the use of body condition scores for sheep.

The difference between the nominal and the ordinal scale therefore is that the ordinal includes not only equivalence but also the 'greater than' and 'less than' property. This property is:

irreflexive (for any $x$, it is not true that $x > x$),
asymmetrical (if $x > y$, then $y \not> x$),
transitive (if $x > y$ and $y > z$, then $x > z$).

In the ordinal scale, any transformation must preserve the order. It does not matter what number is attached to a class, as long as the relationship with other classes is consistent. Thus, a carcass condition score scale can include 5 = good and 1 = poor, and equally 1 = good and 5 = poor, as long as the numbers between 1 and 5 maintain the same order of ranking. Although 'stronger' than the nominal scale, the ordinal scale is still a relatively 'weak' form of measurement.

## *Continuous measurements*

### The interval scale

In an interval scale, the distance between the ranked values is known with some accuracy. A good example is body temperature. Two thermal interval scales are commonly used—Celsius and Fahrenheit—each containing the same amount of information. The ratios of the intervals (temperature differences in this example) are independent of the zero point ($0°C = 32°F$) and are equal to the ratios of the differences on the other interval scales. For example:

$$37°C = 99°F \text{ (approximately)}$$
$$22°C = 72°F \text{ (approximately)}$$
$$6°C = 43°F \text{ (approximately)}.$$

Thus (°C) $\dfrac{37-22}{22-6} = \dfrac{15}{16} = 0.9375$

and (°F) $\dfrac{99-72}{72-43} = \dfrac{27}{29} = 0.9310344...$

that is, the ratios are approximately the same (0.9).

The interval scale therefore includes equivalence, 'greater than' relationships, and ratios of intervals. Because the ratios are dependent on the zero point, arithmetic calculations can be performed only on differences between numbers. The interval scale is a relatively 'strong' form of measurement.

## The ratio scale

The ratio scale is an interval scale with a true zero point. Weight is a ratio scale. The various weight ratio scales may have units of kilograms, grams, pounds or ounces, but they all start from the same zero point. This means that arithmetic operations can be performed not only on the ratios of differences but also on the numbers themselves. The ratio scale may be bounded. Prevalence, for example, can take values only between 0 and 1 (0 and 100%). (Note that a ratio scale is not associated necessarily with ratio measurements; weight, for instance, is a ratio scale that is not a ratio measure.)

In terms of suitability to statistical investigation, most statistical tests can be used with interval and ratio scales. However, not all tests can be applied to the other two scales. This point will be expanded in Chapters 13 and 16.

## *Further reading*

HALL, S.A. (1978) Farm animal disease data banks. *Advances in Veterinary Science and Comparative Medicine*, **22**, 265–286

LEECH, F.B. (1980) Relations between objectives and observations in epidemiological studies. In: *Veterinary Epidemiology and Economics*. Proceedings of the Second International Symposium, Canberra, 7–11 May 1979. Eds Geering, W.A., Roe, R.T. and Chapman, L.A. Pp. 254–257. Australian Government Publishing Services, Canberra

# 10

---

# Sources of data

Epidemiological investigations utilize data relating to disease and its determinants, performance and population size. These data can be collected from many sources, including veterinary practices, farms, diagnostic laboratories, abattoirs and university clinics. These organizations can supply data that they already have recorded, for use in retrospective studies. They can also cooperate in the collection of data in prospective studies.

The collection of data always incurs a cost. This includes postal charges when the data are collected by postal questionnaire (*see* Chapter 14) and laboratory examination charges. The value of data therefore has to be judged in the context of the cost of collecting them.

## Some general considerations

### Nature of data

Data from some sources may be unsuitable because they are inaccurate. Also, they may be of the wrong type. For example, a record which just notes 'lameness' would be useful in a general estimation of the prevalence of bovine foot problems but would be of little value to a detailed study of the various lesions and their causes that produce lameness (*see* Chapter 9).

### Cooperation

The lack of cooperation can pose a problem to epidemiological investigations. There are several reasons why people may not be willing to supply data.

The reasons for undertaking a study or survey may not be clear to potential suppliers of data, and so they may be discouraged. This emphasizes that the objectives of an investigation should be explained to all who are involved with it. Cooperation is more likely if the investigation is part of a planned animal health programme than if it is undertaken in isolation. For example, Sudanese farmers cooperated in a survey of mortality due to schistosomiasis, conducted by interview, because this survey was part of an investigation of the financial viability of a new vaccine against *Schistosoma bovis* (McCauley *et al.*, 1983a,b). However, surveys in Haiti, conducted without a concomitant animal health programme, eventually met with resistance from local animal owners (Perry and McCauley, 1984). Some studies, particularly prospective ones, may also take several years to complete, during which time motivation may be difficult to maintain.

The collection of information may risk a breach of confidentiality, for example if practitioners' records containing details of financial transactions of practices are examined. This, too, may prevent cooperation.

Cooperation is unlikely if data collection is laborious or time-consuming, for instance, completing a complex or cumbersome questionnaire. The method of data collection, therefore, should be as simple as possible, within the constraints of the requirements of the investigation.

### Trace-back

Data on the geographical distribution of disease may be difficult to gather because of an inability to trace animals back to their origin. This can be a major problem at abattoirs where carcasses may not be clearly identified. Trace-back can be very valuable. An obvious example is tracing contacts with rabid dogs. Similarly, the control of chlamydiosis in Californian parakeets has been facilitated by a state law requiring all parakeets to be banded with details of their year of birth and breeding establishment (Schachter *et al.*, 1978).

## Bias

Sources of veterinary data may be biased (*see* Chapter 9), a common problem being selection bias. The bias in the sources of data listed below is indicated when each source is described.

## The cost of data collection

In most countries the collection of information on diseases of national importance is supported by government funds. Similarly, in many countries funds are available for research on diseases of economically important livestock. However, investigation of companion animals' diseases, especially if they are not demonstrably of public health significance, relies on the limited financial support available from welfare societies and charities. Lack of funds, therefore, can restrict companion animal data collection.

## Problems unique to developing countries

Data collection in developing countries may face additional difficulties (Broadbent, 1979). There may be poor laboratory diagnostic support and insufficient manpower. The terrain may be difficult. In these cases, it is often advisable to collect as much information and as many specimens (e.g. faeces for the counting of helminth eggs, and serum for antibody titration) as possible during a survey to investigate several diseases at once, thus avoiding the need for repeated journeys to difficult areas. The prevalence of some diseases can be measured directly while conducting surveys, such as tuberculosis using the intradermal test, and trichomoniasis by examining preputial washings.

## Sources of epidemiological data

The organizations and groups described below represent a comprehensive list of possible sources of data. The membership of the list will vary between countries. Some countries, particularly the developed ones, have veterinary infrastructures that facilitate potential or actual data collection from the majority of these sources. The developing countries may be able to utilize only a few of them.

Some organizations record and store data routinely and therefore provide structured collections of data (data bases) to which reference can be made when mounting epidemiological studies. Some of these established pools of data are discussed in greater detail in Chapter 11. The *International Directory of Animal Health and Disease Data Banks* (USDA, 1982) lists and briefly describes epidemiological, laboratory, clinical and bibliographic data bases and data bases of research in progress. These data bases also have been reviewed by Pilchard (1979).

## Government veterinary organizations

Most countries have organized government veterinary services. These services investigate diseases of national importance, particularly those infectious ones for which legislation enforces reporting (the notifiable diseases). Many governments also operate diagnostic laboratories. Reports are sometimes prepared and published routinely, for example, records of diagnoses made at diagnostic laboratories in the UK (Hall *et al.*, 1980). Submissions to diagnostic laboratories from practitioners are often voluntary and may therefore reflect personal interest and motivation, causing selection bias. Reports of notifiable diseases, similarly, depend upon the conscientiousness of observers.

Publications that collate information from a variety of government sources, including 'field' and laboratory investigations, are also available routinely. In some cases routine reports are prepared but are confidential and therefore not readily available. An international bulletin of animal diseases, covering most countries of the world, is published by the Paris-based *Office International des Epizooties* (OIE: Blajan, 1982). The bulletin provides a statement of disease prevalence, as far as it is known, for the member countries of OIE.

Sometimes surveys have been undertaken that use data collated from several sources. A good example is the survey of livestock diseases in Northern Ireland that was undertaken in 1954 and 1955 (Gracey, 1960). This included demographic and disease data relating to a wide range of infectious and non-infectious diseases in cattle, sheep and pigs. It included data collected from 70% of farms in the country by field officers, and abattoir data.

## Veterinary practices

In countries with private veterinary practices (notably the developed countries) practitioners have

**Table 10.1 An example of routine disease reporting in general veterinary practice: categories recorded by practitioners in the Bay of Plenty region of New Zealand. (From MAFF, 1976)**

**Cattle**
*Metabolic:*
  Milk fever
  Ketosis
  Grass staggers
*General:*
  Actinomycosis
  Arthritis
  Bloat
  Blood testing
  Castration
  Dehorning
  Hernia
  Indigestion
  Miscellaneous
  Postmortem examination
  Starvation
  Unthrift
*Respiratory:*
  Upper respiratory tract
  Pneumonias etc.
*Gastroenteritis:*
  Colic
  Colibacillosis
  Parasitic
  Salmonellosis
  Other or unspecified
*Skin:*
  Facial eczema
  Photosensitivity
    (excluding facial eczema)
  Other dermatoses
*Vaccinations:*
  Brucellosis
  Leptospirosis
  Other (including IPV/BVD)

**Calf losses**
**Sheep**
  Dystocias
  Facial eczema
  Foot-rot
*Neonatal losses:*
  ('Brucellosis')
  ('Toxoplasmosis')
  Pneumonia
  Post mortems
  Prolapsed uterus
  Salmonellosis
  Other
*Rams:*
  Palpation

Semen examinations
Other
*Lameness:*
  Feet—foot-rot
  Abscess
  Other .
*Female:*
  Anoestrus
  Calving
  Herd advice
  Induced calving
  Metritis/uterine irrigation
  Paresis
  Pregnancy diagnosis
  Prolapsed uterus
  Retained fetal membranes
  Teat surgery
*Mastitis:*
  Individual
  Herd advice
*Abortion investigations*
  (Total number of accessions)
*Lepto-redwater:*
  Cases
  Farms
  Animals at risk
*Male:*
  Bull soundness
  Semen examinations
  Vasectomies
  Other faults

**Horses**
  Branding
  Castration
  Colic
  Foaling
  Foals
  Tubing
  Wounds
  Other

**Pigs**
  Castration
  Abscesses
  Reproductive
  Respiratory
  Salmonellosis
  Other

**Small animals**
  Road accidents

contact with farm and companion animals, although the extent of contact varies. Farm animal veterinarians have the greatest contact with dairy cattle, less contact with pigs and beef cattle, and the least with sheep. Problems in ruminants tend to be seasonal and related to parturition.

Owners of companion animals usually attend private clinics. Thus the practitioner is a major potential source of small animal and equine data that relate to a reasonably representative cross-section of animals. In companion animal practice the cost of therapy may prevent animals being presented for treatment and so diseases of animals owned by the poor may be under-represented, therefore inducing selection bias.

In large animal practices mild diseases and hopeless cases are not usually brought to the attention of the practitioner by the farmer and so may be under-represented. Similarly, the farmer may treat some animals himself and so some diseased animals may not be recorded.

The data may not be accurate because of incorrect diagnoses. If the purpose of an investigation is unclear to a practitioner and its results are not presented to him with obvious benefit, he is unlikely to participate in data recording, especially over a long period of time, which may be necessary in prospective studies.

Even when information is freely available, it usually exists as separate accumulations of records in the individual practices and may therefore be difficult to collect and collate. Questionnaires can be used (*see* Chapter 14) and modern developments in computer technology (*see* Chapter 11) may increase accessibility of data. The role of the general practice in continuous monitoring is therefore less important than its role in specific surveys and observational studies. Veterinary practitioners have conducted surveys relating to either total clinic populations, for example, nematode infections in dogs (Turner and Pegg, 1977), or in defined cohorts of populations, for example, *Toxocara canis* infection in puppies (Holt, 1976). These surveys are inevitably limited geographically to the vicinity of the practices concerned.

A few continuous monitoring programmes have been instigated using veterinary practice data, for example, those that collect data from several veterinary practices in Minnesota in the USA (Diesch, 1979).

*Table 10.1* lists the categories of data routinely recorded by some practices in the Bay of Plenty region of New Zealand. Most of the data are categorical. They relate to diagnoses (e.g. ketosis), treatments or procedures (e.g. induced calving) and, occasionally, simply to the reason for presentation of the animal (e.g. road accident). The listed diagnoses may be named according to cause (e.g. salmonellosis), lesion (e.g. metritis) or presenting sign (e.g. unthrift). They may be highly refined (e.g. vasectomy) or less refined (e.g. parasitic). They may relate to observations (e.g. prolapsed uterus) or interpretations (e.g. photosensitivity). Also, in all cases referring to diagnoses, accuracy is not indicated, because the criteria on which the diagnoses were based are not cited. In all cases, the numerator in the morbidity and mortality rate calculations (i.e. number affected) is recorded, but in only one instance (lepto-redwater) is the denominator specified.

## Abattoirs

Red meat abattoirs process large numbers of animals for human consumption and identify some diseases during meat inspection. Only clinically healthy animals usually are presented for slaughter, therefore the majority of diseases that are diagnosed at meat inspection are subclinical. Most reports relate to helminth diseases and internal lesions such as hepatic abscesses.

The objective of meat inspection is to safeguard the health of the human population. Traditionally this is practised by preventing the sale of meat and offal that are **obviously** unfit for human consumption. Therefore, most conditions are diagnosed only by macroscopic post-mortem examination; experience has shown that this approach is adequate.

A secondary objective is to record details of abnormalities that are found, because these findings may be of epidemiological value, for example, in associating outbreaks of disease in man with infections in animals (Watson, 1982). Thus, an increase in the prevalence of tuberculosis lesions in cattle at slaughter was the first indication of a human tuberculosis epidemic in Barbados (Wilson and Howes, 1980).

Epidemiological investigations are essentially a subordinate goal of meat inspection at abattoirs, although it is possible to conduct auxiliary investigations of blood, sputum, lymph nodes and other tissues for specific surveys and studies. Thus, in Ireland, bovine kidneys condemned at meat inspection by the usual macroscopic techniques have been subjected to electron-microscopic examination to determine the nature of the lesions (Monaghan and Hannan, 1983). This is an example of using auxiliary aids to increase refinement of a diagnosis. Similarly, a survey of *Cysticercus tenuicollis* infection of sheep in Britain has been undertaken (Stallbaumer, 1983). This was necessary because the condition was not routinely recorded separately but was included in the 'coarse grained' category: 'other conditions'.

Animals examined at meat inspection do not originate from the abattoir; they have travelled there. Trace-back is therefore desirable if the diseases that are identified are to be associated with their farm or area of origin. This is relatively easy in countries that have a simple marketing system. In Denmark, for example, pigs are shipped directly from producers to cooperative slaughterhouses from which data are collectively pooled, thereby allowing rapid trace-back and surveillance of disease (Willeberg, 1980a; Willeberg *et al.*, 1984). In Britain, marketing involves many sellers and purchasers; this makes trace-back difficult when it is epidemiologically desirable (e.g. Sunguya, 1981).

Even when trace-back from the abattoir is possible, improper identification of viscera can be a further problem. Carcasses may be identified by ear tag or tattoo, but viscera containing lesions may not be labelled adequately and it may therefore be impossible to associate them with the carcasses from which they were removed.

Some countries publish routine meat inspection findings. These include Australia, Cyprus, Denmark, India, Luxembourg, New Zealand, Nigeria, Norway, the UK and the USA. The published data may originate from the majority of abattoirs (e.g. in Denmark); from a sample (e.g. in Britain: Blamire *et al.*, 1970, 1980); or from only a single abattoir (e.g. in India: Prabhakaran *et al.*, 1980). These sources have been used for epidemiological surveys; for instance surveys of reasons for condemnation of sheep at Scottish abattoirs (Cuthbertson, 1983) and of numerous diseases identified in animals in English abattoirs (Blamire *et al.*, 1970, 1980).

Abattoir investigations can also be used to indicate faults in husbandry. A survey of hoof and pedal horn lesions in sows at a Budapest abattoir has assisted in the identification of defects in floor construction in pig houses (Kovacs and Beer, 1979).

## Poultry packing plants

In several countries, poultry are slaughtered separately from the larger food animals on poultry packing plants. Post-mortem examination results from these premises constitute another source of information. Again, the population is biased, comprising only young healthy birds, although some culled hens might also be included. Most clinically diseased and dead birds are excluded before slaughter.

## Knacker yards

In some countries, animals that are ill or have died, and are therefore unfit for human consumption, are sent for slaughter to premises other than abattoirs. These premises are called 'knacker yards'. The carcasses may be fed to animals. In Europe, dogs kennelled for hunting (e.g. fox hunting in Britain) are often supplied with flesh from these sources. Knacker yards also handle horses in countries in which horse flesh is not routinely eaten by man.

Data from knacker yards are biased, but in quite a different way from those obtained from abattoirs and poultry packing plants: animals sent to knacker yards are usually either ill or dead—not alive and healthy. Data from this source are difficult to acquire; they are distributed over many premises and would require professional veterinary inspection of lesions to ensure accuracy.

## Serum banks

Stored collections of serum samples are called serum banks. Such samples are often collected routinely during mandatory control and eradication campaigns (e.g. brucellosis eradication) and during specific serological surveys. Much of the serum is not used, particularly now that diagnostic techniques using very small volumes of serum are available, and so the unused serum is usually discarded. Serum samples can provide useful epidemiological information on vaccination priorities, the periodicity of epidemics, the spatial distribution of infections and the origin of newly discovered infectious diseases. Serum banks are described in detail in Chapter 16.

## Registries

A registry is a reference list (more commonly the word describes the building in which the list is kept). In human medicine, registries of diseases (notably of tumours) are maintained using hospital and death certificate data as numerators and census data as denominators in morbidity and mortality rates. There are some veterinary tumour registries but these usually lack census data and so the denominators tend to be biased by non-response. For instance, when using estimates of population size based on the enumeration of licensed or vaccinated dogs (e.g. Cohen *et al.*, 1959), the denominator will tend to be underestimated because of a low public response to licensing and vaccination.

Some registries reduce the non-response bias by utilizing demographic surveys in specified areas. A Californian tumour registry (Dorn, 1966) defines a 'veterinarian using' reference population, counted by household survey, as the denominator. The Tulsa (USA) *Registry of Canine and Feline Neoplasms* (MacVean *et al.*, 1978) defines a 'veterinarian using' reference population, enumerated by a census of all veterinary practices in the Tulsa area, which includes not only sick animals but also healthy animals presented for routine examination, vaccination and elective surgery; the numerator comprises diagnoses made by registry pathologists from specimens submitted by practitioners. Although these registries reduce the selection bias inherent in specialized populations (e.g. of clinical cases), the true population at risk may not be estimated. In the previous example, animals may not attend veterinary practices and therefore would be undetected, and some animals may attend more than one practice, one animal therefore counting twice in the denominator. The extent of these inaccuracies is difficult to assess, but is probably small.

## Pharmaceutical and agricultural sales

The sales records of pharmaceutical companies provide an indirect means of assessing the amount of disease. The sale of antibiotics, for example, is a rough guide to the prevalence of bacterial diseases, although estimates made from this information may be inaccurate. Antibiotics may be used without isolating specific bacteria—indeed, without even positively incriminating a bacterium—and so may be used when a bacterial infection is not present. They may also be used prophylactically, for example following routine surgery. Similarly, they may be used for a purpose other than that for which they were intended: some small animal practitioners, for instance, sometimes use bovine intramammary antibiotics to treat otitis externa. The extent of unjustifiable and unusual use of some drugs is difficult to estimate.

## Zoological gardens

Most zoos maintain detailed records of animals and their diseases, for example on record cards (Griner, 1980) and in computers (Pugsley, 1981). Several zoos send their data to a central registry in Geneva as part of an international data base: the *International Veterinary Record of Zoo Animals* (Roth *et al.*, 1973).

## Agricultural organizations

There are many agricultural bodies associated with the livestock industry that record information on animal production, such as liveweight gain, food conversion and milk yield. Although these data are not related directly to disease, they can provide information on the composition and distribution of populations that can be of value in defining populations that can be studied. For example, the British National Milk Records File has been used to locate Friesian herds for a survey of reasons for culling and wastage in dairy cows (Young *et al.*, 1983).

## Commercial livestock enterprises

The intensification of animal industries mentioned in Chapter 1 has resulted in the establishment of commercial enterprises, particularly in the pig and poultry sector, where large units are common (*see Table 1.5*). These enterprises have their own recording systems, although again some data may be confidential. These sources have been utilized in some surveys, for example mortality in broiler chickens in Australia (Reece and Meddome, 1983), losses in commercially reared rabbits (Hugh-Jones *et al.*, 1975b), unthriftiness in weaned pigs (Jackson and Baker, 1981) and lesions associated with the movement of weaners (Walters, 1978).

## Non-veterinary government departments

There are non-veterinary government departments that collect data relating to animals. These include economic and statistical units. The latter record the numbers and distribution of animals in Britain, enabling the drawing of choroplethic density maps of cattle, sheep and pigs in England and Wales (MAFF/ADAS, 1976a,b,c).

## Farm records

Many farmers, particularly those keeping dairy cattle and pigs, record production data. Some record information on disease. There are several schemes operated by bureaux and universities that record data from several farms. Records from these sources are difficult to unify and compare because they contain varying categories of data of varying degree of refinement. For example, one records lesions of the bovine foot in considerable detail (Russell *et al.*, 1982a) whereas another simply records that lameness is present (Smith *et al.*, 1983). These various data bases have been used in epidemiological studies and surveys of varying refinement, for example surveys of bovine lameness (Russell *et al.*, 1982a; Whitaker *et al.*, 1983a). These 'on farm' recording systems are becoming an essential component of modern herd health and productivity schemes and are discussed in more detail in Chapters 11 and 19.

## Veterinary schools

Veterinary schools have clinics that record the results of consultations. Many have established data bases, often using computerized techniques that allow rapid access to records, for instance the Florida (Burridge and McCarthy, 1979) and Edinburgh (Thrusfield and Hinxman, 1981) schools. The study population is frequently biased, especially when clinicians have specialist interests resulting in a high proportion of referred cases.

## Other sources

Wildlife and animal conservation organizations and pest control centres record data on feral animals, particularly relating to the size of populations. Wildlife can be important sources of infection to domestic animals and man, for example, of rabies (from skunks in the USA and foxes in Europe) and may be potential sources of infection, for example, of *Brucella suis* (from hares in Britain). Routine monitoring of disease in these animals would be expensive. However, *ad hoc* surveys can be undertaken. Demographic data also are valuable when investigating the actual and potential spread of infection (*see*, for example, the discussion of potential fox rabies in Britain in Chapter 17).

Research laboratories record data on primates, lagomorphs, rodents and cavies that are used in experiments. These sources are very specialized, closed communities, and therefore are obviously biased.

Manufacturers of pet food sometimes collect animal demographic data as part of their market research (e.g. Anderson, 1983), although commercial interests may prevent the release of all of these data.

Companion animal breed societies have information on breed numbers and distribution. The extent of cooperation can vary. If a survey could highlight a certain problem in a particular breed then that breed's society may be unwilling to help. This fear is real, although it is based on the false notion that epidemiological investigations just produce incriminating prevalence figures. The main goal of these investigations, however, is to detect causes, with a view to developing beneficial preventive strategies.

## Further reading

HINMAN, A.R. (1977) Analysis, interpretation, use and dissemination of surveillance information. *Bulletin of the Pan American Health Organization*, **11**, (4), 338–343

HUTTON, N.E. and HALVORSON, L.C. (1974) *A Nationwide System for Animal Health Surveillance*. National Academy of Sciences, Washington D.C.

INTERNATIONAL DIRECTORY OF ANIMAL HEALTH AND DISEASE DATA BANKS (1982) National Agriculture Library. United States Department of Agriculture. Miscellaneous Publication No. 1423

KONIGSHOFER, H.O. (1972) *The Organisation of Surveillance of Animal Diseases*. World Health Organization interregional seminar on methods of epidemiological surveillance of communicable diseases including zoonoses and food-borne diseases, Nairobi, 9–20 October 1972. Working Paper No. 8

POPPENSIEK, G.C., BUDD, D.E. and SCHOLTENS, R.G. (1966) *A Historical Survey of Animal-Disease Morbidity and Mortality Reporting*. National Academy of Sciences, Washington D.C. Publication No. 1346

REPORT OF A MINISTRY OF AGRICULTURE, FISHERIES AND FOOD WORKING PARTY (1976) *Animal Disease Surveillance in Great Britain*. MAFF

SCHILF, B.A. (1975) Meat inspection service as an element of epidemiologic surveillance and a component of animal disease control programmes. Seventh Inter-American Meeting on Disease and Zoonosis Control, April 1974. Pp. 149–153. Pan American Health Organization/World Health Organization Scientific Publication No. 295

# 11

# Data storage and retrieval

Earlier chapters have described some of the sources of veterinary data and the methods of collecting them. Data may need to be stored for a long time if they are to be available for future use, for example, in retrospective surveys. This chapter is concerned with the techniques that are used to store and retrieve veterinary data and with some of the established collections of structured data (**data bases**) that can be used for epidemiological investigations. Emphasis will be placed on the suitability of the techniques to epidemiological studies, although some of the standard methods of clinical case recording also will be outlined. Methods of physically storing and ordering records are de-· scribed in detail elsewhere (Duppong and Ettinger, 1983; Thrusfield, 1985b).

## Data base models

A data base containing animal records includes different types of data that comprise different components of the records. The data consist of several categories (**specifier types**), for example breed, sex, age and signs, that are attributes (**features**) of the animal (**item**). Some of these are permanent attributes and therefore are **case-specific**, for example breed and date of birth. Others, such as diagnoses and signs, change from one consultation (and therefore record of consultation) to another, thus being **record-specific**.

The association between the various components of a record can be viewed in several ways, depending on the way in which the data are stored, producing four models of a data base.

### The 'record' model

The **record** model is the traditional way of structuring data. The central component is the

individual record which contains case- and record-specific data. This is a useful approach for the clinician concerned mainly with individual patient care. However, it is difficult to correlate specifier types between records. Correlation is very useful in epidemiological studies, for example, correlation of breed, age and sex with disease.

### The 'hierarchic' model

The **hierarchic** model and the two that follow are used to explain how data are stored and handled in computerized systems. In this model, data components are stored in **nodes** which are arranged in a tree-like structure (*Figure 11.1*). The uppermost

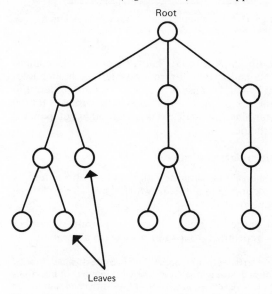

**Figure 11.1** The 'tree' structure of a 'hierarchic' data base.

121

level of the hierarchy has only one node; it is called a **root**. With the exception of the root, every node has one node related to it at a higher level; the latter is called the former's **parent**. No component can have more than one parent. Each component can have one or more components related to it at a lower level; these are called **children**. Components at the end of the branches (i.e. with no children) are called **leaves**. *Figure 11.1* shows a hierarchy with four levels. An example of a hierarchy with only two levels would be one with 'veterinary practice' (the root) and 'veterinary surgeons in the practice' (the children).

## The 'network'* model

Using the terminology of tree structures, if a child in a data relationship has more than one parent, the relationship cannot be a strict hierarchic one. In these circumstances, the structure is described as a **network**. The network model therefore includes and extends the hierarchic model. An example is illustrated in *Figure 11.2*. This model allows

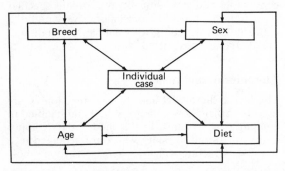

**Figure 11.2** An example of some possible associations in a simple 'network' data base. (From Thrusfield, 1983a)

relationships to occur between many data components and is therefore of considerable epidemiological value because it allows correlation of determinants (e.g. age and sex) with disease if the determinants and diseases are stored as components of the network.

## The 'relational' model

In the **relational** model, all data are represented by two-dimensional tables which have the following properties:

(1) entries in the table are single-valued; neither repeating groups nor arrays are allowable;

*The term 'network' model, in this context, should not be confused with mathematical network models of infectious diseases, described in Chapter 17, or with communications networks, described later in this chapter.

(2) the entries in any one column must all be of the same kind (e.g. one column might contain animals' sexes, and another contain animals' ages);

(3) each column has a unique name and the order of columns is immaterial;

(4) each row of the table is unique and the order of the rows is immaterial.

An example is given in *Table 11.1*.

The relational approach is different from that of the hierarchic and network models. The principal difference is that, in the hierarchic and network models, relationships are expressed explicitly and are predefined. In the relational model, the basic data structure is predefined but record relationships are not defined until they are used. This ability to dynamically reflect relationships, combined with the

**Table 11.1 Structure of data components in a simple 'relational' data base**

| Animal's name | Age | Sex |
|---|---|---|
| Patch | 7 | M |
| Sally | 5 | F |
| Thor | 13 | M |
| . | | |
| . | | |
| . | | |
| Arthur | 4 | M |
| Liz | 15 | F |
| Brenda | 9 | F |
| . | | |
| . | | |
| . | | |

simplicity of the relational model, makes it potentially more flexible than the other models, which it can also represent. The main disadvantage of the relational model is its inefficiency relative to the other two, because, although the model is simple, it is complex to implement on computers. However, with increasing sophistication of computer technology, the model may become more widely used than currently in computerized data recording systems.

# Non-computerized recording techniques

## *Longhand recording techniques*

The recording of data in longhand is a common technique in general veterinary practice where more sophisticated methods, such as computerized storage, may not be available.

## Day books

The day book is a long-established type of longhand record. It is an 'open' record of cases examined during the day, that is it allows any information to be recorded in any form, usually as a narrative description. This type of record now is used infrequently for epidemiological purposes. It is bulky and does not allow either an animal's previous consultations to be located rapidly or correlation of components of different records.

## Record cards

Cards, stored in drawers or boxes, are a common means of storing clinical records. They use a 'record' model of a data base, each card usually referring to one animal. They are usually stored alphabetically according to owners' names. The record-specific data are ordered chronologically on each card, providing a complete history of the patient. Cards may be blank, in which case they can be used to provide an 'open' record. Alternatively, they can be printed as a 'closed' record, that is with a fixed number of options (*see also* Chapter 14: 'Collecting information: questionnaires'). These options commonly include details of specifier types such as breed, sex and date of birth. They are usually partially closed, consisting of a closed section, but with a blank area for the 'open' recording of additional details.

## Pro-formas

A pro-forma is an extension of the partially closed record. It is a mainly closed record, comprising a check list of many features (*Figure 11.3*). This can produce a very detailed record of observational and interpretative data. However, the merits of producing a comprehensive record must be weighed against the unwillingness of busy clinicians to complete them, and against the value of the data. Completion of all components of the record, especially if a 'mandatory' part of the running of a clinic or laboratory, can rapidly lead to rejection of the system (Darke, 1982). Pro-formas should always have an open section to accommodate any salient details that are not included in the closed part. The closed section can be coded and therefore readily entered into a computer or punched card system.

## The 'problem-oriented medical record'

The problem-oriented medical record (POMR) is an attempt to structure a record according to a patient's problems rather than according to diagnostic details. It emphasizes recording of presenting signs, and then works towards identifying lesions and specific causes. The POMR was originally designed for use in American hospitals (Weed, 1970; Hurst and Walker, 1972). Its appearance coincided with the decline of the general medical record as a result of increasing specialization in the 1960s. It has been adapted to veterinary use (Osborne, 1975).

The POMR records four stages in patient care:

(1) establishing a data base;
(2) defining the patient's problems;
(3) formulating plans;
(4) carrying out the plans.

Physical examination of the patient, history and initial laboratory results constitute the data base. Problems can be identified when the data base has been established. These may be overt signs or covert physiological and biochemical changes. The problems are identified as major and minor. Plans are then formulated to resolve them. This involves diagnosing the cause of each problem and developing suitable therapeutic strategies. The fourth stage records the patient's progress by listing **S**ubjective and **O**bjective data, **A**ssessing these data and then **P**lanning future management—abbreviated to the acronym SOAP. Client education is an important component of planning. A master problem list, indicating the dates of occurrence and resolution of the problems, is placed at the front of the record.

The POMR is directed towards solving the problems for which the animal is presented. However, many of the signs detected during completion of the record may be of epidemiological value. The POMR recognizes the inadequacy, on some occasions, of interpretative diagnoses by recording observational data: presenting signs. Some advantages of the POMR are illusory (Feinstein, 1973). The improved patient care that may be associated with the POMR is not a result of the inherent structure of the record; it is caused by the discipline that is imposed on clinicians who use the system, similar to that imposed on pro-forma users. The POMR generates a lot of paper. However, it can be simplified and reduced in size (Lorenz and Schall, 1977). The minimum number of components of a veterinary POMR data base are discussed by Saidla (1983).

## *Punched card recording techniques*

Record cards can have their items (patients) and features (e.g. diagnoses) coded by associating these with holes punched in the cards. This facilitates correlation of features and items. There are two types of punched card: **item** (edge-notched) and **feature** (centre-punched).

### Item cards

Each item card represents an animal. The features (attributes) of the patient are associated with holes

# ROYAL (DICK) SCHOOL OF VETERINARY STUDIES
## UNIVERSITY OF EDINBURGH

100,006

| OWNER | Mr. Mrs. Miss | Surname **CAMPBELL, Mrs.** | Initials **H.** | Address **42, Glenayre Place** |
|---|---|---|---|---|

| | Phone home business | clinician **A.B.Jones** | student | animals name **Petra** |
|---|---|---|---|---|

| ANIMAL | species **Dog** | breed **Shetland Collie** | sex **F.** | age **4yrs.** | colour **Champagne/White** | weight **9kg** |
|---|---|---|---|---|---|---|

**ATTENDANCE** date **1/6/77**  hour    **ADMITTANCE** ☐  **DISCHARGE** ☐  date    hour

**PRIMARY COMPLAINT**  **Pruritus**

**REFERRED BY**  Name                       reply sent    admitting clinician

Address                       phone No.    attending clinician

## MEDICAL HISTORY

**IMMUNISATION** : state age, none or ?  Initial : C.D.                       C.V.H.

Repeats : C.D.                       C.V.H.

Initial : Lep. can/ict.                       Other

Repeats : Lep. can/ict.

**PREVIOUS ILLNESS**, injury or surgery (specify +age, or none)

**DURATION OF ILLNESS**  **1 Month**       Length of time owned  **4 Years**

| | | duration |
|---|---|---|
| **APPETITE** : anorexia  variable  fair  good ✓ excessive  depraved | | |
| **THIRST** : normal ✓ decreased  increased  excessive | | |
| **RESPIRATION** : normal ✓ shallow  dyspnoeic  abdominal  painful | | |
| **SNEEZING** : Nasal discharge  (nature)       Salivation (nature) | | |
| **COUGH** : none  dry  soft  persistent  paroxysmal | | |
| **VOMITION** : none  occasional  frequent  persistent  haematemesis  retching only | | |
| Vomitus : character and when occurs | | |
| **FAECES** : none  normal ✓ soft (not formed)  fluid  blood  mucus  other | | |
| Defaecation : normal ✓ difficult  painful  frequency  colour | | |
| **URINATION** : none  normal ✓ frequent  difficult  painful  incontinent  haematuria | | |
| Volume : normal ✓ decreased  increased  colour : | | |
| **TEMPERAMENT** : normal  listless  depressed  cantankerous  restless  excitable ✓ neurotic | | |
| **NERVOUS** : normal ✓ excitement  hysteria  convulsions  chorea  nystagmus  ataxia  paraplegia | | |
| Paralysis (define) | | |
| **SKIN** : normal  inflamed  pruritus ✓ loss of hair  alopoecia  pigmentation  hyperkeratosis  Licking  rubbing | | |
| Biting (site)       Ectoparasites : | | |
| Wounds (site) | | |
| Tumour (site)       Other lesions : | | |
| **MUSCULO-SKELETAL** : normal ✓ Lameness (limb)       Injuries (site): | | |
| Swellings (site):       Deformities (site) | | |
| **SEXUAL** : Fertility : proven  apparently infertile  unknown | | |
| Libido : normal  none  excessive  unknown | | |
| **OESTRUS** : age of onset  last oestrus  normal  abnormal (define) | | |
| intervals  false preg.  Last litter  No. of litters | | |
| Any discharge (define) | | |
| **EYES** : normal ✓ discharge (specify)       Blindness  Other lesions | | |
| **EARS** : normal ✓ rubbing ear  head shaking  smell  discharge  other | | |
| **DIET** : Daily amount  Meat (specify)       Fish | | |
| Carbohydrate :       Vegetables :       Other : | | |
| **OTHER RELEVANT INFORMATION** :  **Synthetic fibre bedding** | | |

## MEDICAL HISTORY

**Figure 11.3** An example of a clinical case record pro-forma. (From Thrusfield, 1983a)

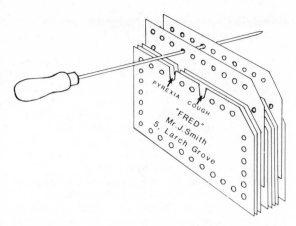

**Figure 11.4** An item (edge-punched) card search. (From Thrusfield, 1983a)

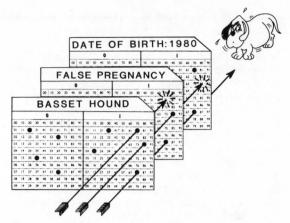

**Figure 11.5** A feature (centre-punched) card search. (After Thrusfield, 1983a)

around the edge of the card. A hole is converted to a notch when the item concerned has the relevant feature. For example, if a dog is male then the hole corresponding **to** male on the dog's item card will be changed to a notch. To search for all items with a particular feature, the cards are held in register and a needle is passed through the appropriate hole. The cards representing items possessing the feature will have been notched in this position so that when the needle is lifted the notched cards fall from the pack. *Figure 11.4* illustrates a search for animals with pyrexia, as an example.

The number of features that can be directly represented by holes is quite small: normally four to each usable inch of card edge. Extra capacity can be obtained only by subcoding, that is, by using combinations of holes. Paired coding, for instance, can produce 15 pairs from 6 holes.

Up to about 500 cards (about 5 inches thickness) can be sorted easily at a time. Beyond this point the method becomes increasingly slow, particularly with the larger and heavier cards.

Item card format is rigid. It is impossible to alter chosen features without altering the coding system.

There are also mechanical problems. When notches occur close together the projecting tab of material between them bends easily and may eventually prevent the card from falling. Also, the card surrounding frequently used holes may tear.

The equipment for an item card system (card tray, needles, cards and notcher), however, is relatively inexpensive.

### Feature cards

In a feature card system, one card is allocated to a single feature. All patients with this feature are each allocated unique reference numbers that are part of a matrix of numbers printed on the card. The

corresponding numbers are centre-punched out of the card when animals possess that feature. *Figure 11.5*, for example, illustrates a feature card search for basset hounds with false pregnancies born in 1980. Only one dog, number 77 (which is punched out), fulfils these criteria.

The search is usually made by laying the cards on an illuminated screen. The equipment for punching holes, which must be aligned accurately, is expensive. The system has been applied to veterinary data storage and retrieval in veterinary schools and zoos (Griner, 1980).

## Computerized recording techniques

Computers are an efficient means of storing, analysing and retrieving data, in addition to acting as complex calculators.

The components of early computers included many valves and transistors and so the machines necessarily were expensive. They were therefore found only in sizeable organizations. The invention and subsequent development of silicon microchips has decreased the size and cost of computers and has made them readily available to a wide range of users, including general veterinary practitioners. Although the initial reason for a practitioner's acquiring a computer may be as an aid to practice management (e.g. Pinney, 1981), the machine can also manipulate clinical data very efficiently.

### *Structure of computers*

#### Basic components

There are two types of computer: **digital** and **analogue**. They allow alternatives to be asked, such as this **and** that, **either or**, **neither nor**, **and**. The digital computer stores information in a discrete fashion, usually in the binary scale (i.e. 0 or 1: 'on' or 'off'). The analogue computer allows quantities to be represented as infinitely variable physical measurements, rather like a slide rule. Most computers with which veterinarians are concerned are digital. The computer comprises **peripheral units** and the **central processing unit** (CPU). The peripheral units include the **input units** and the **output units**.

Information enters through the input unit (paper tape reader, punched card reader, keyboard, etc.) and leaves through the output unit (paper tape punch, card punch, teleprinter, video display unit, line printer, graph plotter, etc.).

The CPU includes:

(1) **a storage (memory) unit**, which records the instructions (program) and information (data);
(2) **the arithmetic unit**, which performs operations (additions, multiplications, comparisons) on data that the program selects from the store;
(3) **the control unit**, which examines the storage unit's instructions sequentially and interprets them.

These physical parts of a computer are termed **hardware.**

The capacity of a computer's data base depends on the size of the memory unit, which gives immediate access to data, and the size of any **auxiliary storage units**, which store information that can be fed into the main memory bank.

### Handling capacity

A computer's storage and handling capacity is measured in **bits** and **bytes**. A bit holds the basic binary doublet: 0 and 1. Bits are formed into bytes. Contiguous bytes are grouped together to form **words** (normally 2 or 4 bytes, depending on the particular computer). A word can be used to store a simple integer or a real number (two words for the latter in the case of a 2-byte word). Complex numbers thus will require either four 2-byte words or two 4-byte words. For the purposes of storing information in auxiliary stores and transferring information between auxiliary storage and the CPU's memory unit, words are formed into **blocks**. The size of a block varies from one computer system to another. In a small computer, typically there are in the order of 500 bytes (i.e. 250 2-byte words) in one block. Two such blocks therefore constitute 1 kilobyte, abbreviated to 1k.

### Auxiliary storage

There are several types of auxiliary storage. Some common ones are paper tape, cards, magnetic drums, magnetic tape, hard magnetic discs (usually stacked vertically), 'floppy' magnetic discs, mini-floppy discs and magnetic tape cassettes.

Large computers use drums, paper tape, cards and discs. Paper tape and cards are becoming obsolescent because they are bulky and easily damaged; drums are also becoming less fashionable.

Floppy discs are about the size of a 45-rpm record, and are flexible. They hold about 484 blocks. Mini-floppy discs have about a quarter of the capacity and are about half the diameter of floppy discs. Smaller discs are also available.

The format also dictates the speed of access. If one wishes to access data at the beginning and end of a tape or cassette, then it is necessary to wind the tape from beginning to end; this can take several minutes. Any part of a disc can be accessed very quickly.

There are currently three main types of computer. Their classification originally was based on their physical size, although, with increasing miniaturization, this is no longer a valid criterion; the distinction now relates to the number of users who can access the computer simultaneously.

(1) The **mainframe** computer has a large capacity CPU and auxiliary store. It can be used simultaneously by many people, often over 100, and can usually run many programs simultaneously. The CPU is usually distant from the many input and output units to which it is connected by electrical cables. Mainframes use drums, hard discs and magnetic tapes as auxiliary stores.
(2) The **minicomputer** is similar to the mainframe, but usually supports fewer users simultaneously. Auxiliary storage is similar to that of the mainframe.
(3) The **microcomputer** is a self-contained unit, with CPU and input and output units (usually a keyboard and video display unit, respectively) located together. The microcomputer is now used by veterinary practitioners because of its relatively low cost and increasing power. Its capacity is sometimes described in terms of RAM (Random Access Memory) which corresponds to the immediate access memory of the mainframe, into which data can be put, and from which they can be extracted. Floppy discs, magnetic tape cassettes and hard discs are used for auxiliary storage.

## Languages

A computer cannot learn; it lacks intelligence. Therefore it must be supplied with a complete set of unambiguous instructions that cause it to perform more or less intelligently. The set of instructions is called a **program**. Programs constitute a computer's **software** (cf. hardware). Problems must be broken down into a form with which the computer will be able to deal, usually by producing a step-by-step sequence of unambiguous rules for the computer to follow. The complete set of rules for solving a problem is called an **algorithm**. This is the basis of a computer program.

It is necessary to communicate with the computer via a resident program, called an **operating system**, that does 'house-keeping' jobs, such as remembering the location of data and arranging for programs to be loaded and run, with access to appropriate input and output units.

Programs have to be written in a recognizable **language**. The most fundamental language, similar to the binary coding, is called **machine code**. In order to avoid the awkwardness of humans reading and writing binary coding, most computers use a fundamental language system similar to the machine codes, but representing the binary notation by mnemonics or acronyms, and numerals in decimal notation, so that the instructions are understood more readily. This type of language is **low level**; a common example is ASSEMBLER.

However, to allow programs to be written more quickly, languages with a more familiar structure have been devised. These are called **high level** languages. Some of them accept ordinary sentences. These languages must be translated into the machine code, and so a translation program, called either an Interpreter or a Compiler, must be used.

Interpreters translate the program line by line as it is executed and are therefore slow to run; translation is performed each time the program is run. Compilers translate the whole program and the machine code is kept to run rapidly whenever required. Although high level languages are easier to use, they slow down the computer and need more space in the memory because of the intermediate compiler program.

There are several types of high level language. These include FORTRAN, which is commonly used by scientists and mathematicians; ALGOL, which is similar to FORTRAN; COBOL, which closely resembles English in appearance and is used in commerce; BASIC, which is used on many home computers; and PASCAL, which is a relatively new multipurpose language. *Table 11.2* indicates the criteria for suitability of some languages for implementation on microcomputers.

## Changing approaches to computing

Since the 1950s, when computers were initially developed, the way in which data are stored and handled inside a computer, and the ways by which data can be accessed, have changed.

### Storing and manipulating data

Initially, programs were written to perform one particular purpose (e.g. 'extract all data about

**Table 11.2 Summary of general criteria for choosing a language for microcomputers. (Modified from Thrusfield, 1983b)**

| *Criteria* | *Languages* | | | | | |
|---|---|---|---|---|---|---|
| | ASSEMBLER | BASIC | FORTRAN | COBOL | ALGOL | PASCAL |
| 1. Embedded in a support environment | − | ++ | − | − | − | +++++ |
| 2. Portable | + | ++ | +++ | +++ | +++ | ++++ |
| 3. Good data structure | − | + | ++ | +++ | ++ | ++++ |
| 4. Support for structured code design | − | − | ++ | ++ | ++++ | ++++ |
| 5. Flexible input/output | − | + | ++++ | ++++ | * | +++ |
| 6. Standardization | + | + | ++++ | ** | ++++ | ++++ |
| 7. Stable | − | − | ++++ | ++++ | ++++ | +++ |
| 8. Easy to teach*** | − | +++ | +++ | ++ | + | +++++ |
| 9. Simple, easy to use and learn*** | − | ++++ | +++ | +++ | ++ | +++++ |
| 10. Flexible storage structures | − | − | − | − | − | +++ |
| 11. Suitability for packages | + | + | ++++ | + | +++ | + |
| 12. Suitable for business data processing (record handling) etc. | − | + | ++ | ++++ | + | +++ |
| 13. Flexible file handling | − | − | +++ | ++++ | + | ++ |
| 14. Suitability for systems programming | ++ | − | − | − | + | + |
| 15. Compiler availability | − | +++ | ++++ | ++ | ++ | ++++ |
| 16. Implemented on mini, micro and mainframe computers | − | +++ | ++++ | +++ | + | ++++ |

*Depends on the system on which the language is implemented.
**Variable, depending on the compiler.
***The grading is subjective and also reflects the aims and capacity of the pupil.
− Language unsuited to criterion.
+ to +++++ Degree of suitability of language to criterion.

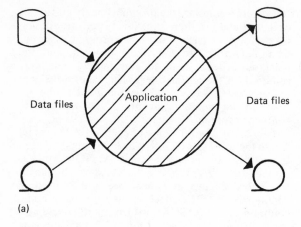

(a)

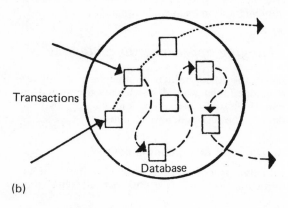

(b)

**Figure 11.6** Approaches to data storage and manipulations: (**a**) the 'systems analysis' approach; (**b**) the 'data base' approach. (From Thrusfield, 1983a)

Hereford cows from the data base'); the programs (**applications**) were considered central to the system, with the data merely passing through the application in a convenient form (*Figure 11.6a*). This 'systems analysis' approach has several disadvantages. The main one is the rigidity of the program. If a new application (e.g. 'extract all data about Charolais cows from the data base') is required, then a new program may have to be written. This means that different correlations often require new programs.

A more recent approach—the 'data base' approach—is more flexible. The data are considered central, and the applications can constantly change (*Figure 11.6b*). This enables flexible querying and correlation of data. This approach is used in constructing network and relational computerized data bases and many of these data base management systems, often with their own special languages, are now available on mainframe and microcomputers.

## Accessing computerized data

*Figure 11.7* illustrates how the approach to computing has developed, and how it affects access to data. In the 1960s, work was run on mainframe computers, usually by inputting work on paper tapes or cards to be run overnight as batch jobs. Response was poor (i.e. the process was slow) and it was very difficult for users to share their data and resources.

In the 1970s, a division took place. Mainframe users began to share time on computers and it was possible to share data and resources, although response varied according to the number of users and the tasks being performed at any one time. Separate 'stand-alone' microcomputer systems developed with good response, but data and resources could not be shared because the systems were not linked.

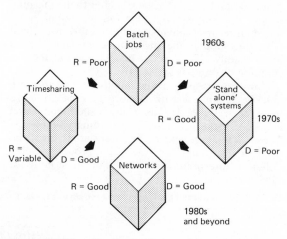

**Figure 11.7** Changing approaches to computerized data access. D = resource and data sharing; R = responsiveness. (From Thrusfield, 1983b)

There have also been developments in communications technology that allow data to be accessed rapidly from several places. Computers can be linked using acoustic signals sent via conventional telephone handsets. However, the rate of data transfer is low. Direct fast links between computers (mainframes and microcomputers) using communications 'networks' are now available.

In some countries, mainframe computers can be shared by many users who can access data bases mounted on the mainframes via their telephones, using a special keyboard as the input unit and a standard television receiver as the output unit. The application of this facility to veterinary epidemiology is discussed by Varley (1984).

Future trends aim at establishing links between many users and speeding up response. The concept is one of a network of individual microcomputers linked to one another and to mainframes by fast communication systems, the mainframes being reserved mainly for complex calculations ('number crunching') and the processing of very large volumes of data.

The development of data base management systems and improved communications technology increase the potential for epidemiological investigation considerably. Data from a wide cross-section of veterinary sources, ranging from veterinary practices to government services, are likely to be more representative because of reduced selection bias, and should therefore produce more accurate morbidity and mortality figures for use in epidemiological surveys. However, collection of this range of data faces several problems, currently including the absence of a standardized recording and coding system (Thrusfield, 1981). The possibility of inaccurate data being recorded can be reduced by stringent validation programs at data entry points, but can never be eliminated completely.

# Veterinary data bases

## *Scales of project recording*

There are three main types of data base, defined according to the method of data collection:

(1) microscale projects (*Figure 11.8a*) concerned with internal disease problems in separated populations such as those on farms and research institutes;
(2) mesoscale projects (*Figure 11.8b*) involved with more widely distributed disease problems, for example data collection at abattoirs, diagnostic laboratories and clinics;
(3) macroscale projects (*Figure 11.8c*) designed to collect data with the purpose of gaining a national view of disease.

### Microscale projects

In the microscale project, information is transferred from the farm to the practice or consulting organization where it is analysed and the results are necessarily fed back to the farm to effect health improvement. With an 'on-farm' system, data may be manipulated and analysed without leaving the farm's confines. Many herd health and productivity schemes are typically microscale. Essentially, they record individual and herd performance and productivity and sometimes disease occurrence, and relate productivity to disease in an attempt to improve the former. These will be considered in greater detail in Chapter 19.

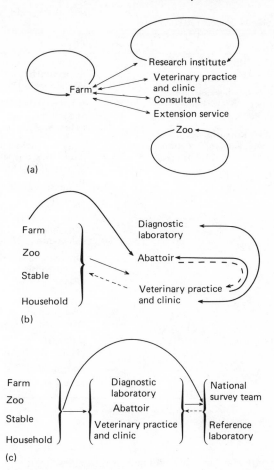

**Figure 11.8** Veterinary data collection projects defined according to flow of data: (**a**) microscale projects; (**b**) mesoscale projects; (**c**) macroscale projects. Solid arrows indicate main paths of data flow. Broken arrows indicate paths of limited or no data flow. (From Thrusfield, 1983b, after Hugh-Jones, 1975)

### Mesoscale projects

In the mesoscale project, data are transmitted from their source to the organizations responsible for analysis. The data are usually of more direct value to the analysing institution than to their source. Therefore, feedback of data is a less important component of the system (although still desirable). Small animal practice records are an example of this type of recording system.

### Macroscale projects

Macroscale projects are designed to gain a national picture and therefore are not designed primarily to help specific animal units. There is thus little flow of data back to their origin. National and international

**Table 11.3 Some veterinary data bases**

| Macroscale | Mesoscale | Microscale |
| --- | --- | --- |
| ANADIS (Roe, 1980) | Danish swine slaughter inspection bank (Willeberg, 1979) | *Checkmate (Booth and Warren, 1984) |
| Danish swine slaughter inspection data bank (Willeberg, 1979) | Edinburgh SAPTU clinical record summary system (Thrusfield and Hinxman, 1981) | *COSREEL (Russell and Rowlands, 1983) |
| Laboratory Management and Disease Surveillance Information System (Christiansen, 1980) | Florida Teaching Hospital data retrieval system (Burridge and McCarthy, 1979) | *DAISY (Pharo, 1983) |
| OIE (Blajan, 1982) | Minnesota Disease Recording System (Diesch, 1979) | *Edinburgh DHHPS (Smith *et al.*, 1983) |
| | Parasitology Diagnostic Data Program (Slocombe, 1975) | *FAHRMX (Bartiett *et al.*, 1982; 1985; FAHRMX, 1984) |
| | Queensland veterinary diagnostic data recording system (Elder, 1976) | *SIRO (Goodall *et al.*, 1984) |
| | Veterinary Recording of Zoo Animals (Roth *et al.*, 1973) | *VAMPP (Noordhuizen and Buurman, 1984) |
| | VIDA II (Hall *et al.*, 1980) | *VIRUS (Martin *et al.*, 1982) |
| | VMDP (Priester, 1975) | |

*These data bases are dairy health and productivity schemes. They can also function to varying degrees as mesoscale systems, supplying information for epidemiological studies.

monitoring and surveillance programmes are typically macroscale.

There is no fundamental reason why microscale projects should not contribute to mesoscale and macroscale projects, thus combining the three into a unified system.

## Some examples of veterinary data bases

Table 11.3 lists some examples of veterinary data bases. A brief outline of seven of them will indicate their scope and the techniques employed in updating and using them.

### ANADIS

ANADIS (the *Australian National Animal Disease Information System*) is operated by the Australian government's veterinary service. This involves a network of computers, situated throughout Australia, which store regional veterinary data. It was concerned originally with the brucellosis and tuberculosis eradication campaigns. Future anticipated

developments include the recording of diagnostic laboratory data, and data relating to outbreaks of exotic diseases, national serum banks and health and productivity schemes. Data are posted periodically to Canberra on floppy discs for central computerized storage and analysis.

### Office International des Epizooties

*Office International des Epizooties* (OIE) runs an international disease reporting system. It was founded in 1924 following an outbreak of rinderpest in Belgium in 1920. It records data on the major animal infectious epidemic diseases throughout the world.

### Danish swine slaughter inspection data bank

This data base contains post-mortem information on pigs collected at slaughter. Most Danish fattening pigs are recorded in the data base, and so not only does the system act as a mesoscale project but it also performs the function of a national macroscale monitoring system.

## Edinburgh SAPTU clinical recording system

This system records clinical case summaries from the veterinary school's *Small Animal Practice Teaching Unit* (SAPTU) on a mainframe computer. It is therefore a mesoscale system. Data are entered as consecutive numeric codes. It uses a network model data base management system, facilitating correlation of case record components.

## VIDA II

VIDA II (*Veterinary Investigation Diagnosis Analyses*) is a mesoscale data base comprising records of specimen submissions to veterinary investigation laboratories in Great Britain. These submissions are voluntary and constitute only a proportion of all post-mortem and laboratory specimens. The initial version used punched cards as a storage medium. The current system stores data on a central mainframe computer. The individual laboratories code diagnostic data on pro-formas using a modification of SNVDO codes (described in Chapter 9), and the pro-formas are then posted to a centre where the data are put into the computer.

## COSREEL

COSREEL (*COmputer System for Recording Events affecting Economically important Livestock*) is a British health and productivity data base. Several dairy farms and their local veterinary practitioners use the system. The data base is maintained on a central mainframe. Data, coded alphanumerically, may be sent on forms by post, or entered via peripheral input/output terminals, using an acoustic telephone link (Rowlands and Russell, 1985). This is a microscale system, because it produces check lists for herd management, but is also mesoscale because data from several farms are available for epidemiological studies.

Other microscale systems use individual mini-computers and microcomputers rather than mainframes, for example DAISY (DAiry Information SYstem) and the Edinburgh Dairy Herd Health and Productivity Scheme.

## VMDP

The VMDP (*Veterinary Medical Data Program*) is a collaborative mesoscale data base involving several veterinary schools in North America. Data are coded using SNVDO codes. The data sources, like many of the others that have been described (*see* Chapter 10), demonstrate selection bias but the data base has provided a considerable amount of material for epidemiological investigations. Several of the observational studies listed in *Table 15.5* used data derived from the VMDP.

## *Further reading*

BROADBEER, R., DE BONO, P. and LAURIE, P. (1982) *The Computer Book*. British Broadcasting Corporation, London

DATE, C.J. (1975) *An Introduction to Database Systems*. Addison Wesley Publishing Company, Philippines

JOLLY, J.L. (1968) *Data Study*. Weidenfield and Nicolson, London

PROCEEDINGS OF THE FIRST SYMPOSIUM ON COMPUTER APPLICATIONS IN VETERINARY MEDICINE. College of Veterinary Medicine, Mississippi State University, 13–15 October 1982

PROCEEDINGS OF THE SECOND SYMPOSIUM ON COMPUTER APPLICATIONS IN VETERINARY MEDICINE. College of Veterinary Medicine, Mississippi State University, 23–25 May 1984

ROBINSON, H. (1981) *Database Analysis and Design*. Chartwell-Bratt, Bromley

THRUSFIELD, M.V. (1985) Data recording in general practice. *In Practice*, **7**, 128–138

VETERINARY COMPUTING (Periodical). Published by American Veterinary Publications Inc., P.O. Drawer, K.K., Santa Barbara, CA, 93102, USA

# 12

# Presenting numerical data

The epidemiologist makes inferences from data collected from groups of animals. The data are frequently quantitative, comprising numerical values. A fundamental characteristic of numerical biological data is their inherent **variability**. The weights of 100 Friesian cows, for example, will not be identical; there will be a range of values. If the 100 cows were a sample of a much larger group—say the national herd—then a different sample of 100, drawn from the same national herd, is almost certain to have a different set of weight values.

Variability is of importance to the epidemiologist in two circumstances: when a sample is taken and when different groups of animals are being compared. In the first case, it is necessary to assess to what extent the sample's values are representative of those in the larger population from which the sample was drawn. This is relevant to surveys which are discussed in Chapter 14. In the second case, it is often necessary to decide whether or not a difference between two groups is due to a particular factor. In epidemiology this frequently involves detecting an association between disease and hypothesized causal factors, and is discussed in the next chapter. For example, if the effect of ketosis on milk yield were being investigated, then two groups of cows—one comprising cows with ketosis and one consisting of cows without ketosis—could be compared with respect to milk yield. A detected difference in yield could be due to:

(1) the effect of ketosis;
(2) inherent natural variation in milk yield between the two groups;
(3) confounding variables (*see* Chapter 3) such as breed: cows of different breed may be present in different proportions in each group, when the different breeds produce different milk yields.

In this example, the second and third reasons for the difference can confuse the investigation by contributing to differences in the milk yields of the two groups. Statistical methods exist to separate the effects of the factors that are being investigated from random variation and confounding. Essentially, these involve estimating the **probability** of an event taking place. Probability may be thought of as the frequency of certain events relative to the total number of events that can occur. Thus, the probability of throwing a 'head' with an unbiased coin is 1/2. The probability of throwing either a 'head' or a 'tail' (i.e. the total probability) is 1. Recall that prevalence is a measure of probability (*see* Chapter 4). Similarly, a specific prevalence value is an estimation of **conditional probability**; a male sex-specific prevalence of 30% means that there is a probability of 0.3 of any one animal having a disease at a given point in time, conditional on its being male.

This chapter deals with the probability distributions of numerical data that are the basis of many statistical tests (some of which are described in Chapter 13) and with the methods of displaying numerical values. The statistical content of this book is not comprehensive; it is designed to give the reader a basic knowledge of some relevant concepts and techniques. The reader who is unfamiliar with elementary mathematical notation should first consult Appendix II.

## Some basic definitions

**Variable**: any observable event that can vary. Variables may be either continuous or discrete (*see* Chapter 9). An example of a continuous variable is the weight of an animal. An example of a discrete variable is the number of cases of disease. In some circumstances, the numerical values of the variable are called **variates**.

**Study variable**: any variable that is being considered in an investigation.

**Response and explanatory variables**: a response variable is one that is affected by another (explanatory) variable; for instance, an animal's weight may be a response variable and food intake an explanatory variable because weight is assumed to depend on the amount of food consumed. In epidemiological investigations, disease is often considered as the response variable, for example, when studying the effects of dry cat food (the explanatory variable) on the prevalence of urolithiasis. There may also be circumstances in which disease is considered as the explanatory variable, for instance when studying the effect of disease on weight. Response variables are sometimes called **dependent** variables; and explanatory variables called **independent** variables.

**Parameter**: a quantity that can differ in different circumstances, but is constant in the case that is being considered. A survey may be designed to detect a minimum disease prevalence, such as 20%. Although prevalence can vary, the minimum detectable prevalence is defined for the objectives of the survey as a single unvarying value, and is therefore a parameter of the survey.

**Data set**: a collection of data.

**Raw data**: the initial measurements that form the basis of analyses.

## Some descriptive statistics

*Table 12.1* lists sample weights of two groups (A and B) of piglets, when weaned at 3 weeks of age. These can be considered as random samples of a much larger group of piglets, namely all piglets at 3 weeks of age. The inherent variability is obvious. The number of piglets with weights within defined intervals (i.e. the group **frequency distribution** of the weights) for group B is recorded in *Table 12.2* and depicted in *Figure 12.1*. This figure, which summarizes the data, is called a **histogram**. The intervals on the horizontal axis are 0.5 kg wide. The number of piglets within each interval is proportional to the area of the vertical bars. If the intervals on the horizontal axis are equal, as in this example, then the number of piglets within each interval is also proportional to the height of the bars. Alternatively, the vertical plots and the midpoints of the horizontal intervals can be joined, rather than constructing bars, in which case a **frequency polygon** is constructed. These data can be summarized further by the use of descriptive statistics that are measures of **position** and **spread** of the histogram.

**Table 12.1 Specimen 3-week weaning weights (kg) of two groups (A and B) of piglets**

*Group A*

| | | | | |
|---|---|---|---|---|
| 4.2 | 5.3 | 5.6 | 6.0 | 6.4 |
| 4.6 | 5.3 | 5.7 | 6.0 | 6.4 |
| 4.7 | 5.4** | 5.7 | 6.1 | 6.4 |
| 4.8 | 5.4 | 5.7 | 6.1 | 6.5 |
| 4.9 | 5.4 | 5.9* | 6.1 | 6.5 |
| 5.1 | 5.4 | 5.9 | 6.1 | 6.5 |
| 5.2 | 5.4 | 5.9 | 6.1** | 6.8 |
| 5.2 | 5.5 | 5.9 | 6.2 | 6.8 |
| 5.2 | 5.5 | 6.0 | 6.3 | 6.8 |
| 5.3 | 5.5 | 6.0 | 6.4 | |

$$n=49; \ \bar{x}=5.76 \text{ kg}; \ s=0.60 \text{ kg};$$
$$Q_2 = 5.9 \text{ kg}; \ SIR = 0.35 \text{ kg}.$$

*Group B*

| | | | | |
|---|---|---|---|---|
| 2.6 | 4.3 | 4.6 | 4.8 | 5.3 |
| 3.4 | 4.3 | 4.6 | 5.0 | 5.5 |
| 3.6 | 4.3** | 4.6 | 5.0 | 5.5 |
| 3.8 | 4.4 | 4.6 | 5.0 | 5.6 |
| 3.9 | 4.4 | 4.7* | 5.0 | 5.6 |
| 4.0 | 4.4 | 4.7 | 5.1 | 5.6 |
| 4.0 | 4.4 | 4.7 | 5.1** | 5.6 |
| 4.1 | 4.5 | 4.8 | 5.2 | 5.7 |
| 4.1 | 4.5 | 4.8 | 5.2 | 6.3 |
| 4.2 | 4.5 | 4.8 | 5.2 | |

$$n=49; \ \bar{x}=4.69 \text{ kg}; \ s=0.67 \text{ kg};$$
$$Q_2 = 4.7 \text{ kg}; \ SIR = 0.40 \text{ kg}.$$

*Median
**Quartiles

**Table 12.2 Grouped frequency distribution for the 3-week weaning weights of piglets in group B of *Table 12.1***

| Weight (kg) | Number of piglets |
|---|---|
| 2.6–3.0 | 1 |
| 3.1–3.5 | 1 |
| 3.6–4.0 | 5 |
| 4.1–4.5 | 13 |
| 4.6–5.0 | 15 |
| 5.1–5.5 | 8 |
| 5.6–6.0 | 5 |
| 6.1–6.5 | 1 |

## Measures of position

A commonly adopted measure of position is the **mean** of the sample, denoted by $\bar{x}$ (pronounced 'x-bar'). It is calculated using:

$$\bar{x} = \frac{\Sigma x}{n}$$

where $n$ is the number of values in the random sample. In *Table 12.1*, $n=49$ in each group, and $\bar{x}=5.76$ kg in group A, and 4.69 kg in group B.

Each sample has been assumed, implicitly, to be drawn from a much larger population; thus the mean of the sample is only an estimate of the true

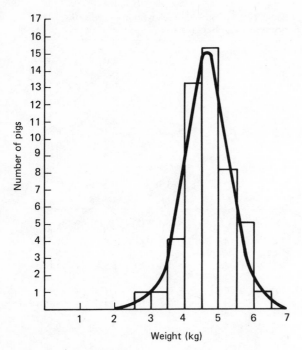

**Figure 12.1** Observed distribution of the weights of the 49 piglets in group B depicted as a histogram (rectangles) and fitted 'Normal' curve (smooth curve). (Data from *Table 12.1*)

population mean, $\mu$ (the Greek letter, mu). Only if all the population is investigated can the parameter $\mu$ be known. As the sample size increases, $\bar{x}$ will be a better estimator of $\mu$.

The **median** of the sample, sometimes denoted by $Q_2$, is the value below which half, and therefore above which half, of the observations lie. Thus, the median is another measure of position. The median values in *Table 12.1* for groups A and B respectively are marked with an asterisk, '*'. If the data set contains an even number of values then the median is defined as the average of the two middle values. Again, the sample median is an estimator of the true population median.

The **lower** and **upper quartiles**, $Q_1$ and $Q_3$ respectively, are defined as the two values that are midway between the lower and upper extreme values and the median. For groups A and B they are marked with two asterisks, '**'.

## Measures of spread

Measures of spread are a little more difficult to calculate than those of position. Two examples of simple measures of spread are the range and the mean of the absolute deviations of the individual

values from the mean. However, these measures often do not distinguish different sets of data.

A commonly adopted measure is the **sample variance**, $s^2$, which is calculated by:

$$s^2 = \frac{\Sigma(x - \bar{x})^2}{n - 1}.$$

This formula may be rewritten in a form that is more easily calculated with small calculators, namely:

$$s^2 = \frac{\Sigma x^2 - \{(\Sigma x)^2/n\}}{n - 1}.$$

The square root of the sample variance is called the sample **standard deviation**. Using the values from *Table 12.1*, group B, and the formula for $s^2$ above, the sample standard deviation $s$ is given by:

$$s = \sqrt{\left[\frac{\Sigma x^2 - \{(\Sigma x)^2/n\}}{n - 1}\right]}$$

$$= \sqrt{\left[\frac{1099.16 - (229.8^2/49)}{48}\right]}$$

$$= \sqrt{\frac{21.45}{48}}$$

$$= 0.67 \text{ kg}.$$

Just as the sample mean is an estimate of the population mean, so the sample variance and sample standard deviation are estimates of the **population variance**, $\sigma^2$ ($\sigma$ is the Greek letter, sigma), and the **population standard deviation**, $\sigma$.

When summary statistics are presented, the sample standard deviation should be presented as well as the sample mean in order to indicate the variability within the population.

Another useful measure of spread that often accompanies the median is the **semi-interquartile range** (*SIR*). This is half of the range between the quartiles, $Q_1$ and $Q_3$:

$$SIR = \frac{Q_3 - Q_1}{2}.$$

This is an estimator for the population semi-interquartile range.

## Interval estimation

The sample mean gives a single estimate for the population parameter $\mu$ and is therefore called a **point estimate**. Repeated sampling of the population will produce different sample means as estimates of the population mean. The square root of the variance of the sample means is termed the **standard error of the mean** (s.e.m.) to avoid confusion with the standard deviation of the individual values. It is given by:

s.e.m. = $\sigma/\sqrt{n}$

This may be estimated by what is termed the **estimated standard error of the mean** (e.s.e.m.), obtained by replacing $\sigma$ by $s$:

e.s.e.m. = $s/\sqrt{n}$

The e.s.e.m. is an indication of the **precision** (*see* Chapter 9) of the sample's estimate of the population mean: the smaller the e.s.e.m., the greater the precision.

It is sometimes more useful to quote a range within which one is reasonably confident that the true mean will lie. This range is known as a **confidence interval**; for example on approximately 95% of occasions that samples are taken from a population of Normally* distributed values, the confidence interval given by the sample mean ± 2 s.e.m. will contain the true population mean. Alternatively, a single calculated confidence interval (sample mean ± 2 s.e.m.) contains the true population mean with probability 0.95. The upper and lower points of a confidence interval are **confidence limits**.

Using the values from group B (*Table 12.1*):

e.s.e.m. = $s/\sqrt{n}$

$= \dfrac{0.67}{\sqrt{49}}$

$= 0.096$

and so the 95% confidence interval is estimated by:

$\bar{x}$ ± 2 e.s.e.m. = 4.69 ± 0.192 kg

$= 4.498 - 4.882$ kg $(4.498, 4.882$

assuming that the 3-week weaning weights are Normally distributed.

## Statistical distributions

### The Normal distribution

If many piglets were weighed, rather than just the 49 in each data set shown in *Table 12.1*, and if the intervals used in the histogram in *Figure 12.1* were reduced, the bars would become narrower. Eventually, the tops would trace a smooth curve. One such curve has been fitted over the bars in *Figure 12.1*, using a computer program which identifies the curve from the weights in *Table 12.1*. The curve has one peak in the middle and is symmetrical. This bell

*The **Normal** distribution is one of several families of statistical distributions, some of which are described later in this chapter.

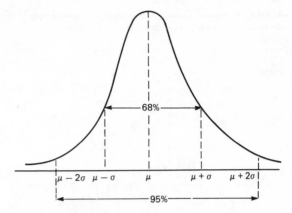

**Figure 12.2** The relationship between $\mu$, $\sigma$ and the proportion of observations for Normally distributed values.

shape is typical of a family of frequency distributions known as the **Normal** family of distributions. It is usually spelled with an upper case N to avoid confusion with other meanings of the word. Another name for this distribution is the **Gaussian** distribution. This distribution is described by two parameters: its mean, $\mu$, and its standard deviation, $\sigma$.

Approximately 68% of all Normally distributed values lie within one standard deviation of the mean of the population from which they were sampled (i.e. $\mu-\sigma$ to $\mu+\sigma$), and 95% within two standard deviations of the mean (i.e. $\mu-2\sigma$ to $\mu+2\sigma$) (*Figure 12.2*).

Many biological variables have a Normal distribution; for this reason it is a very important distribution. However, this distribution cannot be applied to all variables. Measurements to which Normality does not apply (although it can do as an approximation for large samples) are counts (e.g. numbers of ticks on animals) and ordinal data that only have a small number of intervals on the scale.

### The binomial distribution

This distribution relates to discrete data when there are only two possible outcomes on each occasion, for instance, the sex of a calf at birth can only be either male or female. An example is given in *Table 12.3*. The two outcomes may be of any kind but, for convenience, here are termed 'success' and 'failure'. On $n$ occasions, the probability $Pr(r)$ of $r$ successes out of $n$ trials is found to be:

$$Pr(r) = \frac{n!}{r!(n+r)!} \, p^r(1-p)^{n-r} \qquad (r = 0,1,2,\dots n)$$

where $p$ = probability of success on a single occasion assuming **no association** between the outcomes

**Table 12.3 Possible series of calves born to a cow during three successive uniparous gestations (M = male; F = female)**

| First gestation | Second gestation | Third gestation | Total male | Total female |
|---|---|---|---|---|
| M | M | M | 3 | 0 |
| M | M | F | 2 | 1 |
| M | F | M | 2 | 1 |
| M | F | F | 1 | 2 |
| F | M | M | 2 | 1 |
| F | M | F | 1 | 2 |
| F | F | M | 1 | 2 |
| F | F | F | 0 | 3 |

occurring on different occasions. In this example, two males (outcomes, $r = 2$) may be born during three pregnancies (occasions, $n = 3$). If it is assumed that the sex of the first calf does not affect the sex of future calves, and $p = 0.52$, then the probability, $Pr(2)$, will be:

$$Pr(2) = \frac{3!}{2!1!}(0.52)^2(0.48)$$

$$= 0.39.$$

The value of $p$ can vary considerably between 0 and 1, for example, in some genetically determined diseases.

## The Poisson distribution

The Poisson distribution is concerned with counts. It is found when events occur randomly in space or time. Some commonly quoted examples are the distribution of blood cells in a haemocytometer and the number of virus particles infecting cells in tissue culture. This distribution is important in epidemiology because it relates to the spatial and temporal distribution of disease. The random occurrence of cases of disease in unit time or in unit area can follow a Poisson distribution. A significant departure from this distribution therefore indicates temporal and geographical departures from randomness (*see* Chapter 8).

The distribution is characterized by one parameter, $\lambda$ (the Greek letter, lambda): the average count per unit area or per unit time.

The probability of counts of $r = 0, 1, 2, 3, 4$, and so on, is given by the formula:

$$Pr(r) = \frac{e^{-\lambda}\lambda^r}{r!}$$

where $e$ is a constant: the base of natural (Napierian) logarithms = 2.71828. The value of $e^{-\lambda}$ can be found in published tables and is given on many pocket calculators.

For example, suppose that a tissue culture monolayer is being infected with virus particles. If there are $1 \times 10^6$ cells to which are added $3 \times 10^6$ virus particles, then the average count/cell ($\lambda$) is 3. The proportion of cells infected with, for example, 2 particles can be calculated using the formula above, with $\lambda=3$ and $r=2$. Substituting in the formula:

$$Pr(2) = e^{-3}3^2/2!$$

From tables, $e^{-3} = 0.0498$.

Thus: $Pr(2) = 0.0498 \times 3^2/2!$

$$= 0.2241.$$

This means that the expected proportion of cells infected with 2 virus particles is 22.41%.

## Other distributions

There are many other statistical distributions. Some deviate from Normality; some of these deviations are illustrated in *Figure 12.3*. The mean and median are equal when a variable is symmetrically distributed; and the mean and standard deviation provide

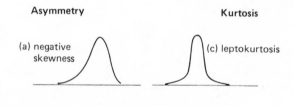

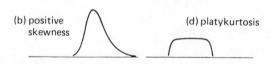

**Figure 12.3** Some deviations from the Normal distribution. (From Sard, 1979)

good measures of position and spread. However, when frequency distributions deviate from Normality, this may not be true. Thus, with a positive skew the mean is located to the right of the peak of the frequency distribution. In such cases, the median and semi-interquartile range are better measures of position and location. Some distributions are neither Normal nor binomial nor Poisson. Two other distributions are compared with the Normal in *Figure 12.4*. If unusual distributions are suspected then expert statistical advice should always be obtained.

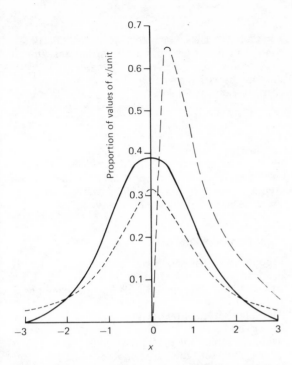

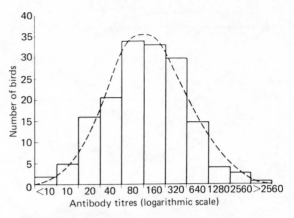

**Figure 12.5** An example of a transformed lognormal distribution. Distribution of the haemagglutination-inhibiting antibody titres of a group of 165 domestic fowls, 6 weeks after having been inoculated with a single dose of an inactivated Newcastle disease virus vaccine. The broken line shows a Normal curve fitted to these results. (From Herbert, 1970)

**Figure 12.4** Two non-Normal distributions compared with the Normal distribution. —— Normal distribution; ------ *t*-distribution; ---- lognormal distribution.

## Transformations

Natural scales of measurement are not always the simplest to analyse and interpret because they may produce non-Normal distributions. However, it is sometimes possible to transform these distributions to approximate Normality by changing the way in which the variables are expressed—usually by raising the variables to a simple power or by converting them to logarithms. The distribution for which the logarithms of the data are Normally distributed is called the **lognormal distribution**. This distribution occurs in biology. It is characterized by a positive skew similar to, but not necessarily the same as, that depicted in *Figure 12.3b*. An example is given in *Figure 12.5* which shows the frequency distribution of antibody titres to Newcastle disease virus in vaccinated birds, plotted on a logarithmic scale. In this case, a transformation was performed by diluting serum samples logarithmically before the titration was performed, initially to base 10 (1/10) and thereafter to base 2 (1/20, 1/40, 1/80 etc.). The application of logarithmic scales to serological investigations is discussed in Chapter 16. Epidemic curves and incubation periods are often lognormal (Sartwell, 1950, 1966; Armenian and Lilienfeld, 1974). In the case of epidemic curves, the data

(numbers of new cases) are discrete, but are treated as continuous measurements because the numbers are frequently large.

## Normal approximations to the binomial and Poisson distributions

When samples are large, and *p* is not too close to 0 or 1, the binomial distribution can be approximated to the Normal. The approximation is better when a 'continuity correction' is applied to binomial data, to allow for the discrete nature of the data, while the Normal distribution relates to continuous data. Similarly, when samples are large, the Normal distribution provides a good approximation to the Poisson distribution. Therefore techniques that are used to analyse Normally distributed data can sometimes be applied to the binomial and Poisson distributions.

Using the Normal approximations for the binomial and Poisson distributions, confidence limits can be defined for the parameters of these two latter distributions, that is, *p* and $\lambda$. The formulae may be found in texts cited in 'Further reading' at the end of this chapter.

## Displaying numerical data

Data should be represented in a form that is easy to interpret and to analyse in detail. This presentation may reveal interesting facts about the data and their distributions. Some of the methods of displaying

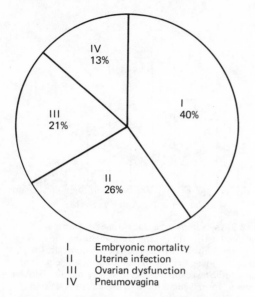

| I | Embryonic mortality |
|---|---|
| II | Uterine infection |
| III | Ovarian dysfunction |
| IV | Pneumovagina |

**Figure 12.6** An example of a 'pie' chart: proportions of principal mare infertilities detected in over 100 clinical cases reported and presented. (From Fraser, 1976)

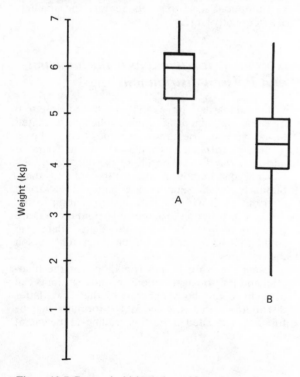

**Figure 12.7** 'Box and whisker' plots of 3-week weaning weights (kg) of two groups (A and B) of piglets. The central horizontal line indicates the median. The upper and lower extremities of the vertical lines (the 'whiskers') mark the maximum and minimum values of the data set. The horizontal sides of the large rectangles (the 'boxes') represent the quartiles. (Data from *Table 12.1*)

data have, of necessity, been described earlier (*see* Chapter 4). These include tables, bar charts and graphs. A further method is the **histogram**, already depicted in *Figure 12.1*. The histogram is used for continuous variates whereas the bar chart is used for discrete data.

## 'Pie' charts

A 'pie chart' is a circle (the 'pie') in which individual characteristics are represented as 'slices', the angle of a segment being proportional to the relative frequency of the corresponding characteristic. An example is given in *Figure 12.6*.

## 'Box and whisker' plots

Frequency distributions can be compared visually using a 'box and whisker' plot (Tukey, 1977; Erickson and Nosanchuk, 1979). An example is shown in *Figure 12.7* using the data in *Table 12.1*. The central horizontal line indicates the median; the upper and lower extremities of the vertical lines (the 'whiskers') mark the maximum and minimum values of the data set; the horizontal sides of the large rectangles (the 'boxes') represent the quartiles. A second example, depicting the distribution of reasons for culling in dairy herds, is presented by Young *et al.* (1983).

## 'Shewhart' charts

The change in a variable's value can be monitored easily over a period of time by plotting values on squared graph paper (or, more likely nowadays, displaying the data graphically, using a computer program) with time as the horizontal axis. This can be of value in detecting undesirable trends in productivity which, in turn, may indicate disease. This technique was developed by Shewhart (1931) to control the quality of manufactured articles. An example is given in *Figure 12.8* which charts the mean of the number of piglets born alive per litter in a herd of pigs over a 2-year period (Wrathall and Hebert, 1983). A decrease in this variable could indicate reproductive disease in the sow, such as parvovirus infection.

Before the means are plotted, a reference value, defining an acceptable target, is chosen and is represented on the chart by a horizontal line. An unacceptable level (the 'decision boundary') is also ruled on the chart. Remedial action is taken if a value of the variable crosses this boundary. In the example, the study variable falls below the decision boundary twice: in September 1977 and March 1978. In the majority of studies, two decision boundaries above and two below the target level are required. The inner pair give 'warning' and the outer pair

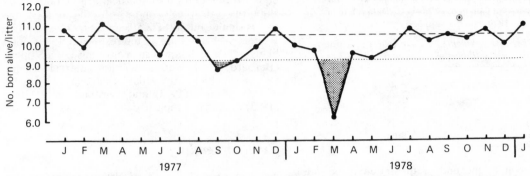

**Figure 12.8** Shewhart chart: number of piglets born alive/litter in a herd of pigs, 1977 and 1978. – – – – Reference value; .....decision boundary. (From Wrathall and Hebert, 1983)

indicate 'action'. Selection of boundaries is discussed by Goulden (1952).

A current problem in veterinary medicine is deciding what are the most useful variables to monitor and which values of these variables should be used as target levels and boundaries. A boundary level cannot be chosen arbitrarily (although this method has been unwisely applied in the past) because individual values may cross the boundary level purely at random. The boundary level should correspond to a suitable multiple of the standard error of the mean, noting that, because the standard error depends on the sample size, it will vary if the sample size varies (this could happen, for example, when monitoring different litters of piglets). If two standard errors are selected, then 2.5% of observations from the population will lie outside the boundary. Therefore remedial action will be taken on 2.5% of occasions when it is not justified. Similarly, if 2.33 standard errors are chosen as the boundary, then action will be unjustifiably taken on approximately 1% of occasions; if three standard errors are chosen, then unjustifiable action will be taken on approximately 0.14% of occasions. While an interval of three standard errors may seem attractive, this is accompanied by a greater probability of failing to take action, when desirable, than if a smaller number of standard errors had been chosen.

### 'Cusums'

'Cusum' is an abbreviation of 'cumulative sum' (Woodward and Goldsmith, 1964). It plots the sum of deviations of the values of the variable being measured from a selected target value. This technique is useful for detecting changes in average levels, determining the point of onset of these changes, obtaining reliable estimates of current average values, and making short-term predictions of future average levels. Cusums detect short-term fluctuations but do not detect steady trends and regular cyclic variations. The cusum chart can detect

smaller changes in a monitored variable than can the Shewhart chart. An example is given in *Figure 12.9* using data from *Table 12.4*. This example relates to the detection of porcine intestinal adenomatosis. The disease does not produce clear clinical signs; the main sign is wasting of piglets. Reduced weight gain therefore can act as an indicator of infection. Column 3 of *Table 12.4* shows the weekly weight gains of a piglet. Note that in this example the sample size, $n$, is only 1, therefore the standard error of the mean equals the standard deviation (1 s.e.m. $= \sigma/\sqrt{n}$). The target level is defined as the mean weight gain per week of the herd: 6.65 lb. Column 4 shows the deviation from the target and column 5 is the cusum. The piglet has a marked

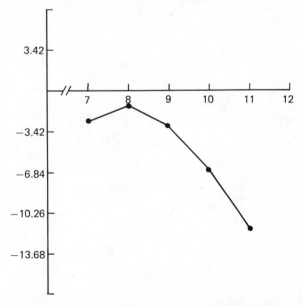

**Figure 12.9** A cusum chart of weekly weight gain (lb) of a piglet during the fattening period. Each vertical interval corresponds to 2 s.e.m. of cusum (s.e.m. = 1.71 lb). (Data from *Table 12.4*)

**Table 12.4 Cusum for weekly gain of a piglet with a target of a weekly weight gain of 6.65 lb/week. (Data relate to Roberts *et al.*, 1979, and are supplied by the authors)**

| Age (weeks) | Observed (lb) | Weight gain (lb/week) | Deviation from 6.65lb | Cusum (lb) |
|---|---|---|---|---|
| 6 | 64 | – | – | 0 |
| 7 | 68 | 4 | −2.65 | −2.65 |
| 8 | 76 | 8 | 1.35 | −1.30 |
| 9 | 81 | 5 | −1.65 | −2.95 |
| 10 | 84 | 3 | −3.65 | −6.60 |
| 11 | 86 | 2 | −4.65 | −11.25 |

cusum deficit at the end of the fattening period, indicating poor weight gain. Subsequent post-mortem examination of this piglet revealed infection with adenomatosis.

A decision must be taken to act when the cusum goes 'too far' beyond the target level. It is not the location of the plot above or below the reference value that indicates abnormality: if the **slope** is greater than 45 degrees from the horizontal then something should be done. The scales of the horizontal and vertical axes must therefore be chosen carefully. If one time period equals one unit on the horizontal axis, and 2 s.e.m. of cusum are equal to one unit on the vertical axis, then a plot's slope of 45 degrees or more will indicate a change that is **significant** at the 2.5% level (*see* Chapter 13). If smaller changes are of interest—and this is quite likely—then techniques such as the use of a V-mask (Barnard, 1959) and a decision interval scheme (Wetherill, 1969) are available. Page (1961), Davies and Goldsmith (1972) and Wrathall and Hebert (1983) discuss this topic in detail.

## *Further reading*

BAILEY, N.T.J. (1981) *Statistical Methods in Biology*, 2nd edn. Hodder and Stoughton, London

DAWKINS, H.C. (1975) *Statforms. 'Pro-formas' for the Guidance of Statistical Calculations*. Edward Arnold, London

ERICKSON, B.H. and NOSANCHUK, T.A. (1979) *Understanding Data*. Open University Press, Milton Keynes

*FRED LEARNS BASIC STATISTICS* (1975) Continua Productions, Macdonald and Evans, Plymouth

MEAD, R. and CURNOW, R.N. (1983) *Statistical Methods in Agriculture and Experimental Biology*. Chapman and Hall, London

SARD, D.M. (1979) *Dealing with Data. The Practical Use of Numerical Information*. BVA Publications, London

# 13

# Demonstrating association

A valuable step in the identification of the cause of a disease is the detection of a statistically significant association between the disease and hypothesized causal factors; this is the basis of the first three of Evans' postulates (*see* Chapter 3). This detection is a useful preliminary pointer to possible causal factors, which can be succeeded by either more detailed observational studies or experimental investigations.

## Some basic techniques

Demonstration of association can be approached in three ways.

(1) The difference, under two different circumstances, between the mean of the probability distribution of a set of values of a variable can be measured. If there is a significant difference between the means in the two circumstances, then the different circumstances may lead to an explanation that reflects a causal association. For example, the weights of two groups of piglets, one group of which has developed neonatal diarrhoea and one group of which has not, can be measured. The effect of diarrhoea on weight can then be assessed by analysing the difference between the mean weights of the two groups.

(2) Variables can be categorized, and a significant association sought between various categories. For example, bitches can be categorized according to whether or not they have physiological urinary incontinence and whether or not they are neutered. Evidence of an association between the syndrome and neutering can then be sought. The study could be further refined by

estimating the degree of association between disease and neutering.

(3) A correlation between variables can be sought. For example, the incidence of lameness in cattle and the amount of rainfall can be recorded to investigate whether increased rainfall is significantly associated with an increased incidence of lameness.

Many of the statistical techniques that adopt these three approaches were developed for use in agricultural science. Although their use is confined to epidemiological investigations in this book, they have a wide application to experimental and observational biological and social sciences, and therefore are described in most general statistics textbooks.

## *The principle of a significance test*

The bell shape of the Normal distribution (*see* *Figure 12.1*) reveals that there is a probability, albeit a small one, of an observation occurring at the extreme tails of the distribution. This distribution may not only be used to describe the frequency distribution of the values of a continuous variable that has a Normal distribution but also of the means of repeated samples taken from that population (here termed the reference population). There is, therefore, a high probability of the mean of a sample being under the peak, and a much lower probability of this mean being close to either of the two tails. If the mean is close to a tail, this indicates either that the sample is one of those improbable samples taken from the reference population, or, more likely, that it has been drawn from a population with a different population mean.

It is necessary to decide when it is improbable that a sample mean has come from the reference population. This decision is taken when the probability, $P$, of obtaining a value for the sample mean at least as extreme as the one observed, **assuming that the sample is drawn from the reference population**, is less than a value corresponding to the **level of significance**. This level is represented by a probability called $\alpha$ (the Greek letter 'alpha'). Conventionally, in biological sciences, $\alpha$ is taken to be 0.05, representing the 5% significance level. In the event of $P<0.05$, the result is reported as 'significant $P<0.05$' and supports the claim that the sample was not drawn from the reference population. The 5% significance level is purely conventional. If more caution in inferring a difference were necessary, the 1% level ($P<0.01$) or 0.1% level ($P<0.001$) could be chosen. Some reporting procedures use *, **, and *** to record significance at levels of 5%, 1% and 0.1% respectively. This decision-making procedure is the principle of a significance test.

## The null hypothesis

In the previous discussion, a statistical test was undertaken on the basis that the sample came from a population with a mean no different to that of the reference population. This constitutes the **null hypothesis**; the null hypothesis thus is one of **no difference**. A significant result indicates that the null hypothesis is rejected in favour of an alternative one which states that the sample has been drawn from a population with characteristics that are different from the reference population. Demonstration of a significant difference implies rejection of the null hypothesis.

Notice that confidence intervals and the outcomes of significance tests are closely related. For example, suppose that the null hypothesis states a particular value for the mean of a Normal distribution. A sample is taken and the significance test rejects the null hypothesis at the 5% level. The corresponding 95% confidence interval (sample mean ± 2 e.s.e.m.) then will **not** contain the value of the mean specified by the null hypothesis. Conversely, if the significance test does **not** reject the null hypothesis at the 5% level then the corresponding 95% confidence interval will contain the value of the mean specified by the null hypothesis.

## Errors of inference

Five per cent of samples from a population lie within the region that would lead to rejection of the null

hypothesis at the 5% level. If this happens it constitutes a rejection of the null hypothesis when the hypothesis is true. This error is an example of a **Type 1 error**: false rejection of a true null hypothesis. The probability of a Type 1 error is just the level of significance discussed above.

A **Type II error** is a failure to reject the null hypothesis when it is untrue. The probability of committing this error is called $\beta$ (the Greek letter 'beta'). Ideally, both $\alpha$ and $\beta$ should be known by the investigator before the study begins.

Depending on the alternative hypothesis, $\beta$ may or may not be determinable. In the previous discussion, if the alternative hypothesis specified the mean of the population from which the sample was drawn, then $\beta$ could be determined for a stated value of $\alpha$ and sample size. However, if the alternative hypothesis only hypothesized that the mean of the population from which the sample was drawn took one of several values, then $\beta$ cannot be calculated. It is known that $\beta$ can be kept small by increasing either $\alpha$ or the sample size. The probabilities of Type I and II errors decrease as sample size increases. For a fixed sample size, the larger the probability of a Type I error is chosen to be, the smaller the probability of a Type II error will be, and vice versa.

Two remaining alternative decisions are possible. These represent correct inferences, rather than errors. The first inference is not rejecting the null hypothesis when it is true. The second is rejecting the null hypothesis when it is false (i.e. demonstrating a significant difference). The probability of the latter is called the **power** of a test; it is denoted by $1-\beta$.

## One- and two-tailed tests

The previous discussion has been concerned with demonstrating any differences between a sample and a reference population, irrespective of the 'direction' of the difference; that is, whether the sample differs because it comes from a distribution with a mean to the left or right of the mean of the reference population. In this case, the investigator is concerned with significant departures towards either of the two tails of the distribution. A test that considers these departures is therefore called a **two-tailed** test.

An investigator may be reasonably certain that significant departures only occur in one direction. An example would be investigating whether diarrhoea depressed weight gain in piglets, rather than either depressed or increased it (the latter is very unlikely). This investigation requires a **one-tailed** test. The 5% significance level in a two-tailed test represents approximately 2 standard errors to either side of the mean. If the same criterion of approximately 2 standard errors were used in a one-tailed test, then the actual significance level would only be 2.5% (corresponding to the tail with which the investigator is concerned). Therefore, rejection of the null hypothesis at the 5% level in a one-tailed test requires a deviation corresponding to that required for rejection at the 10% level in a two-tailed test.

## Student's t-test

The choice of a suitable significance test depends on many factors, such as the type of frequency distribution and sample size. One test, commonly used for small samples of Normally distributed data, is **Student's t-test**. This involves calculation of a test statistic called $t$, which measures departures from the mean that is specified by the null hypothesis. The distribution of this test statistic follows a $t$-distribution (illustrated in *Figure 12.4*)—hence the name of the test. There are three common applications.

The first concerns samples from a single reference population and an hypothesis that the data come from a Normal distribution with mean $\mu$; the variance, $\sigma^2$, is not known. If $\bar{x}$ and $s^2$ are the sample mean and variance, respectively, then the test statistic is:

$$t = (\bar{x}-\mu)/\surd(s^2/n)$$

where $n$ is the sample size. There are $(n-1)$ **degrees of freedom** (these will be discussed later).

The second concerns two samples from different populations and an hypothesis that the data come from Normal distributions with a known difference $\mu_1-\mu_2 = \delta$ (the Greek letter 'delta') between the two population means, $\mu_1$ and $\mu_2$, and common unknown variance, $\sigma^2$. If $n_1$, $\bar{x}_1$, $s_1^2$ are the sample size, sample mean and sample variance from the first population, and $n_2$, $\bar{x}_2$, $s_2^2$ are similar statistics from the second population, then the estimate of the common unknown variance, $\sigma^2$, is:

$$s^2 = \{(n_1-1)s_1^2+(n_2-1)s_2^2\}/(n_1+n_2-2).$$

The test statistic, $t$, is:

$$t = (\bar{x}_1-\bar{x}_2-\delta)/\surd\{s^2(\frac{1}{n_1}+\frac{1}{n_2})\}$$

and there are $n_1+n_2-2$ degrees of freedom.

This test is exemplified using the data in *Table 12.1*:

$n_1 = 49$; $\bar{x}_1 = 5.76$ kg; $s_1 = 0.60$ kg;

$n_2 = 49$; $\bar{x}_2 = 4.69$ kg; $s_2 = 0.67$ kg.

The hypothesis to be tested is that there is no difference in 3-week weaning weights between the two groups of piglets, that is $\delta = 0$.

$$s^2 = \{(48 \times 0.60^2) + (48 \times 0.67^2)\}/96$$

$$= (17.280 + 21.547)/96$$

$$= 0.404.$$

$$t = (5.76-4.69-0)/\surd\{0.404\,(\frac{1}{49}+\frac{1}{49})\}$$

$$= 1.07/\surd 0.0165$$

$$= 8.33.$$

There are 96 degrees of freedom (49+49−2). Appendix III is consulted. It does not have a row corresponding to 96 degrees of freedom, and so the row with the greatest number of degrees of freedom less than 96 is chosen (60 in this instance). This is a conservative procedure. The 0.1% value for 60 degrees of freedom is 3.460. This is considerably less than 8.33. Therefore, in this example, the two groups (A and B) of piglets have mean values that differ significantly at the 0.1% level.

Often, when sample sizes are large, the e.s.e.m.s. are regarded as the true s.e.m.s. and the $t$-test is conducted with degrees of freedom corresponding to infinity ($\infty$). The test then becomes a two-sample $z$-test.

Ninety-five per cent confidence limits can be calculated for the difference $\mu_1-\mu_2$ between the true population means, using the formula:

$$(\bar{x}_1-\bar{x}_2) \pm t_\nu(0.95)\surd\{s^2(\frac{1}{n_1}+\frac{1}{n_2})\}$$

where $t_\nu(0.95)$ is the 95% point of the $t$-distribution with $\nu$ (the Greek letter 'nu') degrees of freedom.

The third application concerns comparisons in which the observations between the two samples are paired. This approach may have the benefit of removing a source of variation, therefore providing a more sensitive test than its unpaired counterpart. For example, the weights of individual calves measured one week, and then a week later, are paired data. The test assumes the difference between the members of each pair is Normally distributed with a mean $\delta$ (usually zero) and an unknown variance, $\sigma^2$. If $\bar{d}$ and $s^2$ are the sample mean and variance, respectively, of the differences then the test statistic is:

$$t = (\bar{d}-\delta)/\surd(s^2/n)$$

where $n$ is the sample size. There are $(n-1)$ degrees of freedom.

### Degrees of freedom

The critical value of the $t$-test leading to rejection or non-rejection of the null hypothesis depends on the sample size and a related figure, known as the **degrees of freedom**. If a sample consists of $n$ **independent** observations (one observation does not influence the value of another) then there are, in a sense, $n$ independent 'pieces of information'.

Calculating the mean in the one-sample and paired comparison *t*-tests uses one piece of information, leaving $(n-1)$ for the variance. This is because knowledge of $(n-1)$ observations and the mean fixes the value of the remaining observation. The number $(n-1)$ is the number of degrees of freedom.

Similarly, in the two-sample case, with sample sizes of $n_1$ and $n_2$, two means are evaluated. There are thus $(n_1+n_2-2)$ 'pieces' of information for calculation of the variance. The number $(n_1+n_2-2)$ is the number of degrees of freedom.

## The $\chi^2$ test of association

The results of an investigation of physiological urinary incontinence (PUI) in bitches are recorded in *Table 13.1*. The question being asked was: 'Does an association exist between the development of PUI and spaying?' The investigators categorized dogs into those with PUI that were spayed, those with PUI that were not spayed, those without PUI that were spayed and those without PUI that were not spayed. These four permutations allow the construction of a two-way table with four 'cells' in it, called a 2 × 2 contingency table.

**Table 13.1 Incidence of physiological urinary incontinence (excluding congenital incontinence) in spayed and entire bitches 6 months of age and older (period of observation = 7 years)**

|  | Urinary incontinence present | Urinary incontinence absent | Totals |
|---|---|---|---|
| Spayed | 34 (*a*) | 757 (*b*) | 791 (*a+b*) |
| Entire | 7 (*c*) | 2427 (*d*) | 2434 (*c+d*) |
| Totals | 41 (*a+c*) | 3184 (*b+d*) | 3225 (*n*) |

The values in the table need to be assessed. A simple method of assessment would be to express the values in each row as percentages of the total of each row. If each row showed similar percentages, this would imply that the row classification did not affect the column classification—that there was no association between the two classifications. This reasoning is sound, but requires large numbers, otherwise sampling variation could affect the result. Taking the data in *Table 13.1*: the percentage of these animals that were spayed and have PUI is 4.3% (34/791); the percentage of those that were not spayed and have PUI is 0.3% (7/2434). This difference could be significant, but it could also merely result from the variation induced by selection of a relatively small sample of the total population at risk.

A common way of conducting a test on these data is to calculate a test statistic called $\chi^2$ ($\chi$ is the Greek

letter 'chi', pronounced with a hard 'ch'). The distribution followed by this statistic is known as the $\chi^2$-distribution. This statistic indicates the extent to which the observed values in the cells diverge from the values that would be expected if there were no association between row and column categories. A table of the $\chi^2$-distribution is then consulted to decide whether the observed $\chi^2$ value is **larger** than that which would be expected, based on a null hypothesis postulating no association.

This example involves only a 2 × 2 contingency table, and the $\chi^2$ equation below is simplified to refer only to this type of table. The test can be performed on contingency tables with several rows and columns (i.e. with several categories). Details can be found in books listed in 'Further reading' at the end of this chapter.

The $\chi^2$ statistic is given by:

$$\chi^2 = \frac{n(|ad-bc| - \frac{n}{2})^2}{(a+b)(c+d)(a+c)(b+d)}$$

where $n/2$ is a continuity correction for 2 × 2 contingency tables, to improve the approximation, because $\chi^2$ is a continuous distribution, yet the data (numbers of animals), and therefore the test statistic, are discrete. The vertical bars, $||$, are **moduli**. They indicate the absolute value of $ad-bc$, that is, the positive value of the difference is always used.

Using the values in *Table 13.1*:

$$\chi^2 = \frac{3225\{|82518 - 5299| - (3225/2)\}^2}{791 \times 2434 \times 41 \times 3184}$$

$$= 73.35.$$

Percentage points of the $\chi^2$-distribution are given in Appendix IV for various significance levels and degrees of freedom. As a rule, the degrees of freedom, $\upsilon$ (the Greek letter 'upsilon'), to be selected are given by:

$$\upsilon = \text{(number of rows} - 1) \times \text{(number of columns} - 1)$$

which, in this example, is:

$$(2-1) \times (2-1) = 1.$$

In a 2 × 2 contingency table, where the row and column totals are all known, knowledge of **one** of the values in the four cells in the body of the table immediately implies knowledge of the values in the other three cells. Similarly in a table with *r* rows and *c* columns, with the row and column totals all known, the knowledge of $(r-1) \times (c-1)$ of the values in the *rc* cells in the body of the table implies knowledge of the values in the other cells. This is the idea behind degrees of freedom, namely the freedom to choose the values in the body of a contingency table when the row and column totals are fixed.

Consulting row 1 (1 degree of freedom) of the table, the observed value, 73.35, is **greater than** the tabulated statistic at the 5% level of significance (3.841) and so an association can be inferred between spaying and PUI. Note that, in this example, the result is also significant at the 1% and 0.1% levels.

## Estimation of risk

The $\chi^2$-test can be used to determine the **significance** of an association between a disease and an hypothesized causal factor. The value of $\chi^2$ cannot be used as a measure of the **degree** of association. This is because $\chi^2$ is a function of the proportions in the various cells and of the total sample size, whereas the degree of association is only really a function of the cell proportions; the sample size has a role to play in detecting significance but not in determining the extent of association.

Detection of association by demonstration of a significant difference using the $\chi^2$-test is frequently insufficient. It may also be desirable to provide a **measure** of the difference between the frequency of disease in a group exposed to a factor or possessing an attribute, and the frequency in a group not exposed to the factor or without the attribute. A measure of the degree of association will give an indication of the extent to which the factor or attribute contributes to the disease's occurrence; in other words, a measure of the extent to which the disease is caused by the factor or attribute. The extent to which a factor causes a disease—the **risk** associated with the factor—is measured in terms of its degree of association with the disease. An extreme situation would be when all animals exposed to a factor developed a disease and all unexposed animals were disease-free. In reality this rarely happens, which is why it is usually possible to construct a 2 × 2 contingency table with values greater than zero in each of the four cells (unless the study population is small). From this a relative measure of risk can be calculated as a ratio of disease incidence in groups exposed to a factor or possessing an attribute, relative to disease incidence in groups not exposed to the factor or not possessing the attribute.

### Relative risk

Consider again the data in *Table 13.1* relating to PUI and spaying, observed as the number of new cases over a defined period of time. Note that when constructing the contingency table, disease is expressed horizontally and the hypothesized causal factor is expressed vertically.

The incidence rate among bitches 'exposed' to spaying ($p_1$) is given by:

$$p_1 = a/(a+b).$$

The incidence rate among 'unexposed' bitches ($p_2$) is given by:

$$p_2 = c/(c+d).$$

The ratio of the two incidence rates—the **relative risk**, $R$—is given by:

$$R = p_1/p_2.$$

Alternatively this may be expressed as:

$$R = \{a/(a+b)\}/\{c/(c+d)\}$$

which, using the data from *Table 13.1*, may be estimated by:

$$R^* = (34/791)/(7/2434)$$
$$= 14.9$$

where * indicates that the value is an estimate.

A relative risk greater than 1 indicates a positive statistical association between factor and disease. A relative risk less than 1 indicates a negative statistical association: possession of the factor may be said to have a protective effect against the disease. A relative risk of 1 suggests no association.

### Odds ratio ($\psi$)

The odds ratio, $\psi$ (the Greek letter, psi), is another measure of degree of association that is commonly used in epidemiological studies. If an event occurs with probability $p$, then the ratio $p/q$ is called the **odds** in favour of the event occurring, where $q = 1-p$. If the odds of disease among exposed animals is $p_1/q_1$, and the odds of disease among unexposed animals is $p_2/q_2$, then the ratio of the odds of disease among exposed animals to the odds of disease among unexposed animals, known as the **odds ratio** ($\psi$), is given by:

$$\psi = (p_1/q_1)/(p_2/q_2)$$
$$= p_1 q_2/q_1 p_2$$
$$= ad/bc,$$

which, using the data from *Table 13.1*, may be estimated by:

$$\psi^* = (34 \times 2427)/(757 \times 7)$$
$$= 15.6.$$

For rare diseases, the risk of disease, $p$, is almost the same as the odds $p/q$, since $q$ is approximately equal to 1; thus, for diseases of low incidence, the odds ratio provides a good approximation to the relative risk. When disease incidence is not low, the values of the relative risk and odds ratio diverge. 'Relative risk' and 'odds ratio' were used interchangeably but their two distinct derivations are now well established.

**Table 13.2 Odds ratio† and 95% confidence intervals† for male dogs, by breed, for canine heart valve incompetence. (Data extracted from Edinburgh University's Small Animal Practice Teaching Unit data base: Thrusfield and Hinxman, 1981)**

| Breed | Cases | Controls | Estimated odds ratio ($\psi^*$) | 95% confidence interval for $\psi$ | |
|---|---|---|---|---|---|
| Beagle | 7 | 84 | 2.18 | 1.03 | 4.64 |
| Cairn terrier | 21 | 255 | 2.11 | 1.34 | 3.32 |
| Chihuahua | 10 | 56 | 4.63 | 2.37 | 9.01 |
| Dachshund | 11 | 144 | 1.97 | 1.07 | 3.62 |
| Basset hound | 3 | 31 | 2.72 | 0.90 | 8.25 |
| Border terrier | 6 | 91 | 1.74 | 0.78 | 3.89 |
| Bulldog | 0 | 9 | 1.28 | 0.07 | 22.06 |
| Cocker spaniel | 14 | 260 | 1.37 | 0.80 | 2.35 |
| Labrador retriever | 13 | 990 | 0.31 | 0.18 | 0.53 |
| German shepherd dog | 4 | 590 | 0.18 | 0.07 | 0.45 |
| West Highland white terrier | 7 | 389 | 1.46 | 0.22 | 0.95 |
| *Totals over all breeds in the study* | 370 | 9028 | | | |

†Calculated using the 'logit' method of Plackett (1981). The value 0.5 is added to the values in each cell of each contingency table because at least one cell can contain the value zero, which leads to problems of estimation of the odds ratio.

These calculations produce point estimates of $\psi$ and $R$. Interval estimates can be calculated although care has to be taken since the odds ratio and relative risk statistics are not Normally distributed and different formulae from those given in Chapter 12 have to be used. It is also possible to decide whether the values of $\psi$ and $R$ differ significantly between groups. The calculations are described in Fleiss (1981), Plackett (1981) and Schlesselman (1982).

If the value of the lower confidence limit of the measure of association, be it odds ratio or relative risk, is greater than 1 at a defined level of significance, then the association between the hypothesized cause and the disease is statistically significant and it can be said that there is evidence of an association. For example, in *Table 13.2*, the positive association between canine heart valve incompetence and breed is significant at the 5% level only for the first four breeds. In the second four breeds, the lower confidence limit is less than 1, and so the association is not significant at the 5% level. In the last three breeds, the upper confidence limit is less than 1, indicating a significant negative association at the 5% level (breed may be said to have a 'protective' effect against the disease).

### Attributable risk ($\delta$)

*Table 13.1* shows that although the incidence rate of urinary incontinence in spayed dogs, $p_1$, is greater than the incidence rate in entire dogs, $p_2$, the spayed dogs are still susceptible to a 'background' risk, corresponding to $p_2$. Put another way, if some of the spayed dogs had not been neutered, then they may still, as entire dogs, have developed urinary incontinence. The extent of the risk associated with spaying is therefore $p_1 - p_2$. This is the **attributable risk**, $\delta$ (the Greek letter 'delta') (Schlesselman, 1982). Thus, in this example:

$$\delta = p_1 - p_2$$
$$= (34/791) - (7/2434)$$
$$= 0.043 - 0.003$$
$$= 0.040$$

This represents an incidence rate of incontinence, attributable to spaying, of 4.0 per 100 during the period of observation.

The attributable risk indicates the extent to which the incidence of incontinence would be reduced by not spaying, **assuming that spaying is causal**.

Attributable risk can be expressed in terms of the relative risk:

$$\delta = p_1 - p_2$$
$$= (\frac{p_1}{p_2} - 1)p_2.$$

Since $\frac{p_1}{p_2} = R$

then $\delta = (R - 1)p_2.$

It is clear that ratios ($p_1/p_2$) of 0.02/0.01 and 0.0002/0.0001 give the same relative risk, even though they represent vastly different incidence ratios. The attributable risk, however, includes the baseline incidence rate, and therefore gives an indication of the **magnitude** of the effect of a causal factor in the population.

The size of the relative risk is a better indication than that of the attributable risk that a causal association exists between exposure to an hypothesized causal factor and disease. However, if a causal relationship is accepted, the attributable risk gives a better indication than the relative risk of the effect of a preventive campaign that removes the factor (MacMahon and Pugh, 1970).

## Aetiological fraction

The **aetiological fraction**, $\lambda$ (the Greek letter 'lambda': Miettinen, 1974), also termed the 'attributable proportion' and, when expressed as a percentage, 'attributable risk percent' (Cole and MacMahon, 1971), is the proportion of all cases attributable to exposure to a causal factor. Therefore it represents the proportion of disease occurrence that would be eliminated if a group exposed to a causal factor has its incidence reduced to the level of the unexposed group.

$$\lambda = \frac{R-1}{R} \times f \quad \text{omit}$$

where $f$ is the proportion of diseased individuals exposed to the causal factor. $(a/a+c)$

Using the figures in *Table 13.1*:

$R = 14.9$
$f = 34/41$
$= 0.829$.

Thus,

$$\lambda = \frac{14.9 - 1}{14.9} \times 0.829 \quad .93$$

$$= 0.77. \quad .93$$

Thus, if spaying is causal, 77% of cases of PUI are attributable to spaying.

In terms of causal model 1 (*see* Chapter 3) the sum of the aetiological fractions of all sufficient causes is 1 (i.e. 100%).

Thus, the aetiological fraction, like the attributable risk, is an indication of the impact that removal of a causal factor would have on reduction in incidence.

There is some inconsistency in the use of this and the preceding term (Markush, 1977); sometimes 'attributable risk' has been applied to the aetiological fraction (e.g. Lilienfeld and Lilienfeld, 1980).

## Differences between measures of occurrence

The odds ratio and relative risk are measures of association based on **ratios** between measures of disease occurrence. Ratios provide a more meaningful comparison than **differences** between measures of disease occurrence because the former relate disease occurrence to a baseline level (the level in the unexposed group). Differences essentially indicate whether or not exposure to a factor results in an increased occurrence of disease.

Thus, using the data in *Table 13.1*, the difference, $D$, between the incidence rate in exposed, $p_1$, and unexposed, $p_2$, animals (which is the attributable risk, $\delta$, defined above) is:

$$D = (a/a+b) - (c/c+d)$$
$$= (34/791) - (7/2434)$$
$$= 0.0429 - 0.0028$$
$$= 0.00401. \quad 0.0401$$

This represents a point estimate of the difference. An approximate 95% confidence interval can be estimated (Miettinen, 1976) using the formula:

$$D(1 \pm 1.96/\chi)$$

(note that $\chi$, not $\chi^2$, is used in this formula).

Using the value of $\chi^2$ estimated above:

95% confidence interval
$$= 0.00401 \, (1 \pm 1.96/\sqrt{73.35})$$
$$= 0.00401 \, (1 \pm 0.2288)$$
$$= (0.00401 \times 0.7712, \, 0.00401 \times 1.2288)$$
$$= (0.00309, \, 0.00493).$$

$$\frac{1.96}{8.56} \quad 4$$

In this example, the lower confidence interval is greater than zero and so there is a difference, at the 5% level of significance, between incidence rates in exposed and unexposed groups.

The confidence interval for differences is symmetric about the point estimate and is therefore constructed in a way similar to that described in the previous chapter.

## *Measuring interaction*

Interaction was introduced in Chapter 5 as occurring between two or more factors when the frequency of disease is either in excess of or less than that expected from the combined effects of each factor. If there is a plausible biological mechanism for the interaction, then **synergism** is said to occur when the frequency is in excess of the anticipated value, and **antagonism** when the frequency is less than the anticipated value.

Two models of interaction were also introduced in Chapter 5: **additive** and **multiplicative**. The choice of model depends on the measure of disease frequency. Generally, the additive model is most appropriate in indicating the impact of interaction on incidence (Kleinbaum *et al.*, 1982). Therefore, an additive model will now be described (details of both types of model are given by Kleinbaum *et al.* (1982) and Schlesselman (1982)). The model is based on additivity of excess risks.

## The additive model

Consider two factors $x$ and $y$. If $p_{00}$ is the incidence rate when neither factor is present, $p_{10}$ the incidence rate when $x$ alone is present, $p_{01}$ the incidence rate when $y$ alone is present, and $p_{11}$ the incidence rate when both are present, then:

$$p_{10} - p_{00} = \text{risk attributable to } x,$$

$$p_{01} - p_{00} = \text{risk attributable to } y.$$

If the combined effect of $x$ and $y$ equals the sum of their individual effects, then:

$$(p_{11} - p_{00}) = (p_{10} - p_{00}) + (p_{01} - p_{00})$$

and there is no interaction.

Lack of interaction can be expressed in terms of the excess relative risk, by dividing the formula above by $p_{00}$:

$$(p_{11}/p_{00} - 1) = (p_{10}/p_{00} - 1) + (p_{01}/p_{00} - 1).$$

The relative risk when both factors are present is denoted by $R_{xy} = p_{11}/p_{00}$; the relative risks when $x$ or $y$ is present alone are denoted by $R_x = p_{10}/p_{00}$ and $R_y = p_{01}/p_{00}$, respectively,

thus $(R_{xy} - 1) = (R_x - 1) + (R_y - 1)$

that is $R_{xy} = 1 + (R_x - 1) + (R_y - 1)$.

If more than two factors, $j$ say, are being considered, then the combined relative risk, $R_m$, for these, is given by:

$$R_m = 1 + \sum_{i=1}^{j} (R_i - 1),$$

where $R_1, ..., R_j$ denote the individual relative risks.

Examples of positive interaction, based on an additive model, are given in *Table 13.4*, using the raw data in *Table 13.3* relating to the feline urological syndrome (Willeberg, 1976).

Hypothesized causal factors in males are the feeding of high levels of dry cat food, castration, and low levels of outdoor activity. The background risk ($R=1$) therefore is represented by entire male cats consuming low levels of dry cat food, and with high levels of outdoor activity.

Consider the two factors: low levels of outdoor activity and high levels of dry cat food intake. The relative risk associated with low levels of outdoor activity and low levels of dry cat food intake in entire males is 3.43 (*a* in *Table 13.3*). The relative risk associated with high levels of dry cat food and high levels of outdoor activity is 4.36 (*b* in *Table*

**Table 13.3 Number of cases of the feline urological syndrome (FUS) and controls, and estimated relative risk values by combinations of categories within the factors, sex, diet and activity. (From Willeberg, 1976)**

| Categories | | | No. of cats | | Estimated relative risk ($R^*$) |
|---|---|---|---|---|---|
| Sex | Level of dry cat food | Level of outdoor activity | Cases | Controls | |
| Entire male | Low | High | 1 | 12 | 1 |
| | Low | Low | 2 | 7 | 3.43 (*a*) |
| | High | High | 4 | 11 | 4.36 (*b*) |
| | High | Low | 2 | 4 | 6.00 (*d*) |
| Castrated male | Low | High | 5 | 12 | 5.00 |
| | Low | Low | 3 | 5 | 7.20 |
| | High | High | 14 | 5 | 33.60*** |
| | High | Low | 28 | 2 | 168.00*** |
| Total no. of male cats | | | 59 | 58 | 12.2** |

$**0.01 > P > 0.001$ ⎫
$***P < 0.001$ ⎬ by common $\chi^2$-method

**Table 13.4 Comparison of estimated and expected relative risk values of the feline urological syndrome (FUS) for male cats for multiple excess risk category combinations based on an additive interaction model. (Adapted from Willeberg, 1976)**

| Categories | | | Estimated relative risk ($R^*$) | Expected relative risk based on additive model ($R_m$) |
|---|---|---|---|---|
| Sexual status | Level of dry cat food | Level of outdoor activity | | |
| Entire | High | Low | 6.00 (*d*) | 6.79 (*c*) |
| Castrated | Low | Low | 7.20 | 7.43 |
| Castrated | High | High | 33.60 | 8.36 |
| Castrated | High | Low | 168.00 | 10.67 |

*13.3*). Therefore, applying the additive model for these two factors (*Table 13.4*):

$$R_m = 1 + (3.43 - 1) + (4.36 - 1)$$

$$= 6.79 \ (c \text{ in } Table \ 13.4).$$

The estimated combined relative risk for these two factors is 6.00 (*d* in *Tables 13.3* and *13.4*).

Thus, there is no evidence for interaction between high levels of dry cat food and low levels of outdoor activity because the estimated combined relative risk (6.00) is similar to the expected combined relative risk assuming no interaction (6.79). Similarly, there is no evidence of interaction between castration and low levels of outdoor activity. However, there is evidence of positive interaction between castration and high levels of dry cat food, and between castration, high levels of dry cat food and low levels of outdoor activity: in each case the estimated combined relative risk is greater than the expected combined relative risk, using the additive model.

A plausible biological mechanism for the interaction can be described, that is, synergism has occurred. Castration and high levels of dry cat food intake (usually associated with overfeeding) may both result in inactivity, thereby reducing blood flow to the kidneys, impairing kidney function, and therefore possibly promoting changes in the urine that are conducive to the formation of uroliths; this constitutes a possible common causal pathway.

## Correlation

*Table 13.5* records the number of cases of lameness in cattle in relation to rainfall for a one-year period on a farm in SW England. The question to be answered is: 'Does the amount of rainfall have an effect on the incidence of lameness?' This is a reasonable question; wet feet could be a causal factor. The values in *Table 13.5* are plotted graphically in *Figure 13.1*, each point being a lameness–rainfall pair. Lameness is measured on the horizontal ($x$) axis and rainfall on the vertical ($y$) axis.

If there were a positive association between increased rainfall and incidence of lameness, most

**Table 13.5 The joint distribution of fortnightly lameness incidence and rainfall on a farm in SW England for a one-year period (1977). (Data supplied by the Institute for Research on Animal Diseases, Compton, UK)**

| Fortnight | Number of lameness incidents ($x$) | Fortnightly rainfall totals (mm) ($y$) |
|---|---|---|
| 1 | 40 | 37.2 |
| 2 | 38 | 48.8 |
| 3 | 55 | 72.0 |
| 4 | 38 | 76.8 |
| 5 | 45 | 14.8 |
| 6 | 42 | 53.2 |
| 7 | 51 | 23.9 |
| 8 | 45 | 11.0 |
| 9 | 41 | 79.9 |
| 10 | 23 | 21.0 |
| 11 | 10 | 2.3 |
| 12 | 29 | 81.1 |
| 13 | 19 | 7.4 |
| 14 | 11 | 31.5 |
| 15 | 11 | 33.2 |
| 16 | 19 | 31.1 |
| 17 | 33 | 109.2 |
| 18 | 47 | 25.0 |
| 19 | 42 | 1.9 |
| 20 | 34 | 28.8 |
| 21 | 17 | 24.4 |
| 22 | 30 | 51.3 |
| 23 | 48 | 38.2 |
| 24 | 59 | 18.0 |
| 25 | 41 | 57.2 |
| 26 | 26 | 33.2 |

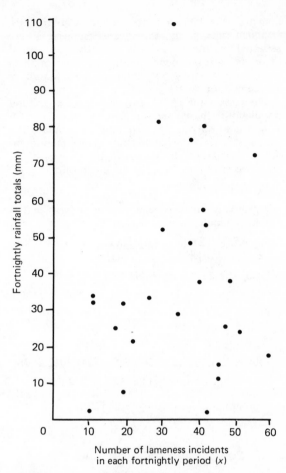

**Figure 13.1** Plot of the joint distribution of fortnightly lameness incidence and rainfall on a farm in SW England for a one-year period (1977). (Data from *Table 13.5*)

entries would be concentrated in a line from the bottom left to the top right of the figure. If there were no association, the pairs would be randomly scattered over the figure. Visually, the results give a slight impression of concentrating along the diagonal, but it is necessary to know whether this clustering is significant.

A useful measure of correlation between $x$ and $y$ is the **correlation coefficient**, $\rho$ (the Greek letter 'rho'). This ranges from +1, representing a complete positive association, to −1, representing a complete negative association. This can be calculated for $x$ and $y$ if they are continuous variables and if they are Normally distributed and successive observations are **independent** of others. These assumptions should always be met. In this example, lameness incidence is assumed to be Normal because lameness is fairly common; if it were rare then it would more likely have a Poisson distribution. Similarly, because there are many incidents of lameness, the data are considered to be continuous, although, technically, they are discrete. It is also assumed that the successive fortnightly observations of rainfall are independent, that is, the rainfall of one fortnight does not influence the rainfall of succeeding fortnights.

The correlation coefficient, $\rho$, refers to the total population; these measurements come from a sample and so can be used only to estimate the sample's correlation coefficient, $r$. Estimation involves calculating the means of the two variables and then estimating $r$, using the equation:

$$\Sigma(x-\bar{x})(y-\bar{y})/\sqrt{\{\Sigma(x-\bar{x})^2\Sigma(y-\bar{y})^2\}}.$$

Alternatively this can be written in a form that is easier to handle during calculation:

$$r = \{\Sigma xy-(\Sigma x)(\Sigma y)/n\}/\sqrt{([\Sigma x^2-\{(\Sigma x)^2/n\}][\Sigma y^2-\{(\Sigma y)^2/n\}])}.$$

Using the data from *Table 13.5*:

$$\Sigma x = 894 \qquad\qquad \Sigma y = 1012.4$$
$$\Sigma x^2 = 35592 \qquad\quad \Sigma y^2 = 57880.04$$
$$\Sigma xy = 36307.5$$
$$n = 26$$

$$\{\Sigma xy-(\Sigma x)(\Sigma y)/n\} = 36307.5-(894)(1012.4)/26$$
$$= 1496.52,$$

$$\{\Sigma x^2-(\Sigma x)^2/n\} = 35592-894^2/26$$
$$= 4852.15,$$

$$\{\Sigma y^2-(\Sigma y)^2/n\} = 57880.04-1012.4^2/26$$
$$= 18458.742.$$

Thus:

$$r = \frac{1496.52}{\sqrt{(4852.15 \times 18458.742)}}$$

$$= \frac{1496.52}{9463.86}$$

$$= 0.158.$$

The significance of this value is obtained by consulting Appendix V. If the value is **greater** in absolute terms (i.e. ignoring sign) than the tabulated value, at a defined significance level, then a significant association is demonstrated. In this example, the value (0.158) is **less** than the tabulated value at the 5% level, which is 0.381. This value is chosen from the table by selecting the number of degrees of freedom, which is $n-2 = 24$. This is one degree of freedom less than might be expected because the calculation of the correlation coefficient uses up one further degree of freedom. The most appropriate row therefore is 25 degrees of freedom. In this example, therefore, there is not a significant association between lameness incidence and rainfall ($P>0.05$).

## Non-parametric tests

Most of the techniques that have been described are based on the Normal distribution. They are called **parametric** techniques because they are concerned with the mean of the distribution, which is one of the distribution's parameters; they assume Normality. Many parametric tests require other assumptions, too. For example, the two-sample $t$-test assumes that if two populations are being compared then they have the same variance, and that variables must be measured on either the interval or ratio scales. If the variances are not equal, then the test must be modified (an example is given in Chapter 16). *Table 13.6* lists some commonly used parametric techniques that test hypotheses relating to the mean. This table is designed to indicate the range of tests that

**Table 13.6 Summary of some parametric statistical techniques for testing hypotheses relating to means of Normally-distributed data**

| Level of measurement | Variance | Parametric statistical test | | | | | Parametric measure of correlation |
| --- | --- | --- | --- | --- | --- | --- | --- |
| | | One-sample case | Two-sample case | | Case with 3 or more samples | | |
| | | | Related samples | Independent samples | Related samples | Independent samples | |
| Interval and ratio | Known | Normal test | Normal test | Normal test | | | Correlation coefficient $\rho$* |
| Interval and ratio | Unknown | $t$-test | $t$-test | $t$-test* (equal variance) | $F$-test (equal variance) | $F$-test (equal variance) | Correlation coefficient $\rho$* |
| | | | | Welch $t$-test (unequal variances) | Welch $F$-test (unequal variances) | Welch $F$-test (unequal variances) | |

*Indicates a test that is exemplified in this chapter.

are available. It does not completely specify either the conditions or the assumptions of the tests. These should be obtained from statistical texts and understood fully before applying the tests.

If the assumptions of a parametric test cannot be met then **non-parametric** techniques could be used. These can be applied to nominal and ordinal data, as well as to interval and ratio data. They do not assume Normality. Most of these tests are **distribution-free**, that is, they do not require assumptions such as the underlying distribution being Normal. The parametric tests are more powerful than the non-parametric tests if the distributional assumptions hold, that is, the former require a smaller sample size than the latter to detect a significant difference of a given magnitude.

The range of non-parametric tests for nominal, ordinal, interval and ratio data is described by Siegel (1956).

## Multivariate analysis

The analytical techniques described concern the study of relationships between two variables. In some cases it is necessary to assess the relationship between a response variable and many explanatory variables. This requires statistical techniques which investigate multiple variables; these are called **multivariate** techniques. They include **cluster analysis**, **factor analysis**, **path analysis**, **discriminant analysis**, **analysis of principal components** and **multiple regression analysis**. These methods are beyond the scope of this book and are described in detail elsewhere (e.g. Chatfield and Collins, 1980). Examples of epidemiological applications include the use of principal components analysis to investigate the association between equine respiratory infections and biochemical and haematological variables (Bryant and Smith, 1981) and the association between pig post-mortem examination variables relating to respiratory disease and a range of microbiological variables (Smith, 1977); factor analysis (Franti *et al.*, 1974) to assess the relationship between losses due to calf diarrhoea and various management and husbandry practices; discriminant analysis to study the association between the incidence of salmonellosis in dairy herds and husbandry and environmental variables, including herd size, source of water supply and method of effluent disposal (Vandegraaff, 1980); cluster analysis to identify prognostic indicators in the 'downer cow' syndrome (Chamberlain and Cripps, 1986); and path analysis to investigate the association between the prevalence of canine echinococcosis and husbandry variables such as mean grazing area/farm, sheep density, and climatic variables such as relative humidity, hours of sunlight and daily maximum and minimum temperatures (Burridge *et al.*, 1977).

## Statistical packages

Collections of computer programs (called 'packages') which perform statistical calculations, including those of the mean, median, standard deviation and standard error, confidence limits, the tests of association and time series analysis, are available on microcomputers and mainframes. Ready-built packages have a variety of names. Those of veterinary value include MINITAB (Ryan *et al.*, 1985), SPSS—Statistical Packages for the Social Sciences (Nie *et al.*, 1977), BMDP (Dixon, 1983) and GLIM (Baker and Nelder, 1978). These are very useful. Complex and lengthy calculations, which would take a long time to perform by hand, can be completed in a few seconds. Data can be directly and graphically represented; for example, using MINITAB, 'box and whisker' plots can be displayed on a VDU from numerical values that are put into the computer.

However, computerized packages can be dangerous. They facilitate easy analysis of data and so tend to encourage the collection of masses of data without a clear objective. It is also easy to try many of the different tests that are available without a knowledge of the tests' underlying principles. These remarks are equally relevant to the use of those pocket calculators that have built-in programs for simple statistical tests.

This chapter has presented some basic statistical concepts and techniques that are used commonly in epidemiology. It has aimed to increase appreciation of and familiarity with statistical method, rather than to produce a veterinary statistician. The latter requires a detailed knowledge of many statistical techniques and, above all, an understanding of the assumptions of the tests. Statistics is a science which is an important part of epidemiology—not just a subordinate adjunct. Quantitative epidemiological investigations therefore frequently require close cooperation between the veterinarian and the statistician.

Expert statistical advice should always be sought if there is any doubt about which analytical technique to use in an investigation. This advice should be obtained **before** the investigation begins, not after it is completed, otherwise time may be spent collecting data, only to discover that they cannot be used to solve the problem that is being posed.

## *Further reading*

BAILEY, N.T.J. (1981) *Statistical Methods in Biology*, 2nd edn. Hodder and Stoughton, London

FLEISS, J.L. (1981) *Statistical Methods for Rates and Proportions*, 2nd edn. John Wiley and Sons, New York

LEECH, F.B. and SELLERS, K.C. (1979) *Statistical Epidemiology in Veterinary Science*. Charles Griffin and Company Limited, London and High Wycombe

MEAD, R. and CURNOW, R.N. (1983) *Statistical Methods in Experimental Biology*. Chapman and Hall, London

SARD, D.M. (1979) *Dealing with Data. The Practical Use of Numerical Information*. British Veterinary Association Publications, London

SOKAL, R.R. and ROHLF, F.J. (1981) *Biometry*, 2nd edn. W.H. Freeman and Company, New York

# 14

# Surveys

Information on disease and its determinants is obtained from **surveys** and **studies** (introduced in Chapter 2). A survey usually involves **counting** members of an aggregate of units and measuring their characteristics such as weight, milk yield, presence of disease, or antibody levels. A study, however, involves **comparison** of groups, and is usually undertaken to elucidate the cause of disease.

If all animals in a population are investigated then the survey or study is a **census**. Demographic censuses of human and animal populations are conducted regularly in many countries to determine the size and structure of the populations. A census is the only means of measuring **exactly** the distribution of a variable in a population. Some prevalence surveys that are 'almost' censuses have been conducted. For example, Jasper *et al.* (1979) surveyed 2400 out of 2800 farms in California to determine the prevalence of mycoplasmal mastitis in dairy cows. Censuses can be expensive and may be difficult or impossible to conduct. However, if a survey is designed well then a reasonably accurate **estimate** of a variable can be made by examining some of the animals in the relevant population, that is, a **sample**.

## Sampling: some basic concepts

The validity of sampling theory is based on the assumption that an aggregate of units can be divided into representative subunits and that characteristics of the aggregate can be estimated from the subunits.

### Some definitions

The **target population** is the total population about which information is required. Ideally, this should be the population at risk.

The **study population** is the population from which a sample is drawn.

Ideally, these two populations should be the same. However, for reasons of practicality, this is often not possible. For instance, if an investigation of periodontitis in Maltese terriers were to be undertaken, then, ideally, all Maltese terriers (the target population) should be sampled, although it may only be possible to investigate animals at dog shows or attending veterinary practices (the study population). If the study population is not 'representative' of the target population, results should not be generalized beyond the study population.

Before a sample is taken, members of the study population must be identified by constructing a list; this is the **sampling frame**. Each member of the sampling frame is a **sampling unit**. Thus, a list of hunting licence receipts was used as the sampling frame to identify hunters in an investigation of the recreational importance of feral pigs in relation to the possible control of African swine fever in the USA (Degner *et al.*, 1983). A register of veterinarians can provide a sampling frame for sampling veterinary practices.

The **sampling fraction** is the ratio of sample size to study population size. Thus, if 10 animals were chosen from 1000 the sampling fraction would be 1%.

Veterinary sampling frames include lists of abattoirs, farms and veterinary practices and can be constructed from some of the other sources of data described in Chapter 10. The objective of sampling is to provide an unbiased estimate of the variable that is being measured in the population. Many veterinary sampling frames (e.g. abattoirs) themselves relate to biased sectors of the total animal population and so caution must be exercised when extrapolating results to other sectors (e.g. farms).

However, biased estimates can also be produced **within** a sampling frame when:

(1) lists of members of the frame are incomplete;
(2) information is obsolescent;
(3) segments of the frame are untraceable;
(4) there is lack of cooperation by some members of the frame;
(5) sampling procedures are not random (*see below*).

These sources of bias are **non-compensating errors** because they cannot be reduced by increasing the size of the sample.

## Types of sampling

There are two main types of sampling:

(1) **non-probability sampling** in which the choice of the sample is left to the investigator;
(2) **probability sampling** in which the selection of the sample is made using a **deliberate**, **random** process.

There are obvious cases when a non-random sample might result in biased estimates. For instance, if a survey were undertaken to estimate the prevalence of lameness in cattle, and if a sample were selected by choosing the first 10 out of 100 animals that entered a milking parlour, the sample would probably underestimate the prevalence because the leading animals would be less likely to be lame than those who entered the parlour last. In other cases, the selection procedure may not induce bias as obviously as in this example, but bias may nevertheless occur. Selection of a **random sample** will ensure that **each animal in a group has an equal probability of being selected** and therefore will reduce selection bias.

There are several ways of selecting a random sample. For instance, each animal in the study population could be represented by a numbered piece of paper in a hat. The desired number of pieces of paper, corresponding to the sample size, could then be drawn from the hat to identify the sample members. This method assumes that selection is random, and could be laborious for large study populations. A more convenient and less haphazard way of random selection uses **random numbers**. These are listed in published tables and can also be generated by computers. Appendix VI includes a random number table and an example of random selection.

A common non-probability sampling technique is **purposive** selection. Two frequently used probability sampling techniques are **simple random** and **systematic** sampling.

### Purposive selection

Purposive selection is the choice of a sample, the averages of whose quantitative characteristics (e.g. weight) or distribution of whose qualitative characteristics (e.g. sex and breed) are similar to those of the target population. The object is to select a sample where characteristics are **balanced** with those of the target population. For example, a veterinarian who is undertaking a tuberculosis test on several herds may be asked to take blood samples from a 'representative' (i.e. balanced) sample for titration of antibodies against various bacteria and viruses. When convenience is the main criterion for selecting a sample, it is very unlikely that the sample will be truly representative of the study population. Purposive selection of so-called 'average' samples can produce a sample, none of whose members is far from the population mean. This sample therefore will only be representative of those collections of sampling units for which none of the members is far from the population mean. The sample will not be representative of all the possible samples that may be taken from the population, some of which will have means far from the population mean. Therefore the variability of the **population** that is being sampled may be underestimated. Additionally, experience and experimental evidence have demonstrated that consciously selected 'representative' samples are always biased. Yates (1981) discusses the disadvantages of purposive selection in detail.

Despite its disadvantages, purposive selection may be the only way of providing information quickly and cheaply, and may be necessary when financial resources are limited. However, care must be taken in extrapolating the results of surveys based on this method of sampling to the target population.

### Simple random sampling

A simple random sample is selected by drawing up a list of **all** animals in the study population, and then selecting the sampling units randomly, for example, by using random number tables.

### Systematic sampling

Systematic sampling involves selection of sampling units at equal intervals, the first animal being selected randomly. For example, if one animal in every 100 were required, the first animal would be selected randomly from the first 100. If this were animal 63, then the sample would comprise animals 63, 163, 263, 363 and so on. Systematic sampling is used frequently in industrial quality control, such as selecting samples of goods on a conveyor belt.

## Simple random v. systematic sampling

A systematic sample does not require knowledge of the total size of the study population. A simple random sample, however, can only be selected when all of the animals in the study population are identified. If lists are available with which to compile the sampling frame (e.g. lists of farms) the random sample can be selected relatively easily. However, if lists are not available it may be difficult—even impossible—to draw up the sampling frame and therefore to select the random sample.

Systematic samples tend to be more evenly spread in the population than random samples. However, the technique can be dangerous if there is periodicity in the sampling frame. For example, if a farmer only sends his animals to slaughter on Tuesdays, and abattoir samples are only selected on Wednesdays, then that farmer's animals will not be represented in the samples.

# Surveys

A survey may be conducted to estimate either a continuous variable, such as weight and milk yield, or discrete events. The commonest application of surveys in epidemiology is estimation of disease prevalence, which is based upon a discrete binomial event (presence or absence of disease). The discussion of surveys in this chapter is therefore limited to estimation of prevalence; the statistics are those used in estimating proportions.

Simple random and systematic sampling can be used to estimate prevalence. In practice, these techniques are used either alone or in combination as part of more complex survey designs. Three main designs are used: **stratified random sampling**, **cluster sampling** and **multistage sampling**.

## Stratified random sampling

A stratified random sample is obtained by dividing the study population into exclusive groups (**strata**), then randomly sampling all of the individual strata. The strata may be different ranges of herd or flock size or different geographical regions. Stratification can improve the accuracy of a sample because it overcomes the tendency of a simple random sample to either over- or under-represent some sections of the sampling frame. For example, if a simple random sample of all herds in a country were being selected then small herds would be just as likely to be included in the sample as large herds; the animals in large herds would therefore be under-represented. Conversely, if a random sample of animals were being selected, animals in small herds would be less likely to be selected than those in large

herds, in which case small herds would be under-represented. Stratification, which ensures that each group in the population is represented, overcomes this problem. Generally, if stratification is practised only to improve the precision of an estimate, then it is not worth having more than five or six strata (Cochran, 1977); two or three are often adequate.

The number of animals selected from each stratum is usually proportional to the number of animals in each stratum. For instance, if a sample of cows were required from the British dairy herd by region, the number of cows selected from each region should be proportional to the number of cows in each region to ensure that cows in regions with large numbers of dairy cattle are not under-represented. *Table 14.1* illustrates this method of selection based on a 5% sampling fraction. This is one method that can be used for determining the number of animals selected from a region, but it assumes equal variability in the measured variables and equal cost in obtaining these measurements. If these assumptions are not true, then other, more complex, methods should be used (*see* Scheaffer *et al.*, 1979).

**Table 14.1 An example of stratification: selection of a stratified random sample of cows from different regions of Great Britain based on a 5% sample of all cows (147 400). (Data extracted from Wilson *et al.*, 1983)**

| Region | Number of cows | Number sampled |
|---|---|---|
| Devon and Cornwall | 302 647 | 302 647 × 0.05 = 15 132 |
| SW England other than Devon and Cornwall | 469 486 | 469 486 × 0.05 = 23 474 |
| S England | 271 225 | 271 225 × 0.05 = 13 561 |
| E England | 119 835 | 119 835 × 0.05 =  5 992 |
| East Midlands | 189 817 | 189 817 × 0.05 =  9 491 |
| West Midlands | 462 826 | 462 826 × 0.05 = 23 141 |
| Wales | 342 346 | 342 346 × 0.05 = 17 117 |
| Yorkshire/Lancashire | 255 626 | 255 626 × 0.05 = 12 781 |
| N England | 273 838 | 273 838 × 0.05 = 13 692 |
| Scotland | 260 366 | 260 366 × 0.05 = 13 018 |
| *Totals* | 2 948 012 | 147 399 |

## Cluster sampling

Sometimes, strata are defined by geographical locations, such as different counties and shires. Sampling of these strata can be time-consuming and costly. This disadvantage can be overcome by selecting a few strata, and sampling the animals only in these strata. Such strata are called **clusters**. This technique is sometimes used when there is an incomplete list of all members of a population. Although the technique is convenient and relatively cheap, information is less precise than if either a systematic or random sample containing the same number of animals were selected, because disease prevalence tends to be more variable **between** groups than **within** them.

### Multistage sampling

Multistage sampling is the selection of a sample in two or more stages, for example randomly sampling dairy herds and then randomly sampling calves in each herd selected.

## *What sample size should be selected?*

The question that must be answered in all sample surveys is: how many animals should be chosen for the survey? The answer cannot be given without considering the objectives and circumstances of the investigation. A survey of disease prevalence can involve:

(1) a single sample, either to determine prevalence or to determine whether or not a disease is present in a group of animals;
(2) two samples, to compare prevalence;
(3) three or more samples (e.g. in experiments to investigate the efficacy of drug therapy).

The first situation is commonly encountered in epidemiological investigations and is discussed in detail in this section.

The choosing of sample size depends on both non-statistical and statistical considerations. The former include the availability of manpower and sampling frames. The latter are the desired **precision** of the estimate of prevalence and the **expected frequency** of the disease.

### Precision of the estimate of prevalence

The ability of an estimator to determine the true population value of a variable (i.e. the estimator's precision) can be expressed in terms of the bound on the error of estimation that can be tolerated. The error can be defined either absolutely or relatively. For example, an acceptable absolute error of ± 2% of a prevalence of 40% represents an acceptable range of 38–42%. A relative error of ± 2% of the same prevalence corresponds to ± 2% of 40%, that is 40% ± 0.8%, representing an acceptable range of 39.2–40.8%.

### Expected frequency of the disease

It may appear paradoxical to suggest that some idea of disease frequency (i.e. prevalence) is necessary before a survey is undertaken, because the objective of the survey is to determine the prevalence. However, a general notion is required: if the prevalence is thought to be close to either 0% or 100% then the confidence interval for a given sample size will be smaller than if the prevalence were close to 50% (*Table 14.2*), that is, fewer animals will be required in the sample to achieve a stipulated width of confidence interval in the former case. Information on prevalence might be obtained from other related surveys. However, frequently this information is not available and so estimates have to be made that may be little more than informed guesses ('guestimates').

## *Estimation of disease prevalence*

### Sampling from a large (theoretically infinite) population

The approximate sample size required to estimate disease prevalence can be determined using *Table 14.2*. The table lists expected prevalence and the desired precision within 10%, 5% and 1% at three levels of confidence (90%, 95% and 99%), the confidence limits indicating the specified bounds within which the estimate will lie with those degrees

**Table 14.2 The approximate sample size required to estimate prevalence in a large population with the desired fixed width confidence limits. (Modified from Cannon and Roe, 1982)**

| Expected prevalence | Level of confidence | | | | | | | | |
|---|---|---|---|---|---|---|---|---|---|
| | 90% | | | 95% | | | 99% | | |
| | *Desired absolute precision* | | | *Desired absolute precision* | | | *Desired absolute precision* | | |
| | *10%* | *5%* | *1%* | *10%* | *5%* | *1%* | *10%* | *5%* | *1%* |
| 10% | 24 | 97 | 2435 | 35 | 138 | 3457 | 60 | 239 | 5971 |
| 20% | 43 | 173 | 4329 | 61 | 246 | 6147 | 106 | 425 | 10616 |
| 30% | 57 | 227 | 5682 | 81 | 323 | 8067 | 139 | 557 | 13933 |
| 40% | 65 | 260 | 6494 | 92 | 369 | 9220 | 159 | 637 | 15923 |
| 50% | 68 | 271 | 6764 | 96 | 384 | 9604 | 166 | 663 | 16587 |
| 60% | 65 | 260 | 6494 | 92 | 369 | 9220 | 159 | 637 | 15923 |
| 70% | 57 | 227 | 5682 | 81 | 323 | 8067 | 139 | 557 | 13933 |
| 80% | 43 | 173 | 4329 | 61 | 246 | 6147 | 106 | 425 | 10616 |
| 90% | 24 | 97 | 2435 | 35 | 138 | 3457 | 60 | 239 | 5971 |

of confidence. The figure quoted for precision is an absolute one. For instance, if the true prevalence were 40% then an estimate precise to within 10% would be one in the interval 30–50%.

As an example of the calculation of sample size, suppose that the true prevalence is thought to be about 40%, and it is desired to estimate this with an absolute precision of 5% at the 95% level of confidence, then 369 animals are required. **Note that the sample size is independent of the total number of animals in the population**. This is because prevalence is a proportion: the larger the study population the greater also the number of diseased animals.

In this example, the use of 40% might be based on prior evidence. In other circumstances the approximate prevalence might not be known. A suitable procedure would be either to choose the 50% figure, or to select the 20% figure and take more samples if necessary.

Appendix VII can also be used. The figures in this appendix give the required sample sizes for various prevalence values at either the 95% or 99% confidence limits. Using the same example of a 40% expected prevalence, the sample would be selected using Figure 5 of the appendix, giving a sample size of approximately 400 (judged by eye from the curve) at the 95% confidence level.

## Sampling from a small (finite) population

*Table 14.2* is constructed using the Normal approximation to the binomial distribution. This is acceptable if the size of the study population is large in relation to the sample. However, as the size of the sample relative to the study population increases, the variance of the estimator of the mean of the study population is decreased and the width of the confidence interval is reduced accordingly. Therefore, in relatively small populations, it is possible to select a smaller sample than one from a theoretically infinite population to achieve the same degree of precision.

The required sample size, $n$, is given by the following formula:

$$\frac{1}{n} = \frac{1}{n_\infty} + \frac{1}{N}$$

where $n_\infty$ is the sample size, based on an infinite population (obtained from *Table 14.2*) and $N$ is the size of the study population.

For example, if prevalence were to be estimated using values similar to those in the example above, but in a small study population, say 900 animals, then:

$$n_\infty = 369$$
$$N = 900$$

therefore

$$\frac{1}{n} = \frac{1}{369} + \frac{1}{900}$$

$$= .00271 + 00111 = .00382$$

$$= \frac{1}{262}$$

Thus, the number of animals required to estimate prevalence to the same degree of precision as the example above (which was based on an infinite population) is 262.

It is difficult to give a strict rule regarding application of this formula; if there is any doubt the formula should be applied and compared with the value given in *Table 14.2*.

## Detecting the presence of disease

If an investigator only wishes to know whether or not a disease is present in a group of animals (rather than determining the prevalence) a suitable sample size can be selected using the formula:

$$n = \text{(approximately) } \{1 - (1-\alpha)^{1/d}\}\{N - \frac{d}{2}\} + 1$$

where:  $N$ = the population size
  $d$ = the number of diseased animals in the population
  $n$ = the required sample size
  $1 - \alpha$ = the desired confidence level (i.e. the probability of finding at least one case of disease in the sample)

*Table 14.3* lists the sample sizes, at the 95% confidence level, for detecting at least one case of disease for various prevalence values and sizes of sampling frame, offering a rapid means of determining sample size, rather than working the formula given above. For example, if the expected prevalence is 25% and the population size is 120, then 10 animals need to be sampled to be 95% certain of detecting at least one case.

If a sample has been selected and no cases have been detected, the upper limit to the number of cases that may be present can be estimated using:

$$d = \{1 - (1-\alpha)^{1/n}\}\{N - \frac{n}{2}\} + 1$$

where $d$, $n$, $N$ and $\alpha$ follow the same notation as above.

*Table 14.3* can also be used for this estimation. For instance, if 25% of 1400 animals were sampled and found to be disease-free, the upper limit of diseased animals, at the 95% confidence level, is 11 Similar tables, constructed for 90% and 9ᶜ confidence limits, are listed in Cannon and (1982).

.1% = 1/1000
.01% = 1/10,000
.001% = 1/100,000
.0001% = 1/1,000,000

**Table 14.3 Sample size required for detecting disease (i); upper confidence limits for number of cases at the 95% level of confidence (ii). (From Cannon and Roe, 1982)**

| Population size (N) | (i) Percentage of diseased animals in population (d/N) OR (ii) Percentage sampled and found clean (n/N) | | | | | | | | | | | |
|---|---|---|---|---|---|---|---|---|---|---|---|---|
| | 50% | 40% | 30% | 25% | 20% | 15% | 10% | 5% | 2% | 1% | 0.5% | 0.1% |
| 10 | 4 | 5 | 6 | 7 | 8 | 10 | 10 | 10 | 10 | 10 | 10 | 10 |
| 20 | 4 | 6 | 7 | 9 | 10 | 12 | 16 | 19 | 20 | 20 | 20 | 20 |
| 30 | 4 | 6 | 8 | 9 | 11 | 14 | 19 | 26 | 30 | 30 | 30 | 30 |
| 40 | 5 | 6 | 8 | 10 | 12 | 15 | 21 | 31 | 40 | 40 | 40 | 40 |
| 50 | 5 | 6 | 8 | 10 | 12 | 16 | 22 | 35 | 48 | 50 | 50 | 50 |
| 60 | 5 | 6 | 8 | 10 | 12 | 16 | 23 | 38 | 55 | 60 | 60 | 60 |
| 70 | 5 | 6 | 8 | 10 | 13 | 17 | 24 | 40 | 62 | 70 | 70 | 70 |
| 80 | 5 | 6 | 8 | 10 | 13 | 17 | 24 | 42 | 68 | 79 | 80 | 80 |
| 90 | 5 | 6 | 8 | 10 | 13 | 17 | 25 | 43 | 73 | 87 | 90 | 90 |
| 100 | 5 | 6 | 9 | 10 | 13 | 17 | 25 | 45 | 78 | 96 | 100 | 100 |
| 120 | 5 | 6 | 9 | 10 | 13 | 18 | 26 | 47 | 86 | 111 | 120 | 120 |
| 140 | 5 | 6 | 9 | 11 | 13 | 18 | 26 | 48 | 92 | 124 | 139 | 140 |
| 160 | 5 | 6 | 9 | 11 | 13 | 18 | 27 | 49 | 97 | 136 | 157 | 160 |
| 180 | 5 | 6 | 9 | 11 | 13 | 18 | 27 | 50 | 101 | 146 | 174 | 180 |
| 200 | 5 | 6 | 9 | 11 | 13 | 18 | 27 | 51 | 105 | 155 | 190 | 200 |
| 250 | 5 | 6 | 9 | 11 | 14 | 18 | 27 | 53 | 112 | 175 | 228 | 250 |
| 300 | 5 | 6 | 9 | 11 | 14 | 18 | 28 | 54 | 117 | 189 | 260 | 300 |
| 350 | 5 | 6 | 9 | 11 | 14 | 18 | 28 | 54 | 121 | 201 | 287 | 350 |
| 400 | 5 | 6 | 9 | 11 | 14 | 19 | 28 | 55 | 124 | 211 | 311 | 400 |
| 450 | 5 | 6 | 9 | 11 | 14 | 19 | 28 | 55 | 127 | 218 | 331 | 450 |
| 500 | 5 | 6 | 9 | 11 | 14 | 19 | 28 | 56 | 129 | 225 | 349 | 500 |
| 600 | 5 | 6 | 9 | 11 | 14 | 19 | 28 | 56 | 132 | 235 | 379 | 597 |
| 700 | 5 | 6 | 9 | 11 | 14 | 19 | 28 | 57 | 134 | 243 | 402 | 691 |
| 800 | 5 | 6 | 9 | 11 | 14 | 19 | 28 | 57 | 136 | 249 | 421 | 782 |
| 900 | 5 | 6 | 9 | 11 | 14 | 19 | 28 | 57 | 137 | 254 | 437 | 868 |
| 1000 | 5 | 6 | 9 | 11 | 14 | 19 | 29 | 57 | 138 | 258 | 450 | 950 |
| 1200 | 5 | 6 | 9 | 11 | 14 | 19 | 29 | 57 | 140 | 264 | 471 | 1102 |
| 1400 | 5 | 6 | 9 | 11 | 14 | 19 | 29 | 58 | 141 | 269 | 487 | 1236 |
| 1600 | 5 | 6 | 9 | 11 | 14 | 19 | 29 | 58 | 142 | 272 | 499 | 1354 |
| 1800 | 5 | 6 | 9 | 11 | 14 | 19 | 29 | 58 | 143 | 275 | 509 | 1459 |
| 2000 | 5 | 6 | 9 | 11 | 14 | 19 | 29 | 58 | 143 | 277 | 517 | 1553 |
| 3000 | 5 | 6 | 9 | 11 | 14 | 19 | 29 | 58 | 145 | 284 | 542 | 1895 |
| 4000 | 5 | 6 | 9 | 11 | 14 | 19 | 29 | 58 | 146 | 268 | 556 | 2108 |
| 5000 | 5 | 6 | 9 | 11 | 14 | 19 | 29 | 59 | 147 | 290 | 564 | 2253 |
| 6000 | 5 | 6 | 9 | 11 | 14 | 19 | 29 | 59 | 147 | 291 | 569 | 2358 |
| 7000 | 5 | 6 | 9 | 11 | 14 | 19 | 29 | 59 | 147 | 292 | 573 | 2437 |
| 8000 | 5 | 6 | 9 | 11 | 14 | 19 | 29 | 59 | 147 | 293 | 576 | 2498 |
| 9000 | 5 | 6 | 9 | 11 | 14 | 19 | 29 | 59 | 148 | 294 | 579 | 2548 |
| 10000 | 5 | 6 | 9 | 11 | 14 | 19 | 29 | 59 | 148 | 294 | 581 | 2588 |
| ∞ | 5 | 6 | 9 | 11 | 14 | 19 | 29 | 59 | 149 | 299 | 598 | 2995 |

The table gives:

(i) the sample size ($n$) required to be 95% certain of including at least one positive if the disease is present at the specified level;

(ii) the upper limit to the number ($d$) of diseased animals in a population given that the specified proportion were tested and found to be negative.

Examples:

(i) expected proportion of positives is 2%; the population size is 480—use 500; from the table, a sample of 129 is required to be 95% certain of detecting at least one positive;

(ii) for a population of 1000, a sample of 10% were all found to be negative; from the table, the 95% confidence limit for the number of positives is 29.

The probability of detecting at least one positive animal, with various sampling fractions, is given in Appendix VIII. The probability of **failing** to detect positive animals for various sample sizes and prevalence values is given in Appendix IX.

## The cost of surveys

Sampling the study population incurs a cost. For example, sampling of cows to determine the prevalence of mastitis by bacteriological examination of milk specimens involves a laboratory cost. The most economic sample size can be determined with defined precision. Alternatively, if a fixed amount of money is available, then the sample size can be determined to maximize precision. Scheaffer *et al.* (1979) describe techniques of estimating sample size for simple random, stratified, systematic and cluster sampling that include **cost functions** in the estimations. An example of estimation of optimum sample size for a fixed cost, relating to a national British bovine mastitis survey, is given by Wilson *et al.* (1983).

## Collecting information: questionnaires

Information that is required for studies and surveys may be available in existing records, for example, those kept at abattoirs, diagnostic laboratories and veterinary clinics. However, there are occasions when the necessary information is not readily available, in which case it must be collected. A common means of collecting information is the **questionnaire**: a set of written questions. Technical information acquired from specialists, such as veterinary practitioners and laboratory staff, is recorded in a standardized fashion on a specialized questionnaire called a **pro-forma**. An example has already been given (*see Figure 11.3*). The person who answers the questionnaire is termed the **respondent**.

## Structure of a questionnaire

The questionnaire is designed to record information:

(1) in a standard format;
(2) with a means of checking and editing recorded data;
(3) by a standardized method of questioning;
(4) with a means of coding.

Questions may be either **open-ended** or **closed**.

### Open-ended questions

These allow the respondent freedom to answer in his or her own words, for example 'What is your opinion of intramammary preparation X?' The chief advantage of the open question is the freedom of expression that it allows: the respondent is allowed to comment, pass opinions and discuss other events that are related to the question's topic. The disadvantages are, first, that the open questions can increase the length of time taken to complete a questionnaire and, secondly, that the answers cannot be coded when the questionnaire is designed, because the full range of answers is not known. A range of answers may be difficult to categorize and code. Continuous variables can be grouped into intervals, for example 0.0–1.9 kg, 2.0–2.9 kg, for coding.

### Closed questions

Closed questions have a fixed number of options of answers. The questions may be **dichotomous**, that is, with two possible answers, such as 'Do you use intramammary tube X for dry cow therapy?—answer yes or no'. Alternatively, the questions may be **multiple choice**, for example 'When did your dog last have a litter?—within the last 3 months, 4–6 months, 7–11 months, or 1–5 years.'

Closed questions are useful for ascertaining categorical, discrete data, such as breed and sex. The advantages of the closed question are ease of analysis and coding because of the limited, fixed response that is allowed. Codes can be allocated when the questionnaire is designed. The closed question is also quick to answer. A major disadvantage is that, because the options of answers are fixed, the answers may not reveal related events that may be significant.

### Coding

Questionnaires are frequently coded to facilitate transcription to computerized recording systems. Coding has already been discussed in detail in Chapter 9. Each question and each possible answer is coded. For example, in the question:

26. What is the sex of your animal?—
enter 1 if male and 2 if female   □

the question is coded as number 26, and the options to the answers to the dichotomous question are coded as either 1 or 2. The name of the respondent may be coded if confidentiality is required. It is also desirable to justify numeric answers to the right for transcription to computerized systems. For example, the date 8 March 1985 is coded as:

| 0 | 8 | 0 | 3 | 8 | 5 |
|---|---|---|---|---|---|

**not**:

| 8 | 3 | 8 | 5 |   |   |
|---|---|---|---|---|---|

to allow for 31 days in the month and 12 months in the year.

## INVESTIGATION OF JOHNE'S VACCINATED HERDS

Conducted by: The Epidemiology Unit, Central Veterinary Laboratory, Weybridge, Surrey.

*PLEASE NOTE ALL INFORMATION WILL BE TREATED AS STRICTLY CONFIDENTIAL*

Herd Owner _____ 1. Herd Code _____

Address _____

_____

2. Present herd type:  Dairy ☐  Beef ☐  Mixed ☐

3. Replacement policy. Entirely home reared. Please write YES or NO _____

4. % breed composition of present adult herd _____

5. Present adult herd size _____

6. Present system of winter housing:  Cowshed ☐  Cubicles ☐  Loose ☐  Outwintered ☐

7. Method of pasture utilization:  Intensive ☐  Extensive ☐

8. Date of approval for use _____ / _____ /19 _____

9. Year in which vaccination started 19 _____

10. If vaccination has been intermittent please give the years in which either vaccine was not used or in which only some of the animals

retained for breeding were vaccinated _____

_____

11. Year in which vaccination ceased. 19 _____  Write NA if not applicable _____

12. Average number of clinical cases of Johne's disease per year prior to vaccination _____ cases

13. Adult herd size at start of vaccination _____

14. Number of clinical cases occurring in each year since vaccination started:

| Years since start of vaccination | Number of clinical cases | Years since start of vaccination | Number of clinical cases |
|---|---|---|---|
| 1 | | 5 | |
| 2 | | 6 | |
| 3 | | 7 | |
| 4 | | 8 | |

If clinical cases occurred 9 years or more after start of vaccination please specify which year(s)

_____

_____

15. Have there been any major changes in breed since vaccination started? Please write YES or NO _____

If 'YES', please specify change with approximate date from _____ to _____ in 19 ____

16. Have there been any changes in herd type since vaccination started? Please write YES or NO _____

If 'YES', please specify change with approximate date from _____ to _____ in 19 ____

17. Have any attempts been made to identify latently infected animals? Please write YES or NO _____

If 'YES', please specify diagnostic methods used:  CFT ☐  Johnin ☐  Microsc. Exam ☐  Faeces Culture ☐

and whether positive animals were called:  Always ☐  Sometimes ☐  Never ☐

18. Please indicate which of the following control measures are practised on the farm:

Please write YES or NO

(a) prompt removal of confirmed clinical cases _____

(b) only 'bucket' rearing of calves (in dairy herds) _____

(c) adequate separation of calves from adults (in dairy herds) _____

(d) removal from herd of calves born of infected dams _____

(e) adequate hygiene of food and water supplies to housed animals _____

(f) piped water supplies to all cattle at pasture _____

(g) prevention of access to ponds and ditches etc. _____

(h) calves grazed on pastures not used by adult cattle _____

19. Have any other changes in management been instituted to control the disease?

_____

_____

_____

20. Do you think the vaccine has had a valuable part to play in the control of Johne's disease in this herd. Please write YES or NO

_____

GENERAL COMMENTS

*THANK YOU FOR YOUR CO-OPERATION IN THIS INVESTIGATION.*

The completed questionnaire should be sent to:

J. W. Wilesmith, B.V.Sc., M.R.C.V.S.
Epidemiology Unit,
Central Veterinary Laboratory,
New Haw,
Weybridge,
Surrey KT14 3NB.

**Figure 14.1** A questionnaire: survey of Johne's disease in vaccinated cattle in Great Britain. (From MAFF, 1976)

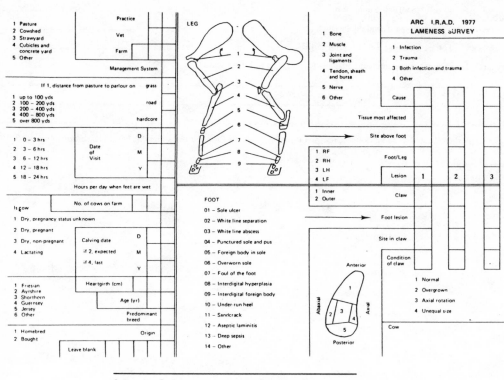

| Code | Term | Description |
|------|------|-------------|
| 01 | Sole ulcer | Circumscribed pododermatitis at sole-heel junction, with or without protrusion of granulation tissue through horn defect |
| 02 | White line separation | Breakdown of integument of white line, usually abaxially, and impaction of foreign material into crack |
| 03 | White line abscess | Breakdown of integument of white line, usually abaxially, and occurrence of septic laminitis of wall |
| 04 | Punctured sole and pus | Traumatic penetration of solar horn with infection of laminae and pus production |
| 05 | Foreign body in sole | Self-explanatory |
| 06 | Overworn sole | Sole which is obviously flexible, horn usually not more than 3mm thick, often discoloured laminae due to haemorrhagic bruising |
| 07 | Foul of the foot | Interdigital necrosis affecting skin and, or, subcutaneous tissues |
| 08 | Interdigital hyperplasia | Thick interdigital skin fold, often with localised areas of pressure necrosis or ulceration as secondary feature |
| 09 | Interdigital foreign body | Self-explanatory |
| 10 | Underrun heel | Separation of heel horn axially towards sole-heel junction, usually with some exposure and infection of sensitive laminae; erosion of heel horn |
| 11 | Sandcrack | Vertical split in wall horn at coronet or lower down, involving sensitive tissues |
| 12 | Aseptic laminitis | Generalised digital pain and heat, often involving more than one foot, and without break in integument |
| 13 | Deep sepsis | Self-explanatory |
| 14 | Other | |

**Figure 14.2** A questionnaire: survey of lameness in cattle in Great Britain. Respondents were requested to indicate which categories were appropriate to their farm and cattle. (From Russell *et al.*, 1982a)

## *Designing a questionnaire*

The success of a questionnaire depends on careful design. Ideally, everyone who is issued with a questionnaire should complete it. The proportion of those who respond is the **response rate** (usually expressed as a percentage). The **non-response rate** is therefore 100 − response rate (%); for example, a response rate of 70% represents a non-response rate of 30%. Non-response from a respondent may be either total, in which the questionnaire is not returned, or partial, in which some questions are not answered but the partially answered questionnaire is returned. Good questionnaire design decreases both types of non-response.

### Initial presentation

The title of the questionnaire should be brief and accurate. A polite letter, explaining the reason for producing the questionnaire and the value of the results deriving from its completion, should be enclosed. The inclusion of a reply-paid envelope should increase the response rate.

### Wording

Wording should be unambiguous, brief, polite, unemotional, and (unless a pro-forma is used) non-technical. If technical terms are used they should be defined simply. Common ambiguous terms include 'often', 'occasionally', 'severe', 'mild', 'heavy' and 'light'. Double negatives should be avoided. Each question should contain only **one** idea. Sensitive, emotive and emotional questions should be avoided.

### Question sequence

Related questions may need to be separated because the answer given to one question may influence that given to the succeeding question, producing the phenomenon termed 'carry over'. General questions should be presented first, and specific ones later. The questionnaire can be made more interesting by 'branching out' from one question to another, for example, 'If you answer yes to question 2, then move to question 8'.

### Question structure

Closed questions must be **mutually exclusive** and **exhaustive**. For example, the age of animals may be expressed as:

Age (please tick): under 6 months ☐
6–12 months ☐
over 12 months ☐

In this case, there is no overlap of ages between categories (they are mutually exclusive) and all possible ages are included (the options are exhaustive). To ensure exhaustiveness, it may be necessary to include **dumping categories** that accommodate all possibilities remaining after the specified options are considered. For example, 'other' is a dumping category in:

Against what infections has your dog been vaccinated? (please tick)
distemper ☐   parvovirus ☐   hepatitis ☐
leptospirosis ☐   other ☐

Lack of confidentiality may increase the non-response rate. Total anonymity ensures confidentiality but prevents the tracing back of information (e.g. of diseased animals to a farm). A limited degree of confidentiality can be ensured by preventing identification of respondents by the majority of the data processing staff. Three ways of doing this are:

(1) by having a separate sheet of paper for the respondent's name and address, with a code identifying the respondent on the questionnaire;
(2) by using a coded strip down one side of the questionnaire, which can be detached;
(3) by using carbon-impregnated paper (NCR paper), allowing duplicates to be produced, but with the respondent's name masked off most of the copies.

*Figures 14.1* and *14.2* are two examples of questionnaires. In the first example (a survey of Johne's disease in vaccinated herds) the following concepts can be demonstrated:

(1) closed questions (e.g. No. 2);
(2) open-ended questions (e.g. No. 19);
(3) mutual exclusiveness and exhaustiveness (e.g. No. 17);
(4) a clear title, with a statement of confidentiality;
(5) a polite presentation (e.g. the last portion of the questionnaire that thanks the respondent for his or her cooperation).

In the second example (a lameness survey in cattle), these additional concepts are illustrated:

(1) a dumping category (the inclusion of '6. other' in the description of breeds);
(2) confidential coding of the veterinary practice and veterinarian (2 digits) and farm (3 digits);
(3) a clear description and definition of terms that are used (sites and nature of lesions in this example).

Questionnaires can either be completed by respondents after having been delivered to them (frequently by mail), or be completed by an interviewer who presents the questions, verbally, to the respondents.

## Mailed and self-completed questionnaires

### Requirements

The main requirements for a mailed or self-completed questionnaire are:

(1) a list of respondents to act as the sampling frame (e.g. a register of veterinarians);
(2) great clarity: no-one will be present to cope with any difficulties that may arise;
(3) a covering letter politely explaining the reason for sending the questionnaire.

### Advantages

The main advantages of this type of questionnaire are that:

(1) it is relatively cheap with potential for wide coverage;
(2) it is quick and easy to organize;
(3) it avoids interviewer bias (*see below*);
(4) it allows a highly motivated respondent to 'check the facts' over a period of time;
(5) respondents have the opportunity to reply anonymously, which may produce a high response rate.

### Disadvantages

The disadvantages of this type of questionnaire are that:

(1) clarity of question may be difficult to achieve;
(2) the questionnaire cannot prevent reviewing of questions, which may lead to undesirable modification of previously answered questions;
(3) the non-response rate cannot usually be decreased by issuing more questionnaires.

### Factors influencing the response rate

Factors influencing the response rate are:

(1) the sponsor—a respected sponsor should enhance the likelihood of obtaining a high response rate;
(2) the nature of the respondent population—a well-educated group should produce a higher response rate than a poorly educated group.
(3) the subject and aim of the study—if the study is of obvious direct relevance to the respondent, then he is likely to reply;
(4) appearance and length of the questionnaire—if it is attractive and concise, then response should be good;
(5) confidentiality.

## Interviews

A personal interview can overcome the disadvantages of mailed and self-completed questionnaires described above, and is particularly useful where illiteracy of the respondent is a problem. However, interviews can be costly to organize, involving training, payment and travelling expenses of interviewers. The tone of the interviewer's voice may also bias the respondent's answer, by implying a desirable answer (interviewer bias). The use of veterinary interviews is discussed by Ruppanner (1972) and, in developing countries, by Perry and McCauley (1984). Examples of their use include surveys of schistosomiasis in the Sudan (McCauley *et al.*, 1983b), swine fever in Honduras (McCauley, 1985), bovine health and productivity in Zambia (Perry *et al.*, 1984a) and sheep diseases in New Zealand (Simpson and Wright, 1980).

## Testing a questionnaire

Several drafts of a questionnaire are usually required following testing. There are normally two stages to testing: **informal** and **formal**.

### Informal testing

Informal testing is carried out on colleagues who can detect trivia, ambiguities and defects in questionnaire design.

### Formal testing

Formal testing is undertaken on a small random sample of the population on which the full survey will be conducted. This testing is called a **pilot survey**. The size of the sample is chosen using the guidelines given in the first part of this chapter, relating to surveys. The pilot survey exposes further defects in questionnaire design. This survey should **never** be used as part of the full survey, and respondents used in the pilot survey should never be used again in the full one.

## Criteria for success of a questionnaire

The two main criteria for the success of a questionnaire are **reliability** and **validity** (*see* Chapter 9).

### Reliability

A questionnaire, like a diagnostic test, is reliable if it produces consistent results (*see Figure 9.4*). The reliability of a questionnaire can be assessed by issuing the same questions to the same respondents more than once.

## Validity

Validity is a measure of the degree to which answers, on average, reflect the truth (*see Figure 9.4*). Validity is therefore achieved by comparing the results of the questionnaire with an independent reliable criterion, enabling calculation of the sensitivity and specificity of the questions. For example, Selby *et al.* (1973, 1976) compared the results of a mailed questionnaire with information derived from farm records and diaries, when investigating congenital abnormalities in pigs. Similarly, Perry *et al.* (1983), in a survey of several animal diseases in Zambia, compared the results obtained from an owner interview survey with those obtained from an investigation of sentinel herds. Unreliability often means invalidity. However, reliable questions may not always be valid (*see Figure 9.4b*).

Further details of veterinary questionnaires are given by Waltner-Toews (1983).

## *Further reading*

ADEQUACY OF SAMPLE SIZE. Health Statistical Methodology Unit. World Health Organization. Publication HSM/73.1. WHO, Geneva

ATKINSON, J. (1971) *Handbook for Interviewers*. Great Britain Office of Population Census and Surveys. Social Survey Division. Her Majesty's Stationery Office, London

BARNETT, V. (1974) *Elements of Sampling Theory*. The English Universities Press Limited, London

BENNETT, A.E. and RITCHIE, K. (1975) *Questionnaires in Medicine*. Published for the Nuffield Provincial Hospital Trust by the Oxford University Press, London

CASLEY, J.D. and LURY, D.A. (1981) *Data Collection in Developing Countries*. Clarendon Press, Oxford

CANNON, R.M. and ROE, R.T. (1982) *Livestock Disease Surveys: A Field Manual for Veterinarians*. Australian Government Publishing Service, Canberra

LEECH, F.B. and SELLERS, K.C. (1979) *Statistical Epidemiology in Veterinary Science*. Charles Griffin and Company Limited, London and High Wycombe

MOSER, C.A. and KALTON, G. (1971) *Survey Methods in Social Investigation*, 2nd edn. Heinemann Educational Books Limited, London

SARD, D.M. (1979) *Dealing with Data. The Practical Use of Numerical Information*. British Veterinary Association Publications, London

WOODS, A.J. (1985) Sampling in animal health surveys. In: Proceedings of a meeting held at the University of Reading on 27, 28 and 29 March 1985. Ed. Thrusfield, M.V. Pp. 36–54. Society for Veterinary Epidemiology and Preventive Medicine

# 15

# Observational studies

Observational studies (introduced in Chapter 2) are used to identify risk indicators and to estimate the quantitative effects of the various component causes that contribute to the occurrence of disease. The investigations are based on analysis of natural disease occurrence in populations. Observational studies differ from experimental studies in that in the former the investigator cannot randomly allocate factors (disease and hypothesized component causes) to individuals, whereas in the latter the investigator is free to allocate factors to individuals at random.

## The three types of observational study

There are three types of observational study: **cross-sectional**, **case-control** and **cohort**. Each classifies animals into those with and without disease and those with and without exposure to hypothesized causal factors. Therefore, they each generate a 2 × 2 contingency table for each disease/factor relationship (*Table 15.1*). However, the methods of generation differ between the types of study.

The cross-sectional study involves the selection of a total of *n* individuals from a larger population, and then the determination, for each individual, of the presence or absence of attribute A and the **simultaneous** presence or absence of attribute B. In the context of a causal investigation, attribute A would represent a disease, and attribute B would be an hypothesized causal factor (inherent attribute, concomitant exposure to an infectious or non-infectious agent, diet, etc.). At the beginning of a cross-sectional study, only the total number of animals (*n* in *Table 15.1*) is predetermined. The numbers of animals with and without disease A, and

possessing or not possessing attribute B, are not known initially.

A cross-sectional study is usually designed to select a random sample of the target population. This contrasts with cohort and case-control studies which involve stratified sampling of the target population.

In a case-control study, cases and controls are selected at the beginning of, or during, the study. Therefore $a + c$ and $b + d$ in *Table 15.1* are predetermined. Cross-sectional and case-control studies categorize the number of existing cases and therefore are based on the measurement of prevalence. Case-control studies may utilize incidence of prevalence values.

In a cohort study, a group (cohort) of animals exposed to an hypothesized causal factor and a group not exposed to the factor are selected and observed to record development of disease in each group. Therefore, incidence is measured, and $a + b$ and $c + d$ are predetermined.

**Table 15.1 The 2 × 2 contingency table constructed in observational studies to determine the cause of disease**

|  | Diseased animals | Non-diseased animals | Totals |
|---|---|---|---|
| Hypothesized causal factor present | $a$ | $b$ | $a + b$ |
| Hypothesized causal factor absent | $c$ | $d$ | $c + d$ |
| Totals | $a + c$ | $b + d$ | $a + b + c + d = n$ |

In **cross-sectional studies** only $n$ can be predetermined.
In **case-control studies** $(a + c)$ and $(b + d)$ are predetermined.
In **cohort studies** $(a + b)$ and $(c + d)$ are predetermined.

These three types of study attempt to identify a cause by applying the first three of Evans' postulates (*see* Chapter 3; postulates 1 and 3, rephrased here, using 'prevalence' and 'incidence' in their definitions):

(1) the prevalence of a disease should be significantly higher in individuals exposed to the supposed cause than in those who are not (evidence supplied by a cross-sectional study);
(2) exposure to the supposed cause should be present more commonly in those with than those without the disease, when all other risk factors are held constant (evidence supplied by a case-control study);
(3) the incidence of disease should be significantly higher in those exposed to the supposed cause than in those not so exposed (evidence supplied by a cohort study).

## Nomenclature of observational studies

A variety of alternative names have been applied to case-control and cohort studies. Both of these studies consider two events—exposure to an hypothesized causal factor or factors and development of disease—that are separated by a period of time. Because of this temporal separation of the two events, each of these studies is sometimes termed **longitudinal**.

The case-control study compares diseased animals (cases) with non-diseased animals (controls) and therefore has variously been called a **case-comparison**, **case-referent** and **case history study**. This study selects groups according to presence or absence of disease and **looks back** to possible causes; it has therefore sometimes been described as a **retrospective study** (looking back, from effect to cause).

A cohort study selects groups according to presence or absence of exposure to hypothesized causal factors, and then **looks forward** to the development of disease. It has therefore sometimes been called a **prospective study** (looking forward, from cause to effect). *Table 15.2* lists the types of observational study and their synonyms.

The groups may be selected as 'exposed' and 'unexposed' now, and then observed over a period

**Table 15.2 Nomenclature of observational studies**

| Cross-sectional | Longitudinal | |
|---|---|---|
| | *Case-control* | *Cohort* |
| Synonym: | Synonyms: | Synonyms: |
| Prevalence | Retrospective | Prospective |
| | Case-referent | Incidence |
| | Case-comparison | Longitudinal |
| | | Follow-up |

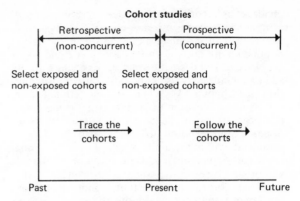

**Cohort studies**

**Figure 15.1** The selection of cohorts in concurrent and non-concurrent cohort studies ('retrospective' and 'prospective' used in the temporal sense). (Modified from Lilienfeld and Lilienfeld, 1980)

of time to identify cases; such a cohort study is termed concurrent (*Figure 15.1*). Alternatively, if reliable records relating to exposure are available, groups may be selected according to presence or absence of previous exposure, and traced to the present to determine disease status; this constitutes a non-concurrent study.

Some investigators use 'retrospective' to refer to any study that records data from the past, and 'prospective' to refer to any study designed to collect future data. Therefore a non-concurrent cohort (prospective, in the causal sense) study alternatively may be termed a retrospective (in the temporal sense) cohort study. Similarly a concurrent cohort study can also be called a prospective (in the temporal sense) cohort study (*Figure 15.1*).

This classification of observational studies into three types is somewhat simplistic. Some studies show characteristics of more than one type. The range of 'hybrid' studies is described by Kleinbaum *et al.* (1982).

## Measures of association used in observational studies

Association between disease and an hypothesized causal factor can be measured in terms of either the absolute **difference** between disease occurrence in 'exposed' and 'unexposed' groups or relatively as the **ratio** of disease occurrence between the two groups. Ratios generally are used because they are more meaningful than absolute differences (*see* Chapter 13). Therefore, the measures of association that are commonly estimated in observational studies are the relative risk and odds ratio.

The relative risk in the study population can be estimated directly in a cohort study, because incidence is recorded in 'exposed' and 'unexposed' groups. However, in case-control studies, the frequencies of *a* and *b*, and *c* and *d* in the target population are not known (because *a* + *c* and *b* + *d* are selected) and so the relative risk can only be estimated indirectly using the odds ratio approximation (*see* Chapter 13). When a cross-sectional study selects a random sample of the target population, the proportions in the target population that are diseased and exposed to factors can be directly estimated, within the limits of sampling error. Thus, the target population's odds ratio can be estimated. Cohort and case-control studies, however, involve a stratified, non-random selection of individuals from the target population; therefore the proportions in the target population cannot be estimated.

## Interpreting results

If the value of the lower confidence limit of the measure of association, be it odds ratio or relative risk, is greater than one, at a defined level of significance, then the association between the hypothesized cause and the disease is statistically significant and it can be said that there is evidence of a positive association. Alternatively, significance can be demonstrated at a defined level using the $\chi^2$-test. The conventional level of significance used in experimental investigation is 5%. This has the effect of restricting the probability of a Type I error—accepting an association when one does not exist— to 0.05. A value for this probability as small as 0.05 is desirable when a particular causal association relating to one factor and a disease is being investigated. This is the so-called 'searchlight' approach which focuses on one factor and is a common aim of cohort studies. However, if a study is undertaken to 'trawl' for any possible causes, the so-called 'bucket' approach to data collection, then the Type II error—the incorrect rejection of a true association—is more important. This is a common aim of case-control studies. In this latter case, a higher level of significance, for example 10% or 20%, with a corresponding lower value for the probability of a Type II error, would be more appropriate in order to reduce the risk of not recognizing true associations.

There is some debate as to whether significance levels or confidence intervals should be used (Jones and Rushton, 1982). A level of significance provides a clear-cut decision boundary which is somewhat artificial. It is now generally accepted that it is better to construct a confidence interval (Rothman, 1978). The interval gives a range that will contain the true value of the measure of association with a certain prespecified probability. The interval provides more than the significance test: it also provides, in an easily interpretable way, a measure of the variability of the data; the wider the interval the more imprecise the inferences to be drawn from the data; the narrower the interval the more precise the inferences are.

Demonstration of a statistically significant association using each of the three observational approaches can fulfil one of Evans' postulates. The credibility of cause is strengthened by fulfilling others of Evans' postulates. Thus, Jarrett's (1980) demonstration of an association between exposure to bracken and the development of intestinal cancer in cattle is more credible because a carcinogen has been isolated from bracken (Wang *et al.*, 1976) (Evans' postulate 10).

## Bias in observational studies

Observational studies are subject to **bias** (*see* Chapter 9). Although many types of bias can occur in observational studies (Sackett, 1979), three are particularly pertinent to observational studies:

(1) selection bias;
(2) misclassification;
(3) confounding.

### Selection bias

Selection bias results from systematic differences between characteristics of the study population and the target population from which it was drawn. Most observational studies use data gathered from convenient populations such as veterinary clinics, abattoirs and particular farms. Willeberg's investigation of the feline urological syndrome in Denmark (Willeberg, 1977), for instance, utilized data collected at a veterinary school's clinic. Ideally, a sample should be selected from the target population (all cats in Denmark in this example), but this is rarely possible. It was stated in the previous chapter that the inferences from investigations that might be biased by selection need to be made with care if they are to be extrapolated to the target population. Consideration should be given to the likelihood of the study population being biased with respect to the disease and factors that are being investigated. Selection bias is unlikely if:

(1) exposure to a factor does not increase the likelihood of an animal being present in the study population;
(2) the likelihood of inclusion of cases and controls in the study population is the same.

For example, Darke *et al.* (1985) investigated the association between the presence of an entire tail (the hypothesized causal factor) and tail injuries (the disease) in a veterinary clinic population to determine whether docking reduces the risk of tail damage. It is improbable that docking or otherwise affects attendance at a veterinary clinic and so selection bias was unlikely in this study.

## Misclassification

Misclassification is a type of measurement bias; it occurs when either diseased animals are classified as non-diseased, or animals without a particular disease are classified as possessing it. The likelihood of misclassification depends on the frequency of disease, the frequency of exposure to the hypothesized causal factor and the sensitivity and specificity of the diagnostic criteria used in the study (*see Figure 9.3*). For example, Thrusfield *et al.* (1985) studied the association between breed, sex and heart valve incompetence in dogs. Animals were classified as being diseased if they had either audible cardiac murmurs or signs of congestive cardiac failure. However, murmurs and cardiac failure can be produced by lesions other than heart valve incompetence—cardiomyopathy and anaemia are examples. Therefore, in order to prevent dogs with the latter two lesions being incorrectly classified as having heart valve incompetence (in which case they would constitute 'false positives') their case records were scrutinized in detail to ascertain the exact nature of their murmurs. Similarly, early heart valve incompetence may not produce audible murmurs, and clinicians may miss the murmurs, in which case animals would be classified incorrectly as disease-free (i.e. 'false negatives').

Two types of misclassification can occur: **non-differential** and **differential**. The former occurs if the magnitude and direction of misclassification are similar in the two groups being compared (i.e. either cases and controls, or exposed and unexposed individuals). Non-differential misclassification produces a shift in the estimated relative risk and odds ratio towards zero (Copeland *et al.*, 1977), depicted in *Figures 15.2a* and *15.2b* respectively. *Figure 15.2a* illustrates that specificity is more important than sensitivity in determining bias in the estimate of relative risk. Even when sensitivity and specificity are seemingly acceptable (90% and 96% respectively, exemplified in *Figure 15.2a*) the relative risk can be severely biased. However, sensitivity plays a more important part as a source of bias in estimation of the odds ratio (*Figure 15.2b*).

Differential misclassification occurs when the magnitude or direction of misclassification is different between the two groups being compared. In this case, the odds ratio and relative risk may be biased in either direction (*see* Copeland *et al.*, 1977, for numerical examples). Therefore, misclassification can not only weaken an apparent association but also strengthen it.

If a simple valid (i.e. highly specific and sensitive) test is not available then there can be difficulty in defining a case in the absence of a rigorous definition. For example, in an investigation of the relationship between enzootic bovine leucosis (EBL) and human leukaemia (Donham *et al.*, 1980), cattle were defined as being exposed to EBL virus when post-mortem examination revealed alimentary lymphosarcoma, even though this lesion may develop without exposure to the virus, and exposure to the virus may not produce alimentary tumours.

Similarly, it may be difficult to define and quantify an hypothesized causal factor to which an animal is

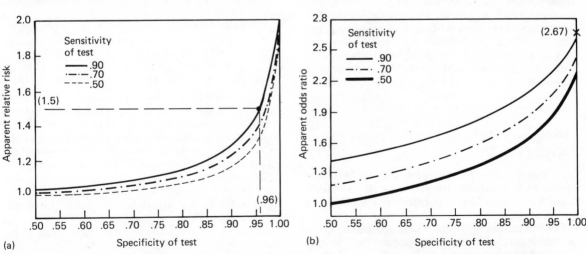

**Figure 15.2 (a)** Cohort study: bias in the estimation of relative risk as a function of sensitivity and specificity. Disease incidence (cumulative) in exposed and unexposed cohorts is 0.10 and 0.05 respectively. True relative risk (exposed and unexposed) equals 2.0. **(b)** Case-control study: bias in the estimation of odds ratio as a function of sensitivity and specificity. Exposure rate in cases and controls 40% and 20% respectively. True odds ratio equals 2.67. (From Copeland *et al.*, 1977)

exposed. For example, if 'inadequate feeding' were the factor, then the investigator may have to rely on an opinion based on owners' descriptions of diet, rather than using the more rigorous results of an examination by a nutritionist.

## Confounding

Confounding has been discussed in detail in Chapter 3 where its effect on the inferring of causal associations has been exemplified. In reiteration, a confounding variable (confounder) is any factor that is either positively or negatively correlated with both the disease and hypothesized causal factors that are being considered. For example, size of herd is a confounding variable in relation to porcine respiratory disease (*see Figure 3.7b*). If fan ventilation were being considered as the factor under study, then the results would be confounded (biased, confused, rendered unrepresentative) if the herds that were fan ventilated and that had respiratory disease comprised all large herds (which are likely to develop the disease), and the herds that were not fan ventilated and were non-diseased comprised all small herds (which are much less likely to develop the disease). The uneven proportion of large and small herds in each group will therefore confound the association between fan ventilation and disease, thereby distorting the estimation of the odds ratio and relative risk.

Confounding is particularly important in case-control studies because animals are chosen according to presence or absence of disease: therefore cases may have a whole range of factors in common, some of which may be causal and some of which may be statistically significant but non-causal, because of an association with a confounder.

Confounding is not an 'all-or-none' event, but occurs to varying degrees. Tests for confounding are discussed by Schlesselman (1982); assessment of the extent of confounding is described by Miettinen (1972) and Ejigou and McHugh (1977). A pictorial representation of confounding is given by Rothman (1975).

## *Controlling bias*

### Selection bias

It is often not possible to control selection bias; this results from inherent characteristics of the study population, and a less biased study population may not be available.

Control can be attempted during either the design or the analysis of the investigation. The former essentially involves avoiding the bias by selecting animals from a population that will not produce the bias. This may be impractical and obviously depends on the investigator being aware of the potential bias.

Control during analysis requires a knowledge of the probability of selection in the study population and the target population. Kleinbaum *et al.* (1982) provide formulae for this correction.

## Misclassification

The control of non-differential and differential misclassification are described by Barron (1977) and Greenland and Kleinbaum (1983) respectively. Essentially, control is effected by algebraic manipulation during analysis, although this is never as satisfactory as using a highly sensitive and specific test to determine diseased and non-diseased animals.

## Confounding

There are two main methods of controlling confounding:

(1) by adjusting for the confounding variable in the analysis, for example by using adjusted rates specific to the confounder (*see* Chapter 4) or by producing a summary relative risk for the combined relative risks of each confounder (Mantel and Haenzel, 1959);

(2) by 'matching' the two groups during the design of the survey; matching can be performed in two ways:

    (a) **frequency matching** in which the groups to be sampled are divided so as to contain the same proportion of the variable, for example, if there are four times as many males as females in the 'case' group, then the 'control' group should also be selected to contain four times as many males as females; this technique therefore is a form of **stratification** (*see* Chapter 14);

    (b) **individual matching** in which each case is matched with a control with respect to the variable, for example, a 6-year-old dog with bladder cancer is paired with a 6-year-old dog without bladder cancer (matching for age).

As a general rule, if the confounding variable is unevenly distributed in the population (e.g. age in relation to chronic nephritis) then it is better to match cases or controls when the study is designed, rather than correct for them in the analysis (all young control animals would, in a sense, be wasted when considering chronic nephritis). It may be cumbersome to match for many possible confounding variables. It is usual to match for the main possible ones: age, sex and breed (i.e. common determinants: *see* Chapter 5). However, it is dangerous to overmatch (Miettinen, 1970). If the effect of a factor is in doubt, it is best not to match but to control it in subsequent analysis; when a factor is matched it cannot be studied separately. It is important to note that when matched studies are conducted they should be analysed as such; the relevant methods are described in Schlesselman (1982). Matching criteria and stratum sizes are discussed by Greenland *et al.* (1981).

These three causes of bias (selection bias, misclassification and confounding) should not be considered in isolation but as an interconnected complex that can distort results.

## Selection of sample size in cohort and case-control studies

Four values should be specified to determine optimum sample size in a cohort study:

(1) the desired level of significance ($\alpha$: the probability of a Type I error—claiming that exposure to a factor is associated with a disease when in fact it is not);
(2) the power of the test ($1-\beta$: the probability of claiming correctly that exposure to a factor is associated with disease, where $\beta$ is the probability of a Type II error);
(3) the incidence of disease in unexposed animals in the target population;
(4) an hypothesized relative risk (odds ratio) that is considered important enough from the point of view of the health of the animal population.

The first, second and fourth values, similarly, should be specified in determining optimum sample size in a case-control study. However, in this study, the third value is the proportion of the target population exposed to the factor.

If a disease is rare, then a cohort study requires a considerable number of animals in the 'exposed' and 'unexposed' groups to detect a significant difference, especially when the relative risk is small. *Table 15.3* illustrates this point. There are various formulae for the calculation of sample size (Snedecor and Cochran, 1980; Schlesselman, 1982) that involve different assumptions about the variance of disease incidence when the relative risk is either 1 or a different value. The figures in *Table 15.3* have been generated using a formula which assumes that:

(1) when the relative risk is 1, the variance is based on the incidence rate in the unexposed population;

**and**

(2) when the relative risk is different from 1, the variance is based on the two incidence rates in the exposed and unexposed populations.

Tables of the smallest and largest detectable relative risks, for different values of these parameters, are given by Walter (1977). A program for determining sample size, which can be used on pocket calculators, is provided by Rothman and Boice (1982). Sample size estimations that include cost functions are described by Pike and Casagrande (1979).

## Multivariate techniques

In case-control studies, if matching is practised to adjust for confounding, then there may be many 2 × 2 contingency tables, for example for different combinations of age, sex and breed. If the disease being investigated is rare then the number of animals in each cell may be very small, resulting in inestimable or large confidence intervals—possibly statistically insignificant—for $R$ and $\psi$. Similarly, if $R$ varies considerably between each contingency table, then the summary relative risk may be small, even though the individual table values are large: information is lost (Bender *et al.*, 1983). These problems can be overcome by using **multivariate** techniques that consider many factors simultaneously. Common methods use a **logistic model** for discrete and continuous variables and a **log linear model** for discrete variables and grouped continuous data. An example is the study of the association between benign and malignant neoplasms in dogs (Bender *et al.*, 1982). Multivariate techniques are not described in this book; details may be found in Kleinbaum *et al.* (1982) and Schlesselman (1982).

## Comparison of the types of observational study

A logical requirement of demonstration of cause is that an animal is exposed to a causal factor **before** disease develops (*see* Chapter 3). The design of cohort studies ensures that this temporal sequence is detected. However, cross-sectional and case-control studies may not detect the sequence. For example, if the association between neutering and urinary incontinence in female dogs were being investigated using a cross-sectional study (neutering being the hypothesized risk factor), then neutered dogs with incontinence may be identified; however, incontinence may have developed before neutering in some of the cases, in which instance neutering could not

**Table 15.3 The estimated number of individuals in each group (exposed and unexposed) for detecting a statistically significant relative risk in a cohort study by relative risk and the incidence rate of disease in the unexposed group.\* (Figures are given to no more than three significant figures)**

| Relative risk | Incidence rate in control group for period of study | | | |
| | 1 per 10 000 | 1 per 1000 | 1 per 500 | 1 per 100 |
|---|---|---|---|---|
| 2 | 143 000 | 14 300 | 7 140 | 1 410 |
| 3 | 40 200 | 4 010 | 2 000 | 396 |
| 4 | 19 700 | 1 960 | 980 | 193 |
| 5 | 12 000 | 1 200 | 599 | 117 |
| 10 | 3 230 | 322 | 160 | 31 |

*Based on the probability of detecting a difference between the two groups of 80% and a significance level of 5%.

**Table 15.4 Comparison of the advantages and disadvantages of cross-sectional, case-control and cohort studies. (Based on Schlesselman, 1982)**

**Cross-sectional studies**
*Advantages*
(1) When a random sample of the target population is selected, proportions exposed and unexposed in the target population can be estimated
(2) Relatively quick to mount and conduct
(3) Relatively inexpensive
(4) Require comparatively few subjects (unless disease is rare)
(5) Current records occasionally can be used
(6) No risk to subjects
(7) Allow study of multiple potential causes of disease
*Disadvantages*
(1) Moderate sample sizes are required to study rare diseases
(2) Control of extraneous variables may be incomplete
(3) Incidence in exposed and unexposed individuals cannot be estimated
**Case-control studies**
*Advantages*
(1) Well-suited to the study of rare diseases or of those with long incubation periods
(2) Relatively quick to mount and conduct
(3) Relatively inexpensive
(4) Require comparatively few subjects
(5) Existing records occasionally can be used
(6) No risk to subjects
(7) Allow study of multiple potential causes of a disease

**Case-control studies (continued)**
*Disadvantages*
(1) Exposed and unexposed proportion in target population cannot be estimated
(2) Rely on recall or records for information on past exposures
(3) Validation of information is difficult or sometimes impossible
(4) Control of extraneous variables may be incomplete
(5) Selection of an appropriate comparison group may be difficult
(6) Incidence in exposed and unexposed individuals cannot be estimated
**Cohort studies**
*Advantages*
(1) Incidence in exposed and unexposed individuals can be calculated
(2) Permit flexibility in choosing variables to be systematically recorded
*Disadvantages*
(1) Exposed and unexposed proportion in target population cannot be estimated
(2) Large numbers of subjects are required to study rare diseases
(3) Potentially long duration for follow-up
(4) Relatively expensive to conduct
(5) Maintaining follow-up is difficult
(6) Control of extraneous variables may be incomplete

**Table 15.5 Some veterinary observational studies**

| Species | Disease | Hypothesized risk indicators | Source |
|---|---|---|---|
| Ox, horse, pig, dog, cat | Congenital umbilical and inguinal hernias | Breed, sex | Hayes (1974a) |
| Ox, horse, dog, cat | Nervous tissue tumours | Breed, sex, age | Hayes et al. (1975) |
| Ox, horse, dog, cat | Oral and pharyngeal cancer | For dogs: sex, age, size of urban area | Dorn and Priester (1976) |
| Ox, horse, dog, cat | Pancreatic carcinoma | For dogs: breed, sex, age | Priester (1974b) |
| Ox, horse, dog, cat | Various tumours | Breed, sex, age | Priester and Mantel (1971) Priester and McKay (1980) |
| Cat | Cutaneous and oral squamous cell carcinoma | Sex, skin colour, exposure to sunlight | Dorn et al. (1971) |
| Cat | Urolithiasis | Breed, sex, age, neutering, season of year, diet, weight, level of activity, time of diagnosis | Willberg (1975a,b,c; 1976; 1981) Willeberg and Priester (1976) |
| Dog | Bladder cancer | Breed, sex | Hayes (1976) |
| Dog | Bone sarcoma | Body size | Tjalma (1966) |
| Dog | Heart valve incompetence | Breed, sex | Thrusfield et al. (1985) |
| Dog | Ectopic ureter | Breed | Hayes (1974b) |
| Dog | Elbow disease (mainly dysplasia) | Breed, sex | Hayes et al. (1979) |
| Dog | Heartworm infection | Breed, breed grouping (e.g. working, sporting, toys), sex, age | Selby et al (1980) |
| Dog | Intervertebral disc disease | Breed, sex, age site of involvement | Goggin et al. (1970) |

**Table 15.5 (continued)**

| Species | Disease | Hypothesized risk indicators | Source |
|---------|---------|------------------------------|--------|
| Dog | Malignant neoplasms | Benign neoplasms | Bender *et al.* (1982) |
| Dog | Mesothelioma | Domestic and owner's exposure to asbestos, urban residence, management, flea repellants | Glickman *et al* (1983) |
| Dog | Oral and pharyngeal neoplasms | Breed, sex, age | Cohen *et al.* (1964) |
| Dog | Progressive retinal atrophy | Breed, sex, age | Priester (1974a) |
| Dog | Renal tumours | Breed, sex, age | Hayes and Fraumeni (1977) |
| Dog | Respiratory tract neoplasms | Environment (urban v. rural) | Reif and Cohen (1971) |
| Dog | Tail injuries | Undocked tails | Darke *et al.* (1985) |
| Dog | Testicular neoplasia | Breed, sex, age, cryptorchidism | Hayes and Pendergrass (1976) Reif *et al.* (1979) |
| Dog | Thyroid neoplasms | Breed, sex, age | Hayes and Fraumeni (1975) |
| Dog | Urinary incontinence | Spaying | Thrusfield (1985c) |
| Horse | Potomac fever | Premises, husbandry and management variables, previous history of the syndrome on premises | Perry *et al.* (1984b; 1986) |
| Horse | Sweet itch | Breed, age, sex, coat colour, topographical location, rainfall, extracts of *Culicoides* spp. | Braverman *et al.* (1983) |
| Ox | Brucellosis | Herd size, stabling, registration status, history of previous reactors, time of exposure, vaccination level, farm density herd type, insemination methods | Kellar *et al.* (1976) |
| Ox | Infertility (female) | Exposure to high voltage transmission lines | Algers and Hennichs (1985) |
| Ox | Calf mortality | Various management and husbandry variables, e.g. corn silage feeding, penning, vaccination | Martin *et al.* (1982) |
| Ox | Ketosis | Metritis, low milk yield before calving, long dry period | Markusfeld (1985) |
| Ox | Mastitis caused by *Streptococcus agalactiae* | Herd size, herd location, participation in a dairy herd improvement scheme | Thorburn *et al.* (1983) |
| Ox | Respiratory disease | Immune status, antibody level to various infectious agents | Pritchard *et al.* (1983) |
| Ox | Salmonellosis | Several management, environmental and production variables | Vandergraaff (1980) |
| Pig | Enzootic pneumonia | Sex, age, clinical disease, ventilation, herd size, replacement policy, diarrhoea | Aalund *et al.* (1976) Willeberg *et al.* (1978) |
| Pig | Reproductive failure | Antibodies to *Leptospira interrogans* subgroup *Australis* | Pritchard *et al.* (1985) |
| Sheep | Abomasal bloat (in young lambs) | Geographical area, type of floor, diet | Lutnaes and Simensen (1983) |
| Sheep | Intestinal adenocarcinoma | Exposure to herbicides | Newell *et al.* (1984) |

have been a component cause in those animals. For this reason, and for the reason that a cohort study measures incidence, the cohort study is a better technique for assessing risk and identifying cause than the other two types of study.

A comparison of cross-sectional, case-control and cohort studies is given in *Table 15.4*. Cross-sectional and case-control studies are conducted relatively frequently in veterinary medicine. Cohort studies are relatively rare; an example is an investigation of the association between testicular tumours and cryptorchidism in dogs (Reif *et al.*, 1979). Examples of observational studies, mainly cross-sectional and case-control, are listed in *Table 15.5*.

## *Further reading*

BRESLAW, N.E. and DAY, N.E. (1980) *Statistical Methods in Cancer Research, Vol. 1: The Analysis of Case-Control Studies*. IARC Scientific Publications No. 32. International Agency on Cancer Research, Lyon

FEINSTEIN, A. (1977) *Clinical Biostatistics*. The C.V. Mosby Company, Saint Louis

FLEISS, J.L. (1981) *Statistical Methods for Rates and Proportions*, 2nd edn. John Wiley and Sons, New York

KLEINBAUM, D.G., KUPPER, L.L. and MORGANSTERN, H. (1982) *Epidemiologic Research. Principles and Quantitative Measures*. Lifetime Learning Publications, Belmont

SCHLESSELMAN, J.J. (1982) *Case-Control Studies: Design, Conduct, Analysis*. Oxford University Press, New York and Oxford

WILLEBERG, P. (1980) The analysis and interpretation of epidemiological data. In: Proceedings of the Second International Symposium on Veterinary Epidemiology and Economics, Canberra, 7–11 May 1979. Eds Geering, W.A., Roe, R.T. and Chapman, L.A. Pp. 185–198. Australian Government Publishing Service, Canberra

# 16

# Serological epidemiology

Serological epidemiology is the investigation of disease and infection in populations by the measurement of variables present in serum. A range of constituents of serum can be measured, including minerals, trace elements, enzymes and hormones. One of the main constituents of serum that is frequently measured is the specific antibody activity of globulins. Alternative terms for antibody measurement are 'titration' and 'assay'. Antibodies provide evidence of current and previous exposure to infectious agents; their assay is commonly employed in veterinary medicine as a relatively efficient and cheap means of detecting this exposure. This chapter describes methods of measuring antibodies and comparing their levels in groups of animals, and discusses the interpretation of results. Finally, serum banks are described. The analytical methods are equally applicable to other diagnostic tests, such as those that detect enzymes and minerals, in which case, however, results can be compared with normal reference levels. Although values for the latter are available in published tables (e.g. Kaneko, 1980), each laboratory should establish its own norms. If the values are Normally distributed, or can be transformed to Normality, then a one-sample $t$-test can be applied to compare a population's values with those of a reference population.

The serological diagnosis of disease based on the detection of circulating antibodies is one of the techniques available for the identification of current and previous exposure to infectious agents. This and other methods are listed in *Table 16.1*. A range of tests to detect antigen/antibody reactions has been developed over the last 100 years and more are being added to the range. Descriptions of these techniques are found in standard immunology texts

**Table 16.1 Methods of diagnosing infectious disease**

*Evidence of recent infection*
Isolation of agent
Clinical signs
Pathognomonic (characteristic) changes
Biochemical changes
Molecular changes (e.g. nucleic integration and novel cell surface antigens in some virus infections)
Demonstration of an immune response

*Evidence of past infection*
Clinical history
Pathognomonic changes
Demonstration of an immune response

(e.g. Rose and Friedman, 1980; Hudson and Hay, 1981; Tizard, 1982; Roitt, 1984) and a basic knowledge of them is assumed.

## Assaying antibodies

### Methods of expressing amounts of antibody

The concentration of antibody is expressed as a **titre**. This is the highest dilution of serum that produces a test reaction. Thus, if the highest dilution that produces a test reaction is 1 in 32, then the titre is 1/32. Alternatively, the reciprocal, 32, can be quoted, indicating that the undiluted serum contains 32 times the antibody for the reaction. Animals with detectable antibody titres are **seropositive**; animals with no detectable antibodies are **seronegative**. Animals previously seronegative and now seropositive have **seroconverted**.

## Logarithmic transformation of titres

Serum is usually diluted in a geometric series, that is, with a constant ratio between successive dilutions. The commonest ratio is 2. Thus, serum is diluted 1/2, 1/4, 1/8, 1/16, 1/32, and so on. This suggests that the titres should be measured on a logarithmic scale. There are two reasons for this measurement:

(1) the frequency distribution of titres is often lognormal (*see Figure 12.5*); statistical tests that assume Normality may therefore be applied;
(2) geometric dilution series are equally spaced on a logarithmic scale; thus serum may be diluted geometrically 1/2, 1/4, 1/8, 1/16 and so on, corresponding to log transformation to base 2, the respective logs to base 2 of the reciprocals of the dilutions being 1, 2, 3, 4 and so on; the dilution can be coded as the value of these logarithms to base 2 (*Table 16.2*).

In some cases, high concentrations of serum that react non-specifically are avoided by initially diluting by $\log_{10}$, and then continuing in $\log_2$ dilutions, thus:

1/10, 1/20, 1/40, 1/80.

**Table 16.2 Antibody titres expressed as reciprocal dilutions (X) and coded titres ($\log_2 X$)**

| Reciprocal dilution (X) | Code titre ($\log_2 X$) |
|---|---|
| 1 (undiluted serum) | 0 |
| 2 | 1 |
| 4 | 2 |
| 8 | 3 |
| 16 | 4 |
| 32 | 5 |
| 64 | 6 |

## Mean titres

If several coded titres are recorded, their **arithmetic mean** can be calculated. This is simply the sum of the coded titres divided by the number of titres. For example, if five titres are 1/2, 1/4, 1/2, 1/8, and 1/4, then the coded titres are 1, 2, 1, 3, and 2 respectively. The arithmetic mean therefore is $(1+2+1+3+2)/5 = 1.8$.

The **geometric mean titre** (*GMT*) is the antilog$_2$ of the coded mean. This can be obtained either from tables of logarithms to base 2 (Finney *et al.*, 1955) or, more commonly, by using logarithms to base 10 (many pocket calculators have a logarithm function key on them). For example, if the arithmetic mean of several coded titres is 4.7, then $\log_2 GMT = 4.7$; thus $GMT = 2^{4.7} = 26$. Applying $\log_{10}$ values:

$$\log_{10} GMT = 4.7 \times \log_{10} 2$$
$$= 4.7 \times 0.301$$

$$= 1.415.$$

Antilog $1.415 = 26$.

Thus the *GMT* is 26.

If an initial $\log_{10}$ dilution has been carried out, subsequently followed by $\log_2$ dilutions, values are divided by 10 before taking logarithms to base 2. For example, dilutions of 1/10, 1/20, 1/40, 1/80 would be coded as 0,1,2,3 (1/10 is coded 0 because it is equivalent to undiluted serum), giving a mean of 1.5. Then:

$$GMT/10 = 2^{1.5},$$
$$\log_{10}(GMT/10) = 1.5 \times 0.301 = 0.45,$$
$$GMT/10 = \text{antilog } 0.45,$$
$$= 2.8.$$

Thus $GMT = 28$.

The logarithm of zero cannot be expressed because it is 'minus infinity'. Therefore, when calculating means of coded titres, seronegative animals have to be excluded because their reciprocal titres are zero and therefore cannot be coded; **mean titres can be calculated only for seropositive animals**. Thus, when comparing coded antibody titres in populations, two parameters must be considered before inferences are made: the relative proportion of seropositive animals, irrespective of titre, and the *GMT*s of the seropositive populations. For instance, it might be found that in two dairy herds approximately 20% of cows in each herd were seropositive to *Leptospira*, serovar *pomona*, but that the *GMT* in one herd was 40 while in the other it was 640. Such circumstances might indicate a recent epidemic in the second herd and merely the persistence of antibodies in convalescent animals in the first. Conversely, a serological survey of workers in two different abattoirs might reveal similar *GMT*s of complement fixing antibodies to *Coxiella burneti* in each group of seropositive workers, but at one abattoir 30% of workers had titres, while at the other only 3% were seropositive. Such results would indicate a much greater probability of infection at the first abattoir, although the *GMT*s of the groups were similar.

## *Quantal assay*

A quantal assay measures an 'all-or-none' response, for example, agglutination or no agglutination, infected or non-infected. Two systems frequently used are:

(1) single serial dilution assay;
(2) multiple serial dilution assay.

The first is the commoner. Both techniques utilize geometric (logarithmic) dilutions, the range of dilution depending on the sensitivity of the test. Sensitivity here refers to the ability of the system to detect amounts of antibody and antigen: the more sensitive the test, the smaller the amount of antibody and antigen it will detect. (Thus 'sensitivity', in this context, should not be confused with the validity parameter 'sensitivity', described in Chapter 9.)

## Single serial dilution assay

In a single serial dilution assay, each dilution is tested once. For instance, in a virus haemagglutination-inhibition test, the highest dilution that prevents agglutination of erythrocytes on a test plate is the antibody's haemagglutination-inhibition titre. This is a relatively **weak** form of measurement (*see* Chapter 9). If the titre is 1/32 it implies that 1/31 would not produce the effect. However, since 1/16 is the next lowest dilution that is tested, the actual titre could lie between 1/17 and 1/32. Thus, this type of titration, which tests only dilution intervals, actually divides the dilutions into blocks. The blocking is more marked when titres are expressed as 'less than' or 'greater than' (e.g. <1/8 or >1/256). The data therefore are essentially **ordinal**.

## Multiple serial dilution assay

In a multiple serial dilution assay each dilution is tested several (preferably at least five) times. The object is to achieve a 'strong' measure. The end-point is the dilution of a substance at which a specified number of members of a test group show a defined effect, such as death or disease. The most frequently used and statistically useful end-point is 50% (Gaddum, 1933). Thus, in pharmacology, the toxicity of a drug can be expressed as an $LD_{50}$ (lethal dose$_{50}$): the amount of drug that will kill 50% of test animals. An amount of drug can therefore be expressed in terms of the number of $LD_{50}$s that it contains.

Fifty per cent end-point titrations can also be used to estimate antibody concentrations, in which case antibody titres are expressed in terms of the dilution

of serum that **prevents** an effect in 50% of members of a test group, the effect being produced by the infectious agent responsible for the induction of the antibodies that are being titrated. For example, the dilution of serum that prevents infection of 50% of cell culture monolayers with a standard concentration of virus can be estimated: an 'effective dose$_{50}$' ($ED_{50}$). Several methods of calculating 50% end-points are available, including the Reed–Muench and Spearman–Kärber methods, and moving averages. The Reed–Muench method is not recommended (Finney, 1978) because precision cannot be assessed, there is no validity test, and the method is less efficient than some of the alternatives. The second method (Spearman, 1908; Kärber, 1931), which involves relatively simple calculations, is described below.

## Example of a Spearman–Kärber titration

The antibody titre to a virus is required. The defined measured response is a cytopathic effect (CPE) in cell culture monolayers. The test serum is diluted (usually in twofold geometric increments). One tenth of 1 ml of each dilution is inoculated into groups of five cell culture monolayers, each of which has been inoculated with a fixed, potentially lethal, dose of the virus. *Table 16.3* depicts the results. The 50% end-point is the dilution of serum that prevents a CPE in 50% of the monolayers in a group, that is, in two and a half monolayers (note that this is a statistical estimation).

According to the Spearman–Kärber formula:

$$\text{Log } ED_{50} = L - d(\Sigma P - 0.5)$$

where $L$ = log highest dilution at which all monolayers survive intact,

$d$ = log of the dilution factor (i.e. the difference between the log dilution intervals),

$\Sigma P$ = sum of the proportion of 'positive' tests (i.e. intact monolayers) **beginning** at the highest dilution showing a positive result.

**Table 16.3 Example of a 50% end-point titration (Spearman–Kärber method)**

| Serum dilution | $Log_{10}$ dilution | Monolayers showing cytopathic effect | Intact monolayers | Proportion 'positive' (intact) P | 1 − P |
|---|---|---|---|---|---|
| 1/1 | 0.0 | 0 | 5 | 1.00 | 0.00 |
| 1/2 | −0.3 | 0 | 5 | 1.00 | 0.00 |
| 1/4 | −0.6 | 0 | 5 | 1.00 | 0.00 |
| 1/8 | −0.9 | 1 | 4 | 0.80 | 0.20 |
| 1/16 | −1.2 | 1 | 4 | 0.80 | 0.20 |
| 1/32 | −1.5 | 3 | 2 | 0.40 | 0.60 |
| 1/64 | −1.8 | 4 | 1 | 0.20 | 0.80 |
| 1/128 | −2.1 | 5 | 0 | 0.00 | 1.00 |

From *Table 16.3*:

$$L = 0.6$$
$$d = \log_{10}2$$
$$= 0.3$$
$$\Sigma P = 1.00 + 0.80 + 0.80 + 0.40 + 0.20$$
$$= 3.20.$$

Thus

$$\log_{10}ED_{50} = -0.6 - \{0.3(3.2 - 0.5)\}$$
$$= -0.6 - (0.3 \times 2.7)$$
$$= -0.6 - 0.8$$
$$= -1.4$$

Therefore $ED_{50}$ = antilog $(-1.4)$
$$= 1/(25.1).$$

Thus 0.1 ml of serum contains 25.1 $ED_{50}$s, and 1 ml contains 251 $ED_{50}$s.

The estimated standard error (e.s.e.) is calculated using:

$$\text{e.s.e.}(\log_{10} ED_{50}) = d\sqrt{[\Sigma\{P(1-P)\}/(n-1)]}$$

where $n$ = number of animals in each group.
Substituting the values from *Table 16.3*:

$$\log_{10} \text{e.s.e.} = 0.3\sqrt{[\{(0.8 \times 0.2) + (0.8 \times 0.2) +}$$
$$(0.4 \times 0.6) + (0.2 \times 0.8)\}/(5-1)]$$
$$= 0.3\sqrt{\{(0.16+0.16+0.24+0.16)/4\}}$$
$$= 0.13.$$

Thus the titre may be quoted as $10^{1.4 \pm 0.13}$ $ED_{50}$s per 1/10 ml or $10^{2.4 \pm 0.13}$ $ED_{50}$s per ml.

When comparing titres between groups of animals, an $ED_{50}$ is a continuous variable that is an **interval** measure (*see* Chapter 9) and may be analysed statistically using parametric methods. Further, since antibodies are usually lognormally distributed, standard tests that assume Normality can be used.

# Serological estimations and comparisons in populations

## *Detecting the presence of antibody*

Detection of the presence of antibody in an animal population, without particular regard to the significance of antibody titre, requires application of the basic survey sampling theory described in Chapter 14. Animals are categorized as either 'positive' or 'negative'. Whether or not a test detects antibody depends not only upon exposure to specific antigen but also upon the ability of the test to detect antibodies (*see below*, 'Negative results').

## *Comparison of antibody levels*

### Comparison of two different populations

If a comparison of two populations in terms of presence and absence of antibody (i.e. 'positive' or 'negative' animals) is required, then the $\chi^2$-test can be used. A continuity correction is needed because the data are discrete.

If the frequency distribution of antibodies in two populations are to be compared, and the scale of measurement is 'strong' (i.e. on the interval or ratio scale), a parametric test can be used.

An $ED_{50}$ is an interval measurement. The following example uses the data in *Table 16.4* relating to vaccination titres in two groups of five dogs, one group vaccinated with killed rabies virus of porcine origin, and the other with vaccine of feline origin. The comparison is between the titres in each group, 60 days after vaccination. Log titres are

**Table 16.4 Serum antibody titres (SN$_{50}$: 'serum neutralizing dose$_{50}$') of dogs, for two types of rabies vaccine, before and 60 days after vaccination. (From Merry and Kolar, 1984)**

| Vaccine | Dog number | Pre-vaccination titre | | Titre 60 days after vaccination | |
|---|---|---|---|---|---|
| | | Reciprocal | $\log_{10}$ | Reciprocal | $\log_{10}$ |
| Killed vaccine | A653 | 3 | 0.48 | 214 | 2.33 |
| feline cell origin | A616 | 3 | 0.48 | 182 | 2.26 |
| | 2C10 | 2 | 0.30 | 280 | 2.45 |
| | 2B39 | 2 | 0.30 | 267 | 2.43 |
| | 2B47 | 2 | 0.30 | 198 | 2.30 |
| Mean: | | 2.4 | 0.372 | 228 | 2.354 |

$\Sigma x_1 = 11.77$; $n_1 = 5$; $\Sigma x_1^2 = 27.7339$; $\bar{x}_1 = 2.354$; $s_1 = 0.086$

| Vaccine | Dog number | Pre-vaccination titre | | Titre 60 days after vaccination | |
|---|---|---|---|---|---|
| Killed vaccine | A603 | 3 | 0.48 | 10 | 1.00 |
| porcine cell line | A654 | 2 | 0.30 | 51 | 1.71 |
| origin | A618 | 2 | 0.30 | 9 | 0.95 |
| | 2C16 | 2 | 0.30 | 16 | 1.20 |
| | 2C3 | 2 | 0.30 | 38 | 1.58 |
| Mean: | | 2.2 | 0.366 | 25 | 1.288 |

$\Sigma x_2 = 6.44$; $n_2 = 5$; $\Sigma x_2^2 = 8.763$; $\bar{x}_2 = 1.288$; $s_2 = 0.342$

used; this transformation allows the assumption of Normality. Student's *t*-test for independent samples can be used (*see* Chapter 13) assuming unknown variance. Using the same notation as that in Chapter 13:

$$n_1 = 5, \bar{x}_1 = 2.354, s_1 = 0.083,$$

$$n_2 = 5, \bar{x}_2 = 1.288, s_2 = 0.342.$$

The hypothesis to be tested is that there is no difference in 60-day antibody titres between the dogs vaccinated with killed rabies virus of porcine origin and dogs vaccinated with vaccine of feline origin.

Let $\mu_1$ and $\mu_2$ be the mean 60-day titres in the two groups, and let $\delta = \mu_1 - \mu_2$. The hypothesis may then be written as $\delta = 0$.

First it is necessary to check that $s_1^2$ and $s_2^2$ are estimates of a common population variance. This is done by calculating the ratio of the two variances, where the numerator is the greater of the two. This ratio is then compared with the appropriate percentage points of an *F*-distribution (Appendix X) with a pair of degrees of freedom, the first being one less than the sample size used in calculating the variance in the numerator, and the second being one less than the sample size used in calculating the variance in the denominator. In this particular case:

$$s_2^2/s_1^2 = 17.0$$

with (4,4) degrees of freedom.

The 1% point of the corresponding *F* distribution is 16.0. The sample value of 17.0 is greater than this value. The sample value is therefore significant at the 1% level and there is strong evidence to suggest that the variances of the $\log_{10}$ of 60-day antibody titres differ between groups.

The test statistic in this situation now is:

$$t = (\bar{x}_1 - \bar{x}_2 - \delta)/\sqrt{\{(s_1^2/n_1) + (s_2^2/n_2)\}}$$

with approximate degrees of freedom, $\nu$, given by:

$$\nu = (\nu_1 + \nu_2)^2/(\nu_1^2/\nu_1 + \nu_2^2/\nu_2),$$

where:

$$\nu_1 = s_1^2/n_1$$

and

$$\nu_2 = s_2^2/n_2$$

to take account of unequal variances (Snedecor and Cochran, 1980).

For this example:

$$t = (2.354 - 1.288 - 0)/\sqrt{\{(0.083^2/5) + (0.342^2/5)\}}$$

$$= 1.066/\sqrt{(0.00138 + 0.02339)}$$

$$= 6.773.$$

Thus:

$$\nu = (0.00137 + 0.02341)^2/(0.000000466 + 0.000137)$$

$$= 4.47.$$

Rounding $\nu$ down to the nearest whole number, when using the *t*-table (Appendix III) there are only 4 degrees of freedom because the variances differ significantly. From Appendix III, the 5% value for 4 degrees of freedom is 2.776, which is less than 6.773. Therefore, the two groups of dogs have significantly different mean titres at the 5% level. Note that the result is also significant at the 2% level and the 1% level.

The more common geometric dilution titrations, which define a titre as the highest dilution producing a test reaction, present a more difficult choice of statistical test because the titres are ordinal data. This is particularly evident when a large proportion of the titres are expressed as 'less than' or 'greater than' a particular dilution. If there are no 'less than' or 'greater than' titres and there is a reasonable spread of titres, then the log titres can be regarded as crude approximations to Normally distributed measurements, and a *t*-test for unrelated samples can be used. Otherwise, a non-parametric test should be used. Standard texts on non-parametric statistics (e.g. Siegel, 1956) describe suitable tests.

## Comparison of different estimates on the same population

If a population is sampled twice over a period of time, a suitable comparison can be made using a *t*-test for related samples—again using log titres to assume Normality. The test is described in standard statistical texts. Again, if the measurement is ordinal then the appropriate non-parametric test should be used.

# Interpreting serological tests

## *Refinement*

Infectious agents have a variety of antigens on their surfaces and in their interiors. Additionally, non-structural antigens can be detected in the early stages of virus replication. Some of the antigens are shared by several groups of isolates and are the basis of division into broad categories. Other antigens are unique to a particular group of isolates. For instance, influenza type A viruses are distinguished from types B and C by their core nucleoproteins and matrix proteins. Influenza A viruses are divided into subtypes on the basis of their surface haemagglutinin and neuraminidase antigens. Similarly, subtypes are divided further into strains according to more refined differences in the antigenic composition of the haemagglutinins and neuraminidases (*Table 16.5*). This refinement in antigenic definition is also termed specificity (not to be confused with specificity as a validity parameter of a diagnostic test). The epidemiological value of a serological test, for

**Table 16.5 The classification of some influenza A viruses. (Source: WHO, 1980)**

| Haemagglutinins (H) and neuraminidases (N) | Strains |
|---|---|
| H1 N1 | A/PR/8/34 |
| H1 N1 | A/Weiss/43 |
| H1 N1 | A/swine/Iowa |
| H1 N1 | A/duck/Alberta/35/76 |
| H3 N2 | A/Hong Kong/1/68 |
| H3 N2 | A/Port Chalmers/1/73 |
| H3 N2 | A/swine/Taiwan/1/70 |
| H3 N2 | A/turkey/England/69 |

example, when tracing the spread of a particular infection, increases in relation to its ability to detect more refined antigenic differences.

Serological tests vary in their ability to detect subtle antigenic differences. *Table 16.6* illustrates varying refinement of serological tests for influenza A viruses. The complement fixation test (CFT), using virus extracted from chorioallantoic membranes as antigen, will detect antibody against virus nucleoprotein and therefore is specific only to the level of virus type. However, the use of whole virus as antigen results in a CFT that is specific for subtypes because it will detect particular subtypes of haemagglutinins and neuraminidases. Identification of specific strains is possible if carefully selected reference strains are used as antigens; the titre of antibodies to haemagglutinins and neuraminidases is highest when the antibodies are directed against the strain-specific antigens. It should be emphasized that one type of test is not always more refined than another (e.g. radial immunodiffusion v. complement fixation) for **all** antigen/antibody reactions, and that refinement also depends on the nature of the antigen that is used in the test.

## *Accuracy*

In common with other diagnostic tests, false positives and false negatives can occur. *Table 16.7* lists the reasons for positive and negative results in serological tests.

**Table 16.7 Reasons for positive and negative results in serological tests**

| | |
|---|---|
| *Positive results* | |
| Actual infection | true +ve |
| Group cross-reactions | |
| Non-specific inhibitors | false +ve |
| Non-specific agglutinins | |
| *Negative results* | |
| Absence of infection | true −ve |
| Natural or induced tolerance | |
| Improper timing | |
| Improper selection of test | |
| Non-specific inhibitors e.g. anticomplementary serum; tissue culture toxic substances | false −ve |
| Antibiotic induced immunoglobulin suppression | |
| Incomplete or blocking antibody | |
| Insensitive tests | |

**Table 16.6 Summary of tests for influenza serology. (From Stuart-Harris and Schild, 1976)**

| Test | Test antigens | Antibody detected | Recommended use[θ] | |
|---|---|---|---|---|
| | | | Serosurvey | Serodiagnosis |
| HI | Whole virus | HA[ζ] | ++++ | ++++ |
| NI | Whole virus | NA[ζ] | ++++ | |
| CF | CAM extract | NP | | ++ |
| | Whole virus | HA, NA | | +++ |
| SRD | Whole virus* | HA, NA | +++ | ++++ |
| | Disrupted virus* | NP, MP | | +++ |
| IDD | Disrupted virus* | HA, NA | + | ++ |
| | Disrupted virus* | NP, MP | + | ++ |
| N-IHA | NA | NA | ++++ | |

HI    =  haemagglutination inhibition
NI    =  neuraminidase inhibition
CF    =  complement fixation
SRD   =  single radial immunodiffusion
IDD   =  immuno-double-diffusion
N-IHA=  neuraminidase-indirect haemagglutination
HA    =  haemagglutinin
NA    =  neuraminidase
NP    =  nucleoprotein
MP    =  matrix protein
CAM  =  chorioallantoic membrane
[θ]The usefulness of the test for the indicated purpose is expressed on a scale of + (least useful) to ++++ (most useful).
[ζ]Serum containing high antibody titre to the second surface antigen (HA or NA) may at low dilutions and under certain conditions cause inhibition.
*Test refinement (specificity) achieved by selecting viruses or recombinant viruses with the required antigenic composition.

## Positive results

A true positive result derives from actual infection.

False positive results occur for a variety of reasons. **Group cross-reactions** can occur between an infectious agent and antibodies to different organisms with similar antigens. For example, infection with *Yersinia enterocolitica*, serotype 9, can produce antibodies that cross-react with *Brucella abortus* antigens.

**Non-specific inhibitors** present in serum may inhibit reactions that are normally associated with the action of intact antigens that are not specifically bound to antibody. These inhibitors therefore mimic the effects of antibody in the latter's absence. An example is non-specific inhibitors in haemagglutination tests against influenza viruses. Agglutination of antigen by **non-specific agglutinins** similarly mimics the effect of antibodies that are agglutinins.

## Negative results

A true negative result indicates absence of infection.

Again, false negative results can occur for several reasons. Some animals show **natural or induced tolerance** to antigens and therefore do not produce antibodies when challenged with the agent. Thus, exposure of the bovine fetus to bovine virus diarrhoea virus in the first half of gestation results in offspring that do not produce detectable antibodies when challenged with the same strain of virus (Coria and McClurkin, 1978).

**Improper timing** may result in a test's failure to detect infection. For instance, sampling of some cows before abortion, using the CFT, may not detect *Br. abortus* because detectable complement fixing antibodies may not appear until after abortion (e.g. Robertson, 1971).

Some tests may be **unsuitable** for detecting infection. Thus, infection by African swine fever virus cannot be detected using a serum neutralization test because infected pigs do not produce detectable levels of neutralizing antibodies (De Boer, 1967); an immunofluorescence test, however, will detect antibodies.

Some **non-specific inhibitors** will produce false negative results by their mode of action (cf. those above that produce false positive results). Some sera, notably contaminated and haemolysed specimens, are anticomplementary; thus complement cannot be fixed in the CFT and the test is therefore assumed to be negative although antibodies may be present. This can occur with CFTs for *Br. abortus* infections (Worthington, 1982). Similarly, substances that are toxic to tissue culture monolayers may mimic the effects of un-neutralized virus, giving the impression that neutralizing antibodies are absent when they may be present.

**Table 16.8 Relative sensitivity of assays for antigens and antibodies. (From Stites *et al.*, 1982)**

| Technique | Approximate sensitivity (per dl) |
|---|---|
| Total serum proteins (by biuret or refractometry) | 100 mg |
| Serum protein electrophoresis (zone electrophoresis) | 100 mg |
| Analytic ultracentrifugation | 100 mg |
| Immunoelectrophoresis | 5–10 mg |
| Single radial diffusion | <1–2 mg |
| Double diffusion in agar (Ouchterlony) | <1 mg |
| Electroimmunodiffusion (rocket electrophoresis) | <0.5 mg |
| One-dimensional double electro-immunodiffusion (counterimmunoelectrophoresis) | <0.1 mg |
| Nephelometry | 0.1 mg |
| Complement fixation | 1 $\mu$g |
| Agglutination | 1 $\mu$g |
| Enzyme immunoassay | <1 $\mu$g |
| Quantitative immunofluorescence | <1 pg |
| Radioimmunoassay | <1 pg |

Some antibodies are **incomplete** and so cannot take part in antigen/antibody test reactions. A common type of canine autoimmune haemolytic anaemia is characterized by incomplete antibodies on the surface of red blood cells, which can only be detected by an antiglobulin test (Halliwell, 1978). Occasionally **blocking antibodies** prevent antigen/antibody reactions occurring. This occurs sometimes when conducting CFTs for bovine *Br. abortus* infection (Plackett and Alton, 1975), as a result of excess $IgG_1$ blocking $IgG_2$ (the latter being responsible for complement fixation) at low concentrations: this is the 'prozone' effect.

Finally, a serological test may be too **insensitive** to detect antibody. Sensitivity in this context again refers to the ability of a test to detect amounts of antibody or antigen. *Table 16.8* lists some common serological tests and their approximate sensitivities.

## *The relationship between sensitivity and specificity*

Sensitivity and specificity were introduced in Chapter 9 as measures of the validity of diagnostic tests; the terms are used in the remainder of this chapter in this sense. Although the description is in the context of serological investigations, it is equally relevant to other types of diagnostic test and their application, for example in genetic screening.

There is an inverse relationship between sensitivity and specificity in a particular test. This is illustrated in *Figure 16.1* in which the upper graph

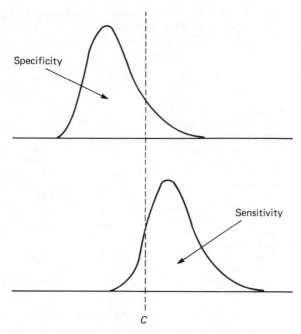

**Figure 16.1** The relationship between sensitivity and specificity (*see* text for explanation). Upper graph = frequency distribution of a variable in a healthy population; lower graph = frequency distribution of the variable in a diseased population; $C$ = cut-off point defining the boundary between healthy and diseased individuals.

represents the frequency distribution of a variable in a healthy population and the lower graph represents its frequency distribution in a diseased population. The frequency distributions differ between the two populations and so measurement of this variable can be used as a diagnostic test. Individuals for whom the variable's value is to the right of the cut-off point, $C$, are classified as diseased; individuals for whom the variable's value is to the left of the cut-off point are classified as healthy. Animals with values to the right of the cut-off point in the upper graph are false positives; animals with values to the left of the cut-off point in the lower graph are false negatives. If the area under each curve represents 100% then the marked area to the right of the cut-off point corresponds to the test's sensitivity, whereas the marked area to the left of the cut-off point corresponds to the test's specificity. If fewer false positives are required, $C$ is moved to the right: specificity increases and sensitivity decreases. However, if fewer false negatives are required, $C$ is moved to the left: sensitivity increases and specificity decreases.

When a large cross-section of a population initially is tested to detect disease (e.g. in screening), interpretation of the test is directed towards increased sensitivity at the expense of specificity. This is because initial tests are not usually intended to provide definitive diagnoses but are designed to detect as many cases as possible. Therefore, a high proportion of false positives (resulting from increased sensitivity) is not as critical as a high proportion of false negatives (resulting from increased specificity).

## *The predictive value of serological tests*

### Calculation of predictive value

When using either serological or other screening tests to determine the presence of disease in a population it is important to know the probability that an animal, 'positive' according to the test, is actually positive; alternatively that a test-negative animal is a true negative. These probabilities are the **predictive values** of the test. The parameter most often quoted as the predictive value of a test is the predictive value of a positive (as opposed to negative) test result.

The predictive value depends on specificity and sensitivity **and prevalence**. Sensitivity and specificity are innate characteristics of a test and do not vary, but the prevalence of a disease in a population being tested will affect the proportion of test-positive animals that are actually diseased.

If the proportion of a population classified as having a disease in a test is $P^T$, and the true prevalence is $P$, then there are two components to $P^T$:

(1) the true positives;
(2) the false positives.

The proportion of animals, $P^T$ is then:

$$P \times \text{sensitivity} + (1-P) \times (1-\text{specificity}).$$

For example, if $P = 0.01$ (1%), sensitivity = 0.99 (99%) and specificity = 0.99 (99%), then:

$$P^T = 0.01 \times 0.99 + (1-0.01) \times (1-0.99)$$

$$= 0.02.$$

This represents an overestimation of 100% (the actual prevalence is 0.01 and the estimated prevalence is 0.02). The smaller the prevalence, the larger the proportional overestimation, that is, the lower the predictive value (positive test result).

It follows that if the sensitivity and specificity of the test are known then a corrected estimate of the true prevalence, $P$, can be made by:

$$P = \frac{P^T + \text{specificity} - 1}{\text{sensitivity} + \text{specificity} - 1}.$$

The predictive value (positive test result) is given by:

$$\frac{P \times \text{sensitivity}}{P \times \text{sensitivity} + (1-P) \times (1 - \text{specificity})}.$$

**Table 16.9 Possible results of a diagnostic test**

| Test status | True status | | Totals |
|---|---|---|---|
| | Diseased | Not diseased | |
| Diseased | a | b | a + b |
| Not diseased | c | d | c + d |
| Totals | a + c | b + d | a + b + c + d |

It can be expressed as a value between 0 and 1, but is commonly expressed as a percentage.

Alternatively, the calculation can be expressed more simply in terms of the values in *Table 16.9* which were presented originally in *Table 9.1*. The table categorizes animals into those that are 'true' and 'false' positives and negatives.

$$\text{Sensitivity} = a/(a+c).$$

$$\text{Specificity} = d/(b+d).$$

The predictive value = $a/(a+b)$.
(positive test result)

The predictive value = $d/(c+d)$.
(negative test result)

Four screening tests (or modifications of them) are being used for brucellosis testing in various parts of the world: the tube agglutination test (TAT), the CFT, the Brewer Card Test (BCT), and the milk ring test (MRT). Sufficient data are available to estimate the sensitivity and specificity of the first three tests (MAF, 1977). These are summarized in *Table 16.10*.

**Table 16.10 Sensitivity and specificity of three screening tests for bovine brucellosis**

| | Sensitivity (%) | Specificity (%) |
|---|---|---|
| Tube agglutination test | 62.0 | 99.5 |
| Complement fixation test | 97.5 | 99.0 |
| Brewer Card test | 95.2 | 98.5 |

Assume that the TAT will be applied to 100 000 cattle in three different areas in which the prevalence of brucellosis is 3%, 0.1% and 0.01% respectively. From these data, and the figures in *Table 16.10*, the predictive value (of a positive test result) of the test can be calculated for the populations in each of the three areas. The results are given in *Tables 16.11a, b and c* respectively. As the prevalence of disease declines, so does the predictive value of the test, which could result in, for example, an increasing proportion of healthy animals being destroyed in a test and slaughter programme.

**Table 16.11 Predictive value (positive test result) of the tube agglutination test for bovine brucellosis at three different prevalence levels (sensitivity = 62%; specificity = 99.5%)**

**(a) Prevalence of brucellosis: 3%**

| Test status | True status | | Totals |
|---|---|---|---|
| | Brucellosis present | Brucellosis absent | |
| Brucellosis present | 1860 (a) | 480 (b) | 2340 |
| Brucellosis absent | 1140 (c) | 96 6520 (d) | 97 660 |
| Totals | 3000 | 97 000 | 100 000 |

Predictive value (positive result) $= \dfrac{a}{a + b} = 79.5\%$

**(b) Prevalence of brucellosis: 0.1%**

| Test status | True status | | Totals |
|---|---|---|---|
| | Brucellosis present | Brucellosis absent | |
| Brucellosis present | 60 | 500 | 560 |
| Brucellosis absent | 40 | 99 400 | 99 440 |
| Totals | 100 | 99 900 | 100 000 |

Predictive value (positive result) = 10.7%

**(c) Prevalence of brucellosis: 0.01%**

| Test status | True status | | Totals |
|---|---|---|---|
| | Brucellosis present | Brucellosis absent | |
| Brucellosis present | 6 | 500 | 506 |
| Brucellosis absent | 4 | 99 490 | 99 494 |
| Totals | 10 | 99 990 | 100 000 |

Predictive value (positive result) = 1.2%

If a test with a sensitivity of 0.990 (99%) and a specificity of 0.999 (99.9%) were used in a disease eradication campaign, and if the prevalence were 0.1 (10%), a single test conducted on 10 million animals would record 990 000 true positives and 9000 false positives. The test therefore would be acceptable at the beginning of the campaign. However, as the campaign proceeded, the prevalence would fall. When the prevalence was reduced to 0.0001 (0.01%) the test would record 9900 true positives and 9990 false positives. **The number of false positives would be unchanged after the disease was eradicated.** Therefore acceptable levels of sensitivity and specificity depend on the stage of a control or eradication campaign. Ideally, towards the end of an eradication campaign, a more sensitive and specific test is required if the campaign depends only upon a serological test. In practice, other techniques are used, such as repeated testing, isolation of infected farms and maintenance of disease-free areas.

In some tests there are no false positives, for example, when identifying blood parasites by microscopic examination of blood films. Estimation of true prevalence in this circumstance is discussed by Waltner-Toews *et al*. (1986).

Further discussion of the predictive value of serological and other diagnostic tests is provided by Vecchio (1966), Galen and Gambino (1975) and Rogan and Gladen (1978).

## Antibody prevalence

### Half-life

The presence of detectable antibody indicates that an animal or its dam has been exposed to the antigen that stimulates the antibody's production. In the absence of further challenge, the antibody level will decline. The rate of decline, usually measured in terms of the antibody's **half-life** (the time taken for its level to halve), varies between antibodies. Titres to some antibodies persist because the antibodies have a long half-life or there is persistent infection or repeated challenge. The possession of a long half-life explains why some vaccines can produce lifelong immunity after a single course.

The prevalence of detectable antibody depends on the rate of infection, the rate of antibody loss and the time at which these rates have been effective. A high prevalence therefore may reflect not a high rate of infection but a low rate of antibody loss; recall (*see* Chapter 4) that prevalence, *P*, is related to incidence, *I*, and duration, *D*:

$$P \propto I \times D.$$

It follows that not only the prevalence of detectable antibody in a population but also the titre in the individual is related to the half-life of the antibody.

### Repeatability of tests

The repeatability of serological tests (an indication of their reliability) depends on a variety of factors including the degree of standardization of test reagents and the expertise of the tester; different results might be produced by two different laboratory technicians conducting the same test on the same serum sample. Thus, a twofold difference in antibody titre between samples from the same animal, taken at different times, may reflect either a true change in titre or similar titres associated with low repeatability.

**Table 16.12 Typical titres of sera from 100 individuals tested twice. (From Paul and White, 1973)**

| First reading (reciprocal titre) | Second reading (reciprocal titre) | Frequency |
|---|---|---|
| <8 | <8 | 24 |
| <8 | 8 | 2 |
| 8 | 16 | 2 |
| 16 | 8 | 2 |
| 16 | 32 | 3 |
| 32 | 16 | 3 |
| 32 | 32 | 8 |
| 32 | 64 | 6 |
| 64 | 32 | 4 |
| 64 | 64 | 16 |
| 64 | 128 | 1 |
| 128 | 64 | 3 |
| 128 | 128 | 6 |
| 128 | 256 | 2 |
| 128 | 512 | 2 |
| 256 | 128 | 4 |
| 256 | 256 | 6 |
| 256 | 1024 | 2 |
| 512 | 256 | 2 |
| 512 | 512 | 2 |

Generally, a geometric fourfold change in antibody titre (e.g. from 1/16 to 1/64) is assumed to reflect a real change; a twofold change is not considered to be significant. *Table 16.12* illustrates the reasoning behind this decision. The table shows typical results when sera from 100 individuals are tested twice. Each of the two readings should be identical for a single serum sample. However, the table shows that this is true only for 62 samples. Of the remaining 38 samples, 34 show a twofold shift and 4 show a fourfold shift. The shift is caused by the value of the test's repeatability not being 100%. Note also that the fourfold shift in titres occurs with high dilutions. If these titres are typical of the test then, when future samples are drawn from the study population, 4% of the animals might be expected to show a fourfold shift in titre which does not represent a true change. Since this shift can be caused by the second sample showing either a higher or a lower titre than the first, then, when evidence of a **rising** titre is required from two samples taken from the same animal at different times, 2% of the animals can be expected to show spurious fourfold increases in titre. This degree of error is generally acceptable.

## Serum banks

A serum bank is 'a planned catalogued collection of serum forming a random sample that is as representative as possible of a population and that is stored to preserve its immunological and biochemical characteristics' (Moorhouse and Hugh-Jones, 1981, after Timbs, 1980).

## Applications of serum banks

The general principles of serum banks are discussed in two World Health Organization Technical Reports (WHO, 1959, 1970), and by Moorhouse and Hugh-Jones (1981). Additionally, the last two authors describe a computerized data base for storing serum bank information.

In the context of identifying and titrating antibodies, a serum bank can aid the following goals in relation to infectious diseases:

(1) identification of major health problems;
(2) establishment of vaccination priorities;
(3) demarcation of the distribution of diseases;
(4) investigation of newly discovered diseases;
(5) determination of epidemic periodicity;
(6) an increase in the knowledge of disease aetiology;
(7) evaluation of vaccination campaigns;
(8) assessment of economic losses due to disease.

## Sources of serum

*Table 16.13* lists the potential sources of serum and some of their characteristics. This indicates that each source has its own advantages and disadvantages. The accuracy of results obtained from a serum bank depends on:

(1) the sensitivity and specificity of the test performed on the serum;
(2) the quality of the survey design used in collecting the serum;
(3) the degree of degradation that has occurred in the serum during storage.

The first component is an inherent characteristic of the tests employed. The third component is related directly to the means of storage.

## Collection and storage of serum

### Collection

Samples should be taken aseptically. Blood should be allowed to clot for 1–2 hours at room temperature, stored horizontally overnight at 4°C, and then the serum should be separated by centrifugation at 2000–3000 rpm for 10–15 minutes. Blood can also be collected on filter paper discs; the serum can then be eluted later, although the amount of serum that is stored is small and only allows semiquantitative investigations.

### Storage

The reactivity of antibodies to serological tests can be severely impaired by prolonged storage as a result of damage to immunoglobulin molecules. Two storage techniques are available: **deep freezing** and **lyophilization (freeze-drying)**. Four options are available for the former:

(1) liquid phase of liquid nitrogen: −196°C;
(2) vapour phase of liquid nitrogen: −110°C;
(3) ultra-deep freeze: −70°C to −90°C;
(4) standard deep freeze: −20°C to −40°C.

Prolonged storage at −20°C may allow deterioration of antibodies. Refrigeration at 4°C is satisfactory for short-term storage. Lyophilization is a better technique than deep freezing, but is relatively expensive and technically complex. The following facts should be remembered in relation to freezing:

(1) prolonged storage of antibodies can lead to the production of monovalent Fab fragments, resulting in a decline in specific antibody;
(2) repeated thawing and refreezing are deleterious;
(3) the use of cryoprotectants and/or enzyme inhibitors will reduce or eliminate deterioration;
(4) uninterrupted storage at −20°C appears to be a satisfactory procedure with very little loss of specific activity for at least 2 years; however, precise indications of the longevity of whole serum stored under serum bank conditions are not available;
(5) rapid freezing of samples is required;
(6) sterility is important;
(7) samples should be tested immediately after being thawed;
(8) delays will lead to increased rates of proteolysis.

Table 16.13 Potential sources of samples for serum banks and some of their characteristics. (From Moorhouse and Hugh-Jones, 1981)

| Source | Potential no. of samples | Selection bias in study population | Cost to serum bank | Ease of collection | Standard of documentation |
|---|---|---|---|---|---|
| *Ad hoc* field visits | High | Low | High | Low | High |
| Other field visits | High | Low-high | Low | High | Moderate-high |
| Slaughter houses | High | High | Low | High | Low |
| Livestock marketing chain | High | High | Low-moderate | Moderate | Low |
| Veterinary diagnostic laboratories | Low | High | Low | High | Moderate-high |
| Private individuals | Low | High | Low | Moderate | Moderate-high |
| Existing collection | Low-high | Low-high | Low | High | Low-high |

Despite a recommendation, over 25 years ago, for the establishment of veterinary and medical serum banks (WHO, 1959) this recommendation has not been heeded widely in veterinary medicine. Established banks include one in Canada, using serum collected during the bovine brucellosis eradication campaign (Kellar, 1983) and others in Louisiana, USA (Moorhouse and Hugh-Jones, 1981), and New Zealand (Timbs, 1980).

## Further reading

FINNEY, D.J. (1978) *Statistical Method in Biological Assay*, 3rd edn. Charles Griffin and Company Limited, London and High Wycombe

PAUL, J.R. and WHITE, C. (Eds) (1973) *Serological Epidemiology*. Academic Press, New York and London

MOORHOUSE, P.D. and HUGH-JONES, M.E. (1981) Serum banks. *Veterinary Bulletin*, **51**, 277–290

RICE, C.E. (1968) Comparative serology of domestic animals. *Advances in Veterinary Science*, **12**, 105–162

WORTHINGTON, R.W. (1982) Serology as an aid to diagnosis: uses and abuses. *New Zealand Veterinary Journal*, **30**, 93–97

# 17

# Modelling

Modelling is the representation of physical processes, designed to increase appreciation and understanding of them. Thus, two causal models were described in Chapter 3, and two models of interaction in Chapter 5. Similarly, the Normal distribution (*see* Chapter 12) is sometimes termed the Normal probability model. A more specific meaning of modelling is the representation of events in quantitative mathematical terms so that predictions can be made about the events. Modelling, in this sense, is applied to many disciplines, including engineering, agriculture and medicine. In epidemiology, models are constructed to attempt to predict patterns of disease occurrence and what might happen if various alternative control strategies are adopted. Accurate models can be useful guides to choosing the most efficient disease control techniques as well as increasing understanding of life-cycles of infectious agents. This chapter outlines the main types of model, giving examples relating to infectious diseases, and keeps mathematical equations to a minimum. A more mathematical introduction is given by Thrusfield and Gettinby (1984).

Modelling dates back to the 19th century. William Farr predicted the course of the 1866 British rinderpest epidemic using a simple mathematical model which involved fitting a curve to observed data (Farr, quoted by Brownlee, 1915). During the early part of this century, Farr's approach was applied to human diseases such as smallpox. Since the early work, there has been a division into the theoretical approach, which is concerned with epidemic theory, and the practical approach, which attempts to be of direct value to disease control campaigns. The early models, which founded general theory, described natural epidemics of infectious disease. Successive models have attempted to become more realistic, incorporating the effects of control techniques, such as vaccination, in order to evaluate alternative strategies for disease control.

Veterinary medicine has entered the field of disease modelling more recently than human medicine and, logically, models incorporating economic factors have become important. Many techniques use computers to simulate situations, although they are not always necessary.

A model can be utilized effectively only if it is sound. This is not always easy to assess. Affirmative answers to three questions, however, will support the model's validity:

(1) have all the known determinants that influence outbreaks of the disease been included?
(2) can the value of these determinants be assessed with accuracy?
(3) does the model make biological 'common sense'?

Models cannot stand alone in determining efficient control strategies, but should be used in conjunction with accurate field data and experimental techniques. They then provide a useful means of investigating diseases where experiments and field observations may be impracticable. Thus, a model may be constructed to investigate the dissemination of foot-and-mouth disease virus in countries that are free from the infection.

## Types of model

### Density and prevalence models

Veterinary modelling has been directed towards infectious diseases, although non-infectious ones

187

can also be modelled. Infectious agents can be classified into two groups according to their generation dynamics: **microparasites** and **macroparasites**. The microparasites multiply when inside the hosts, increasing the level of parasitism. Microparasites include viruses, bacteria and protozoa. Although macroparasites may reproduce within or on the host as part of their life-cycle, the level of parasitism is not usually increased. Macroparasites include helminths and arthropods. These two different dynamic patterns lend themselves to two different types of modelling.

**Density models** consider the absolute number of infectious agents in each host, and are commonly used in macroparasitic infections where numbers of infectious agents can be estimated either in the host or in the environment. Enumeration of absolute numbers of microparasites is impracticable because of their rapid rate of replication, and so these cannot be modelled readily using density models. Microparasitic infections are frequently studied using **prevalence models** which consider the presence or absence of infection in various host cohorts, for example young and mature, immune and susceptible. The density model is potentially the more refined of the two techniques because it attempts to enumerate the amount of infectious agent with which a host is challenged.

### Deterministic and stochastic models

The values of parameters put into a model can be fixed. The output generated by the model will then comprise point estimates that are governed solely by the input values. Such models are **deterministic**.

Alternatively, the probability of the occurrence of events can be built into a model, for example the probability of one animal infecting another. This means that a range of input values can be used and that a range of output values will be generated, producing both point and interval estimates of output parameters. Such models are **stochastic**, the word being derived from the Greek adjective *stochastikos*, meaning 'skilful in aiming at, able to guess'.

### Sensitivity analysis

Sensitivity analysis is a method of determining to what extent changes in an input parameter affect output parameters. If minor changes in values of an input parameter induce major changes in output parameters then the model is highly sensitive to that input parameter. Conversely, if major changes in an input parameter induce only minor changes in output parameters then the model is relatively insensitive to the input parameter.

# Forecasting systems

It is useful to be able to forecast animal disease morbidity so that suitable prophylactic measures can be instituted. There are three possible ways of doing this: by using **empirical models**, **explanatory models**, or time series analysis of past morbidity data (*see* Chapter 8). This last method is the more convenient of the three because it relies only on past morbidity data from recorded statistics; the first two require the recording of current information. Time series techniques have been used only occasionally in veterinary medicine. Examples include diseases of cattle, horses, fowl and pigs in Japan (Takizawa and Ito, 1977), and foot-and-mouth disease in Paraguay (Peralta *et al.*, 1982: Chapter 8). They depend on accurate animal morbidity records which are frequently unavailable.

## *Empirical models*

Empirical models utilize **indicators that are obtained by analysing the relationship between morbidity and any associated variables**. Frequently used variables are those relating to climate. These models are not strictly mathematical models because they do not attempt to analyse the dynamics of agents' life-cycles; they simply quantify associated phenomena. Nevertheless, empirical models have been used widely in veterinary medicine; examples include studies of fascioliasis and nematodiriasis.

### Fascioliasis

Fascioliasis has been modelled empirically in Britain (Ollerenshaw and Rowlands, 1959; Ollerenshaw, 1966; Gibson, 1978). The life-cycle of *Fasciola hepatica* is complex, involving stages inside a final host and an intermediate host, and on herbage. Two important meteorological factors in the development of the parasite are temperatures above 10°C and the presence of free water. In the late 1950s, Ollerenshaw suggested that development therefore is usually impossible during the winter (too cold) and that there may be insufficient water during some of the summer months (too dry). This is the basis of the '*Mt*' forecasting system for fascioliasis. *Mt* is a monthly index of wetness given by:

$$(R - p + 5)n$$

where, on a monthly basis:
$R$ = rainfall in inches
$p$ = potential transpiration
$n$ = number of rain days.

Observations suggested that, because parasite development is also temperature-dependent, the rate of development is similar in June, July, August

**Table 17.1 Associations between ΣMt values* and losses owing to fascioliasis in England and Wales. (Data from Ollerenshaw, 1966)**

| ΣMt | | Losses |
|---|---|---|
| NW England, SE England and N Wales | Other parts of England and Wales | |
| <300 | <400 | No losses |
| 300–450 | 400–450 | Some losses |
| >450 | >450 | Heavy losses |

*See text for explanation.

and September but is halved in May and October, when the *Mt* index should therefore be halved.

A seasonal summation of *Mt* indices (Σ*Mt*) can be calculated by adding the *Mt* values for the 6-month period May to October. This sum can be used to predict losses owing to fascioliasis, so that suitable prophylactic measures can be undertaken (*Table 17.1*). This prediction model uses point values in the equation and is therefore deterministic. The model has been adapted for use in France (Leimbacher, 1978) and Northern Ireland (Ross, 1978).

### Nematodiriasis

Attempts have also been made to predict morbidity rates of some nematode infections using climate as an indicator (Gibson and Smith, 1978a,b; Thomas, 1978). The life-cycle of *Nematodirus* spp. is temperature-dependent. There is a correlation between soil

**Table 17.2 Estimated peak hatch dates of *Nematodirus* spp. eggs in NE England in years of various national disease severities. (From Gibson and Smith, 1978a)**

| Actual national disease severity | Year | Estimated peak hatch date in NE England |
|---|---|---|
| Low | 1957 | 11 April |
| | 1961 | 11 April |
| Below average | 1952 | 16 April |
| | 1959 | 17 April |
| | 1967 | 18 April |
| | 1966 | 20 April |
| | 1960 | 22 April |
| Above average | 1953 | 21 April |
| | 1964 | 28 April |
| | 1968 | 29 April |
| | 1956 | 30 April |
| High | 1951 | 3 May |
| | 1954 | 4 May |
| | 1963 | 4 May |
| | 1965 | 6 May |
| | 1958 | 8 May |
| | 1955 | 12 May |
| | 1962 | 12 May |

temperature (taken 30 cm deep) and larval hatching dates. The mean soil temperature in March is used to predict the date of maximum larval count on the pasture. Additionally, there is a correlation between the estimated peak hatch date in NE England and national disease severity which can be used to predict, semiquantitatively, national prevalence (*Table 17.2*). Again, this is a deterministic model because no consideration is given to random variations.

## Explanatory models

More recently, mathematical models have been formulated that describe the dynamics of the parasite and host populations. These more sophisticated techniques allow the course of a disease to be simulated. They include models for forecasting fluke morbidity (Hope-Cawdery *et al.*, 1978; Williamson and Wilson, 1978), the airborne spread of foot-and-mouth disease (Gloster *et al.*, 1981; Donaldson *et al.*, 1982) and the occurrence of clinical ostertagiasis.

### Ostertagiasis

The level of pasture contamination by infective *Ostertagia ostertagi* larvae can be predicted by simulating the course of events experienced by a cohort of parasite eggs deposited on pasture (*Figure 17.1*: Gettinby *et al.*, 1979). This involves estimating the proportion of eggs that proceed to the first, second and third larval stages, using 'development fractions' which quantify the rate of development of the parasite according to the temperatures that it experiences. In addition, parameters associated with infectivity, fecundity and migratory behaviour of the larvae must be included. A prediction of burdens of infective larvae on herbage, based on a model that incorporates these parameters, can facilitate optimum use of anthelmintics and movement of animals to clean pasture before challenge by large numbers of infective larvae, thereby preventing clinical ostertagiasis.

## Deterministic population models

A population model attempts to quantify the mechanisms that regulate numbers at different stages of an infectious agent's life-cycle in order to describe the dynamics of the host/parasite relationship. Ideally, this requires estimation of absolute parasite numbers and so is more likely to be achieved using a density model than a prevalence model. The object is to gain a better understanding of the natural history of a disease, so that changes in

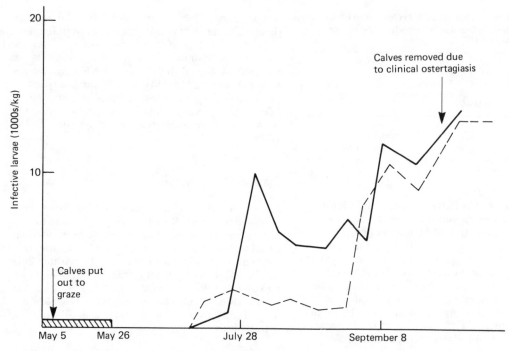

**Figure 17.1** Observed and predicted counts of infective *Ostertagia ostertagi* larvae on pasture in 1975. ——— Observed pasture count; —–—predicted pasture count; ▨ overwintered infective larvae. (From Gettinby *et al.*, 1979)

disease patterns, either natural or as a result of control campaigns, can be **explained**.

The early models of simple epidemics assumed that no infectious individuals were removed from the population during the course of the epidemic. This assumption was incorporated into one of the first models—the Reed–Frost model—which, although described in full only relatively recently (Frost, 1976), formed the basis of many early models. Although this assumption may sometimes be true of human epidemics, it is frequently untrue with animal epidemics: infectious animals are often removed by culling and slaughter. Recently, attempts have been made to model animal epidemics with regard to this difference (Takizawa *et al.*, 1977). Human models that consider the possible removal of infectious individuals from circulation by either death or isolation have also been developed.

The earlier models assumed that a group was of a given size with homogeneous mixing. They also assumed that a susceptible individual was infectious as soon as it was infected, that is, prepatent and latent periods were ignored. Most infectious diseases have prepatent periods and mixing is rarely homogeneous; more recent formulations include these factors.

Additionally, only a few diseases are characterized by interepidemic periods when no cases of disease occur (e.g. rabies and foot-and-mouth disease in Britain). Most diseases are endemic to a varying degree, and it is possible to have recurrent epidemics requiring different models.

The earlier models considered epidemics as processes that occur in continuous time—these were **continuous time** models. **Discrete time** models have been designed which portray disease patterns in fixed intervals of time. For example, if an epidemic starts with a single individual or several simultaneously infected individuals, then new cases will occur in a series of stages separated by time intervals equal to the disease's incubation period. A further discrete time development has been of models that consider individuals as occurring in a variety of states (**multistate** models), for instance susceptible, immune, infected, and dead. Models that consider how individuals can move from one state to another are called **state-transition** models. These are frequently prevalence models.

## Deterministic models using differential calculus

Many models are based on a mathematical technique called differential calculus, which considers the rate of change in a variable with respect to time. Models using this technique are formulated in terms of the rate of change of numbers of parasites with respect to time. Examples of diseases investigated by this type of model include tuberculosis in badgers and rabies in foxes.

## Tuberculosis in badgers

Bovine tuberculosis continues to be a problem in SW England because wild badgers are infected and are a source of infection to cattle. A possible method of control is to reduce the badger population to a level below the threshold density for maintenance of the infection.

The dynamics of bovine tuberculosis in badgers have been investigated using a deterministic state-transition model (Trewhella and Anderson, 1983), which includes three states: susceptible animals, animals incubating the disease, and infected animals (*Figure 17.2*). There is no need to include an immune state because badgers show no immunity to bovine tuberculosis. Parameters include density-dependent regulation of the badger population, natural and disease-induced death rates, the incubation period of the infection, and the rate of transmission.

The model predicts that prevalence increases with badger density (the predicted values being supported by field observations) and that prevalence oscillations occur with a periodicity of 18 years. The model suggests that, in areas of high badger density, considerable effort would be required to control the infection.

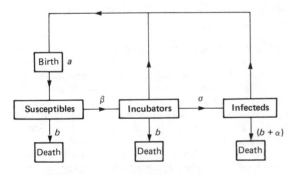

The flow of individual hosts between states is controlled by the rate parameters:

| | | |
|---|---|---|
| $a$ | = | the per capita birth rate |
| $b$ | = | the natural death rate |
| $\beta$ | = | the disease transmission coefficient |
| $\sigma$ | = | the rate at which incubating individuals become infected |
| $\alpha$ | = | the disease induced death rate |

**Figure 17.2** Flow chart of the deterministic model of bovine tuberculosis in badgers. (From Trewhella and Anderson, 1983)

## Rabies in foxes

Foxes are hosts of rabies in North America and Europe, and constitute a serious obstacle to control of the disease. The infection became established in foxes in Poland towards the end of the Second World War. The epidemic has spread slowly westwards at a rate of about 30 km/year. The standard method of control is slaughter of foxes, but results have been disappointing. A mathematical model (Macdonald and Bacon, 1980) suggests that control, other than by slaughter of foxes, may be more successful. The model has two components:

(1) prediction of the course of the disease in fox populations;
(2) evaluation of different control policies.

The model of the disease in fox populations makes plausible assumptions about the host and parasite. Foxes breed once a year in the autumn and fox mortality is highest in the winter, resulting in an annual fluctuation in fox numbers. The virus has a long incubation period and can therefore survive in hosts of high, changing and low densities; in the last circumstance, it can exist for a long time in individuals.

If rabies enters a fox population, the future of the host and parasite will be affected by the number of healthy foxes that are infected by rabid foxes; expressed as a ratio, this is the **contact rate**. If the disease is modelled for various contact rates, then there are different predicted outcomes; these are shown in *Figure 17.3a*. The upper lines of the graphs represent the total fox population, the lower lines the healthy foxes and the shaded areas the number of rabid foxes. The horizontal lines represent the number of foxes which, theoretically, can be carried by the habitat. A contact rate of 0.5 (one rabid fox infecting half a healthy fox) will, according to Kendall's Threshold Theorem (*see* Chapter 8), be insufficient to allow the infection to become established; the model supports this. Higher contact rates result in fluctuation in the fox population and in the number of rabid foxes. A contact rate of 1.4 allows the disease to persist, oscillating annually. A contact rate of 1.9 produces epidemics every 4 years that are severe enough to reduce the population to a level that will not support infection. The infection again becomes epidemic when the fox population recovers. Field surveys have shown that this periodicity is demonstrated in European foxes. Higher contact rates would lead to extinction of the fox population.

The second component of the model considers three control techniques (*Figure 17.3b*):

(1) slaughter;
(2) temporary sterilization;
(3) bait vaccination of foxes.

In case A, a single cull is instituted when rabies is at its earliest detectable level. Although slaughter

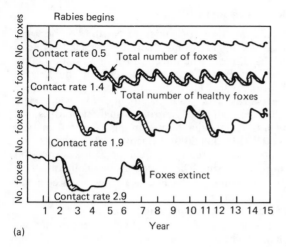

(a)

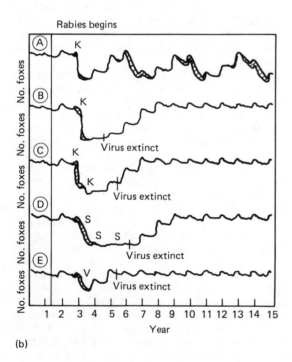

(b)

Control strategies:

K = controlled fox kill

S = temporary sterilization of foxes

V = bait vaccination of foxes

**Figure 17.3 (a)** Merlewood model of rabies in foxes; **(b)** Merlewood model of alternative strategies for controlling rabies in foxes. In each graph the initial level of the fox population is the same. (From Macdonald and Bacon, 1980)

initially decreases the prevalence of the disease, it soon increases again and then follows a pattern similar to that in the graph in *Figure 17.3a* depicting a contact rate of 1.9.

In case B, killing takes place later, probably when rabies is more likely to have been detected. Paradoxically, although initially there are more cases, the disease and the kill work together because more of the foxes that are not killed are incubating rabies and therefore will die. The virus thus becomes extinct as the fox population is dramatically reduced.

Case C represent two killings, separated by 6 months. Again, the virus becomes extinct, but the fox population is reduced below the levels in A and B.

Three applications of temporary sterilizing agent are illustrated in case D. The virus again is extinguished, but the fox population is reduced further.

Vaccination of foxes using vaccine-laden bait, shown in case E, offers the best results: removing the virus from the population and maintaining the number of healthy foxes (with 60% of foxes assumed to be immunized).

This model therefore suggests a more efficient and ecologically acceptable way of controlling fox rabies than the conventional slaughter policy. However, unknown variables may also be at work. Immune carriers may exist, and animals other than foxes may be hosts. Unrecorded behaviour patterns that bring foxes closer together than anticipated may also occur. These possibilities do not invalidate the model; they illustrate that more needs to be known about all relevant variables before an accurate model can be produced.

A defect of models based on differential calculus is the common assumption that parameters remain constant throughout the period of operation; for example, that the survival rate of helminth eggs does not change during a season, whereas, in reality, climatic variations may alter survival rates from day to day. The models frequently analyse 'steady state' conditions which represent parasite levels that may not be obtained in practice. For example, steady state levels of mature *Ostertagia* spp. larvae may not be reached in animals during autumn and winter due to larval inhibition.

## Deterministic matrix models

Some models use mathematical matrix theory. The matrices often take the form of a rectangular array containing numbers of hosts or of parasites in a defined state or stage of development, known as the **state vector**, or containing reproduction or survival rates of hosts or parasites in different states or stages, known as the **transition matrix**. In this way, it is possible to obtain the state of the system from one point in time to another. Stochastic matrix models of populations exist (e.g. Pollard, 1966) but are used less widely than deterministic models.

## Fascioliasis

The population size of the various stages in the life-cycle of *F. hepatica* have been formulated in a density matrix model (Gettinby and McClean, 1979). This is a state-transition model with five states: mature fluke (in sheep), egg (on grass), redia (in snails), metacercaria (on grass), and immature fluke (in sheep). A mortality rate is attached to all stages, and fecundity to the adult fluke and redia, which reproduce sexually and asexually respectively. The matrix includes probabilities of transition from one stage to the next, and fecundity, based upon available field data.

The first part of the model describes the natural infection in sheep in Britain and Ireland. The second part investigates and compares various control strategies: the use of flukicides, molluscicides and land drainage. There are three conclusions. Molluscicides are most effective when applied in early spring. Flukicides eradicate the infection when given monthly and control it when given at 2-monthly intervals. If dosing is only annual, then it is best carried out in August. Good drainage is an effective means of control. Again, in the absence of accurate field data to support the values of the input parameters in the model, the model only indicates possible outcomes.

## Stochastic population models

The first epidemic models considered that **the course of an epidemic must depend on the number of susceptibles and the contact rate between susceptible and infectious individuals**; this is the basic assumption underlying deterministic models. In a deterministic model, the future state of an epidemic process can be predicted precisely if the initial number of susceptible and infectious individuals is known.

Later, it was realized that the deterministic approach was not always applicable: variation and choice (of contact between susceptible and infected individuals) should be considered as part of the epidemic process. **Stochastic** modelling, which includes **the probability of infection**, therefore evolved. Each of these approaches to modelling produces a different result when modelling a simple epidemic. In *Figure 17.4*, the deterministic curve represents absolute point values. The stochastic curve represents the mean of all of the values

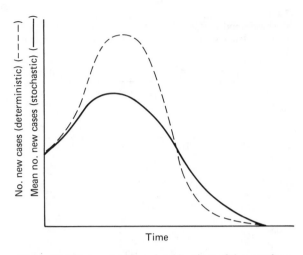

**Figure 17.4** Deterministic and stochastic model curves for a simple infectious epidemic. (After Bailey, 1975)

generated by the various probabilities. The probability of events occurring can be estimated in a variety of ways. One method uses random numbers to decide whether an event either has or has not occurred, somewhat akin to gambling, hence the description 'Monte Carlo' technique. In circumstances where infection can be interpreted simply as being either present or absent (i.e. a binomial event), a chain of newly infected individuals arises, which can be described by 'chain binomial' models.

## *Stochastic models using differential calculus*

### Populations of the sheep tick

The sheep tick, *Ixodes ricinus*, is a three-host tick; the three hosts are usually sheep. A knowledge of the dynamics of the tick population could be of value to control strategies. Field investigations (Milne, 1950) revealed that tick occurrence was patchy: a pasture may have a heavy burden whereas an apparently identical pasture, separated from the first only by a fence, may have no ticks. This suggested that ticks have problems with effective dispersal. One reason may be that at low densities tick population growth is inhibited by a low rate of mating. A stochastic model has been designed to describe incidence of mating (Plowright and Paloheimo, 1977). There are several assumptions: that each adult only mates if it encounters an individual of the opposite sex on the sheep to which it is attached; that each adult only mates once; that each tick has an equal probability of attaching to a sheep; that all ticks have an equal probability of encountering one another. The last two assumptions

**Table 17.3 Comparison of results of deterministic and stochastic models of incidence of mating in *Ixodes* for various parameter values. (From Plowright and Paloheimo, 1977)**

| *p* | Number of ticks | Number of sheep | Total number of matings | |
|---|---|---|---|---|
| | | | *Deterministic model* | *Stochastic model (mean of 600 replications)* |
| 0.05 | 40 | 10 | 3.3357 | 3.4400 |
| 0.05 | 40 | 20 | 4.7532 | 4.7833 |
| 0.05 | 40 | 40 | 5.1271 | 5.1533 |
| 0.05 | 40 | 80 | 3.9683 | 3.8395 |
| 0.05 | 40 | 160 | 2.2143 | 2.2117 |
| 0.05 | 80 | 10 | 8.9590 | 9.0883 |
| 0.05 | 80 | 20 | 13.2866 | 13.4567 |
| 0.05 | 80 | 40 | 15.3686 | 15.5733 |
| 0.05 | 80 | 80 | 12.6488 | 12.8450 |
| 0.05 | 80 | 160 | 7.9323 | 8.0050 |
| 0.01 | 40 | 10 | 0.3021 | 0.2933 |
| 0.01 | 40 | 20 | 0.5528 | 0.5567 |
| 0.01 | 40 | 40 | 0.9282 | 0.9017 |
| 0.01 | 40 | 80 | 1.3279 | 1.2733 |
| 0.01 | 40 | 160 | 1.4345 | 1.4633 |
| 0.01 | 80 | 10 | 1.0342 | 1.0017 |
| 0.01 | 80 | 20 | 1.8993 | 1.9483 |
| 0.01 | 80 | 40 | 3.2270 | 3.0550 |
| 0.01 | 80 | 80 | 4.7108 | 4.5867 |
| 0.01 | 80 | 160 | 5.2683 | 5.3367 |

*p* = probability of a tick attaching to a sheep.

are dubious but do not affect the model appreciably. The total number of matings at various sheep densities, and with varying numbers of ticks on each sheep, can be modelled by applying a Poisson distribution (*see* Chapter 12). *Table 17.3* lists the results and demonstrates the difference between the stochastic and deterministic output. By including a rate of survival in the model, it is possible to predict the growth rate of the tick population for different levels of tick population size and sheep density. When the sheep population is low, the rate of tick population increase is insensitive to changes in the size of the tick population, but highly sensitive to changes in the size of the sheep population. Conversely, when the tick population is low, the rate of tick population increase is relatively insensitive to changes in sheep numbers, but sensitive to changes in tick numbers. This supports the hypothesis that it is difficult for ticks to establish themselves in new pastures. It also suggests that a reduction in host density may not be an effective means of controlling tick infestation because the rate of tick population increase does not always depend on sheep density. The model also predicts that extinction of the tick population takes place over a narrow range of tick population sizes, corroborating field observations of patchy tick distribution.

## Stochastic network models

The inability to alter parameters and inputs during the running of a model, which may be associated with calculus-based methods, can be circumvented by using a **network representation** of a parasite's life history. This comprises interconnected paths that describe the components of the parasite's life-cycle. The various paths can be manipulated separately during the simulation, therefore variables can be altered. This technique is thus more capable of imitating fluctuations in factors during an actual infection. The flexibility of the network representation facilitates the construction of a stochastic model. Deterministic models can also be constructed but do not exploit fully the network approach.

### Ostertagiasis

*Figure 17.5* shows a network model of ostertagiasis in sheep (Paton and Gettinby, 1983; 1985). It allows variations in survival of eggs and adults, fecundity of adult eggs and the proportion of infective larvae that are ingested to be input independently into the model while it is running. Values for these parameters are obtained from available field evidence.

The effects of various anthelmintic strategies can be investigated by altering components of the network that will be affected by the particular strategy. For example, dosing of lambs will reduce the lamb egg input (Z) and dosing of ewes will decrease the ewe egg input (X). The simulation suggests that regular dosing of lambs at 4-weekly intervals for the first 6 months of life is very effective. Similarly, dosing lambs three times in July and August is effective. The single administration of an anthelmintic to ewes at lambing time is the least effective of the anthelmintic strategies.

## Further veterinary applications of modelling

Some theoretical models have been described which relate to natural epidemics under different conditions, for example Gumboro disease (Takizawa *et al.*, 1978a,b; 1980a,b), and consider possible control strategies, for example, bovine virus diarrhoea (Taylor, 1968). However, models that emphasize realism, rather than mathematical rigour, are of greater value to disease control. Four examples are given below.

### Hydatid control in New Zealand

This is a model of a two-host parasitic disease designed to evaluate the probable effect and relative

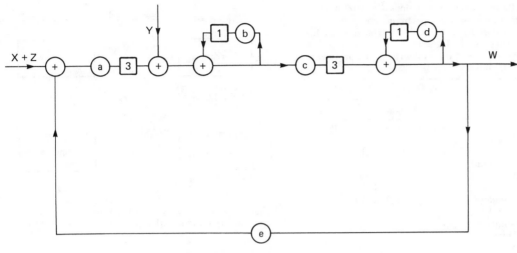

W = adult parasite output

X = ewe-derived eggs

Y = overwintered infective larvae

Z = lamb-derived eggs

a = survival rate of eggs which have undergone a three-week development period

b = proportion of infective larvae surviving until the following week

c = proportion of infective larval population which are ingested weekly

d = survival rate of adult worms from week to week

e = weekly fecundity rate of adult eggs

**Figure 17.5** Network model of the life-cycle of *Ostertagia circumcincta*. Squares denote time delays (in weeks in this example); circles denote scaling parameters. (From Paton and Gettinby, 1983)

merits of canine and ovine anthelmintics and vaccines (Harris *et al.*, 1980). It may be fully described as a deterministic, discrete time, multi-state model. The parasites considered are *Ecchinococcus granulosus*, *Taenia ovis* and *T. hydatigena*. The time period involved is 7 weeks: the appropriate latent period in the definitive canine host for the three parasites. This is also the prepatent period for *Taenia* spp. cysts in the sheep. The prepatent period for *E. granulosus* cysts in the sheep is approximately 20 time periods (140 weeks).

The possible states are uninfected and susceptible; latent infection; patent infection; acquired immunity; and vaccine immunity. There are several simplifying assumptions involved in these state definitions, and the mode of transmission assumes random distribution of infected animals, which is less likely to be true at very low prevalence. The

model simulation therefore excludes prevalence values lower than 0.1%. *Table 17.4* shows the results, simulating various control strategies. The model is designed to determine the relative merits of each type of strategy. The times taken to reduce prevalence are therefore relative, rather than definitive.

The conclusions are:

(1) canine anthelmintics have little effect when administered annually;
(2) canine anthelmintics administered at 7-weekly intervals reduce the percentage of patent canine infections with *T. ovis* and *T. hydatigena* to below 0.1% in 5 and 3 years respectively;
(3) there is less effect on *E. granulosus* than on other cestodes;
(4) ovine infections are reduced below 0.1% in a

**Table 17.4 Results of some simulations of control strategies for reducing the prevalence of patent infections of *Echinococcus granulosus* (E.g.), *Taenia hydatigena* (T.h.) and *Taenia ovis* (T.o.) in dogs and sheep. The figures represent the number of years taken to reduce prevalence to below 0.1%. (From Harris *et al.*, 1980)**

| Strategy | Dogs | | | Sheep | | |
|---|---|---|---|---|---|---|
| | E.g. | T.h. | T.o. | E.g. | T.h. | T.o. |
| No control | 10 | 10 | 10 | 10 | 10 | 10 |
| Dogs dosed every 7 weeks | 10 | 5 | 3 | 10 | 10 | 8 |
| Sheep dosed annually | 7 | 10 | 9 | 8 | 10 | 10 |
| Dogs dosed every 7 weeks and vaccinated annually | 7 | 3 | 1 | 10 | 6 | 5 |
| Sheep dosed and vaccinated annually | 5 | 5 | 3 | 5 | 6 | 3 |
| Dogs dosed every 7 weeks and sheep dosed annually | 2 | 2 | 1 | 4 | 4 | 3 |

simulated 10-year period only in *T. ovis* infections;

(5) annual administration of anthelmintics to sheep is more effective than 7-weekly dog dosing for ovine and canine *E. granulosus* infections;

(6) a combination of anthelmintic and vaccine therapy given annually to sheep is more effective than the use of an anthelmintic alone;

(7) annual vaccination of dogs is as effective as 7-weekly dosing;

(8) a combination of 7-weekly anthelmintic treatment and annual vaccination of dogs is more effective than either strategy alone;

(9) a single control strategy used on both hosts is generally more effective than more intensive strategies used on one host.

### Epidemic foot-and-mouth disease in the USA

This model is designed to predict the outcome of an epidemic of foot-and-mouth disease in the USA, with and without various control strategies (McCauley *et al.*, 1977). It is a state-transition model of a special type—the 'Markov Chain'—in which the transition from one state to another is assumed to be independent of previous transitions. There are four states:

(1) susceptible;
(2) infectious;
(3) immune;
(4) removed.

Transition pathways are summarized in *Figure 17.6*. Basic units are herds rather than individuals. The time period is one week. Probabilities of multiple transitions from one state to others are reset each week as the simulated epidemic proceeds.

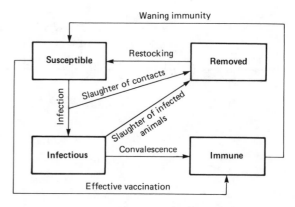

**Figure 17.6** Main pathways of a state-transition model of epidemic foot-and-mouth disease. (From McCauley *et al.*, 1977)

Not all transitions are considered for obvious biological reasons, such as 'infectious' to 'susceptible', 'removed' to 'infectious'. Again, certain features appropriate to the disease have to be built into the system. The herds are separated populations, therefore the concept of spread among a homogeneously mixed population is not valid. The factor 'dissemination rate' is included in the model. This represents the average number of herds to which virus is delivered, irrespective of herd states. The only real data relating to spread came from Britain where the topography is different, and where airborne spread was known to occur. (For a discussion of simulation of the British 1967–68 epidemic, *see* Tinline, 1972.) Dissemination in parts of America (e.g. the midwest) is likely to be greater than in Britain.

Using this model, and including contact slaughter and vaccination as control strategies, the simulation suggests that:

(1) 60% of susceptible herds could be affected within 30 weeks if there was a 'runaway' epidemic;

(2) in the absence of vaccination, the epidemic would reappear after 60 weeks to begin a series of endemic cycles;

(3) even with dissemination rates only slightly greater than those seen in the UK, a 'runaway' situation (1000 herds/week) could be reached within 5 weeks;

(4) if contact slaughter were employed on 18% of potentially infectious herds before excreting virus, an epidemic similar to the 1967–68 UK epidemic could be reduced in size by 50%.

### Brucellosis in a dairy herd in the UK

This is a multistate model to investigate what happens in infected herds and the effects of different control strategies (Hugh-Jones *et al.*, 1976). Reliable laboratory data were available but there were little sound epidemiological data when the model was formulated. Several input parameters (e.g. the risk of contracting infection) were therefore based on expert opinion.

There are three states: 'healthy', 'infected', and 'reactor' (in the serological and legal sense). Animals in the system may be newly born calves, or heifers, or cows. The probability of events occurring is calculated using the Monte Carlo technique.

The model is designed for a dairy herd incorporating usual practices (e.g. selling calves at different ages, buying all replacements, or partly internally replacing). Herd size can vary.

Control is effected by vaccination and several culling policies including:

(1) culling in which the farmer cannot recognize the difference in the health status of animals and therefore randomly selects cows in various states;
(2) culling in which the farmer can detect reactors;
(3) culling in which the herd is retested during the next period, if reactors are found;
(4) culling as in (3), but with a 2-month delay until retesting of the herd.

Again, there are simplifying assumptions, for example, that the test for reactors has a sensitivity and specificity of 100% (which is virtually impossible), that reactors are slaughtered immediately, and that farm disinfection is totally effective.

Results of the simulation trials include:

(1) the probability of converting from 'healthy' to 'infected';
(2) interrelationships between the numbers of 'infected' and 'reactor' cows;
(3) the number and pattern of herd tests;
(4) the effect of a summer start of eradication;
(5) the effect of numbers of 'infected' stock on eradication;
(6) advantages of isolating aborting and calving cows;
(7) the possible benefits of modifying the vaccine protection;
(8) the effect of changing the ability of animals to be infectious;
(9) the effects of making infected cows 'react' sooner in pregnancy;
(10) the ability to control disease related to herd size.

The model concludes that the eradication time would be shorter if eradication were started in the summer (most compulsory schemes began in October and November during the British eradication campaign). There is also a distinct advantage in isolating any aborting cow. Isolation of cows that

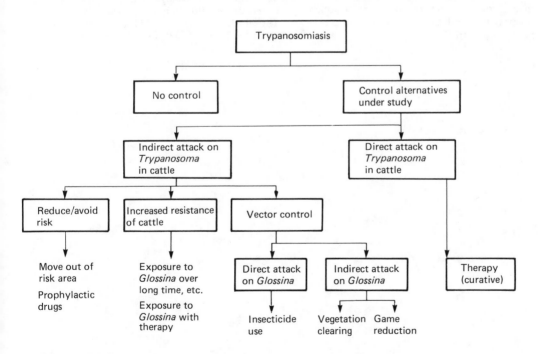

**Figure 17.7** Diagrammatic representation of the disease-vector control alternatives evaluated in a model of African trypanosomiasis. (From Habtemariam *et al.*, 1983a)

may be infectious at calving is also desirable. There are further advantages to control if the maximum number of cows are calved in isolation and if those more than 3 months pregnant are grazed away from the remainder of the herd (a conclusion supported by actual findings in the Netherlands). The British policy of blood-testing animals at 4-monthly intervals during eradication gives the best results in the model. There is little advantage in retesting at shorter intervals when reactors are identified according to the model.

### Trypanosomiasis in Ethiopia

Trypanosomiasis is responsible for serious losses in African cattle and renders some areas uninhabitable for both livestock and man. The protozoan parasite infects not only domestic cattle but also wild game. It is carried by an arthropod vector: the tsetse fly. A model using differential calculus has been constructed to evaluate alternative control strategies for the disease in Ethiopia (Habtemariam *et al.*, 1983c). This model is an extension of models of the natural infection (Habtemariam *et al.*, 1983a,b).

The various control techniques are summarized in *Figure 17.7*. The model evaluates a prevalence of 27.3% (the estimated endemic prevalence of trypanosomiasis in Ethiopia at the time of the model's construction) and is run over a 10-year period with combinations of the various strategies. The simulation predicts that a combination of vegetation clearing, insecticide spraying, resettlement of areas cleared by spraying, and therapy offers the most efficient means of control.

Modelling is one component of the epidemiological approach. It cannot be used effectively without reliable field and experimentally derived data relating to diseases' natural history; the dangers of applying modelling in isolation from field observation are emphasized by Hugh-Jones (1983). However, when used in association with diagnostic and experimental disciplines, modelling is a valuable aid to an increased understanding of disease.

## Further reading

ANDERSON, R.M. and MAY, R.M. (Eds) (1982) *Population Biology of Infectious Diseases*. Report of the Dohlem Workshop on Population Biology of Infectious Disease Agents, Berlin, 14–19 March 1982. Springer-Verlag, Berlin

BAILEY, N.T.J. (1975) *The Mathematical Theory of Infectious Diseases and its Applications*, 2nd edn. Charles Griffin, London

BARTLETT, M.S. (1960) *Stochastic Population Models in Ecology and Epidemiology*. Methuen's Monographs on Applied Probability and Statistics. Methuen and Company Limited, London

CVJETANOVIC, B., GRAB, B. and UEMURA, K. (1978) Dynamics of acute bacterial diseases: epidemiological models and their application to public health. *Bulletin of the World Health Organization*, **56**, Suppl. No. 1

ESCH, G.W. (Ed.) (1977) *Regulation of Parasite Populations*. Academic Press, London and New York

THRUSFIELD, M.V. and GETTINBY, G. (1984) An introduction to techniques of veterinary modelling. In: Society for Veterinary Epidemiology and Preventive Medicine, Proceedings, Edinburgh, 10–11 July 1984. Ed. Thrusfield, M.V. Pp. 114–138. (Also published separately, ISBN: 0 948073 01 2)

# 18

# The economics of disease

Livestock are part of farm enterprise. The effects of disease and the need for disease control therefore have to be considered as part of the economic assessment of farms individually, regionally and nationally. This aspect of assessment is closely allied to epidemiological (biological) studies. A basic knowledge of economic techniques therefore provides a necessary perspective to the veterinarian's activities in large animal practice.

## Production as an economic process

From a technical (i.e. biological) point of view, livestock products are obtained from the conversion of nutrients from feed **inputs** to various **outputs** (e.g. liveweight, milk, eggs, wool). An economist would extend the list of inputs to include those that 'facilitate the process' as well as those that actively undergo physical transformation. The former include land, labour, machinery and managerial skill. Typically, increased production is associated with the use of more inputs. Disease usually reduces productivity and therefore acts as a 'negative input'. If a disease problem exists, the main concern is to recover production; therefore additional inputs of one kind or another will be necessary. This is associated with an economic problem: inputs are normally scarce, therefore each has a price, and prices give rise to costs of production. A condition for economic efficiency is that inputs should be used in a combination that minimizes the cost of producing a given level of output. Similarly, the methods used to recover lost production should be at least cost.

## The nature of economic decisions

Economics is a science of choice. The part of the science that is of greatest importance to animal disease problems is **microeconomics**, which is concerned with efficiency arising from decisions that affect the availability and use of resources and products by the many individual producers and consumers who make up the national economy. Microeconomic analysis is concerned to a large extent with identifying the optimum level of production in relation to total resource use, and achieving the most efficient combination of inputs within that total. The criteria of efficiency are economic rather than technical.

Although initially the idea may seem unusual, technical and economic efficiency are seldom synonymous. Under normal circumstances of diminishing physical returns, they are the same only if inputs are costless. For example, it is efficient in an economic sense for a dairy farmer to aim for maximum milk yield per cow only when the cow's feed is free. If the farmer has to pay for the feed which, of course, is invariably the case, then optimum economic efficiency is obtained when the yield per cow is less than the maximum technical potential. Furthermore, the overall economic optimum (maximum profits) will change with variations in relative prices of both output and inputs and with methods of production. This observation is important in the context of animal disease because the incidence of disease that is acceptable from an economic point of view may well change with relative prices and techniques of production. Additionally, it should not be supposed that reduction of disease depends **exclusively** on veterinary services and medicines. An economist regards these as just particular types of inputs that may have substitutes in the form of greater managerial expertise, use of more land to reduce stocking rate, and so on, all of which may increase economic efficiency by reducing disease. The economist asks the question: what **combination** of veterinary and other inputs will optimize economic efficiency?

## The economic analysis of animal disease

The application of economics *per se* to problems of animal disease is relatively new. The majority of studies that have been undertaken in the past have been concerned with the financial assessment of animal health problems (which is different from the main economic questions about efficiency of real resource use), and especially with applications of **cost-benefit analysis**. Both of these approaches are rather specific and narrowly defined aspects of economic analysis in general. Nevertheless, they are important parts of the whole subject area; the remainder of this chapter, therefore, introduces examples that emphasize the financial and cost-benefit methods. An extended explanation of relevant broad economic principles is provided by Howe (1985).

## The need for economic assessment of disease control

Control campaigns incur a cost, derived from the use of resources ranging from prophylactic and therapeutic drugs to veterinary and agricultural manpower. Before disease control campaigns are instituted it is therefore desirable to assess:

(1) the costs arising from the disease;
(2) the cost of the control campaign.

It is then possible to weigh the **cost** of the control campaign against the **benefits** (e.g. increased production) that would accrue from control of the disease in order to determine the economic viability of the campaign. Clearly, if the control campaign costs more than the losses due to the disease then the campaign is not economically viable.

The traditional animal plagues (e.g. rinderpest and pleuropneumonia) have such marked effects on production that the net financial benefits of control are obvious. However, the complex diseases that are frequently present in systems of intensive husbandry tend to have more subtle effects on production, for instance, the effect of bovine ketosis and mastitis on milk yield (Lucey *et al.*, 1984), and so require precise costing before justifiable control can be undertaken. The cost of control campaigns in intensive units can also involve considerable financial outlay by the producer, for example, a vaccination policy in a 1000-sow pig unit. The significance of financial evaluations in intensive units has been partly responsible for the increased application of economic techniques to animal disease control since the 1960s. The techniques have also assisted in the formulation of national and international control campaigns, for example, brucellosis eradication in England and Wales (Hugh-Jones *et al.*, 1975a), swine fever eradication in Europe (Ellis *et al.*, 1977) and rinderpest control in Nigeria (Felton and Ellis, 1978).

## Methods of financial evaluation

Evaluation can be undertaken in two ways. First, a large number of units can be visited and the extent of the disease and the profitability of a particular unit can be accounted by comparison with the average. This method assumes that an increased profitability is a direct result of a decreased disease prevalence, which is true if other factors, such as husbandry practice, product prices and costs of production, remain unchanged. However, there may be other reasons. Profitable farms may be able to afford preventive measures more than unprofitable farms. Similarly, increased profits and decreased disease prevalence both may be the result of good farm management and efficient allocation of farm resources. The second method of evaluation involves the construction of a model (similar to those described in the previous chapter) that includes prices.

## Assessing the cost of disease

The financial losses caused by disease can be divided into five categories (Beynon, 1964):

(1) the cost of resources that are wasted on animals that die;
(2) the cost of drugs;
(3) the cost of veterinary fees;
(4) excessive expenditure on feed as a result of poor feed conversion efficiency;
(5) losses due to inefficient production.

The last category is different from the first four. Reduced levels of production represent a loss of the opportunities for earning higher revenues. In contrast, the first four categories represent actual financial expenditures.

The following example (Christian *et al.*, 1973) illustrates how the financial costs of disease may be calculated. It relates to all diseases in a British pig fattening unit, and compares 2 years; disease

**Table 18.1 Data used in costing disease in a British pig fattening unit (applied in** *Table 18.2*; **results in** *Table 18.3*). **(From Christian** *et al.*, **1973)**

|  | 1st year | 2nd year |
|---|---|---|
| Pigs purchased | 7 997 | 9 337 |
| Deaths | 572 | 336 |
| Casualty slaughter pigs | 460 | 724 |
| Total condemned carcasses | 14 | 24 |
| Food conversion efficiency | 4.54 | 3.88 |
| Liveweight of unit at end of period | *335 909 lb | 462 150 lb |
| Liveweight sold | 1 488 577 lb | 1 666 073 lb |
| Liveweight of unit at start of period | 251 405 lb | *274 865 lb |
| Liveweight purchased | 539 489 lb | 685 908 lb |
| Average cost of weaners | £8.03 | £8.63 |
| Overhead cost per pig | £2.08 | £1.72 |
| Average liveweight gain of pigs going off fat | 153 lb | 129 lb |
| Cost of food per lb | £0.014 | £0.015 |
| Average liveweight gain of pigs dying | 41 lb | 22 lb |
| Average liveweight gain of pigs sent as casualties | 64 lb | 44 lb |
| Receipts from casualty slaughter | £4 312.00 | £6 465.00 |
| Drugs and disinfectants | £1 650.00 | £1 566.00 |
| Number of pigs sent off fat | 6 965 | 8 277 |

*The difference between these figures is due to a period of one month between the end of the first year of study and the start of the second year.

**Table 18.2 Calculation of the costs of disease in a British pig fattening unit (data presented in** *Table 18.1*)

*Food conversion efficiency: FCE*
$FCE$ = Total amount of food consumed (lb)/total liveweight gain (lb)

*Total liveweight gain: Tlb*
$T = (A + B) - (C + D)$
where:
$A$ = liveweight in unit at end of period (lb)
$B$ = liveweight sold during period (lb)
$C$ = liveweight in unit at start of period (lb)
$D$ = liveweight of pigs purchased during period (lb)

*The cost of producing one fat pig: £P*
$P = E + F (G \times H \times I)$
where:
$E$ = average cost of weaner pigs (£)
$F$ = overhead costs per pig purchased, made up mainly of rent on buildings, labour and services (£)
$G$ = average liveweight increase (lb)
$H$ = overall food conversion efficiency
$I$ = average cost of food per lb (£)

*The cost of mortality: £M*
$M = X\{E + F + (G_1 \times H_1 \times I)\}$
where:
$X$ = the number of dead pigs
$G_1$ = liveweight increase of pigs dying
$H_1^*$ = food conversion efficiency of these pigs

*The cost of casualty slaughter: £S*
$S = Y\{E + F + (G_2 \times H_2 \times I)\} - Z$
where:
$Y$ = number of casualty slaughter pigs (£)
$Z$ = financial return from these pigs (£)
$G_2$ = liveweight increase of pigs sent to casualty slaughter (lb)
$H_2^*$ = food conversion efficiency of these pigs

*Cost of total condemnations at normal slaughter: £N*
$N = W\{E + F + (G \times H \times I)\}$
where:
$W$ = number of condemned carcasses

*Potential loss due to poor food conversion efficiency: a lb*
$a = b - (b/c \times d)$
where:
$b$ = total food used (lb)
$c$ = food conversion efficiency on farm
$d$ = standard food conversion efficiency: defined as 3.5 in this case (Goodwin, 1971a)

*The food conversion efficiency of pigs that die ($H_1$) and casualty slaughter pigs ($H_2$) are different, but are both simplified to $H$ in this calculation.

**Table 18.3 Costs of disease in a British pig fattening unit for 2 years (disease incidence lower in the second year). (Abridged from Christian *et al.*, 1973)**

| | 1st year | | 2nd year | |
|---|---|---|---|---|
| | Total (£) | Cost per pig sold fat (£) | Total (£) | Cost per pig sold fat (£) |
| *Direct cost* | | | | |
| Cost of death | 7 271 | 1.04 | 3 928 | 0.48 |
| Cost of casualty slaughter | 2 208 | 0.31 | 2 947 | 0.36 |
| Cost of total condemnations | 276 | 0.03 | 443 | 0.05 |
| *Total direct cost* | 9 755 | 1.38 | 7 308 | 0.89 |
| *Indirect cost* | | | | |
| Poor food conversion | 11 967 | 1.73 | 4 135 | 0.50 |
| Drugs and disinfectants | 1 650 | 0.24 | 1 566 | 0.20 |
| Cost of third man (primarily concerned with cleanliness of the unit) | – | – | 1 500 | 0.18 |
| *Total indirect cost* | 13 617 | 1.97 | 7 201 | 0.88 |
| *Total cost* | 23 372 | 3.38 | 14 509 | 1.77 |

incidence was much reduced in the second year. The data used in costing disease are presented in *Table 18.1*. The relevant calculations are depicted in *Table 18.2*, and the results are shown in *Table 18.3*. Two assumptions are made in the calculation:

(1) that poor food conversion is only a reflection of disease (rather than of other factors, such as poor quality feed), and is therefore included as a disease cost;

(2) that the cost of employing a third man (*Table 18.3*) is a disease cost, because he was primarily concerned with hygiene within the unit (this is, however, an exceptional situation).

Also, the transitory costs of veterinary time, building alterations, partial condemnations and loss of production during depopulation are excluded from the calculation. Although the cost of casualty slaughter and losses due to condemnations was higher during the second year because of a more active disease control policy, the total costs in the second year, attributable to disease, are approximately 66% of those in the first year.

Other examples of the costing of diseases include financial losses due to abortion in a dairy herd (Bates *et al.*, 1984), salmonellosis in a calf-rearing unit (Peters, 1985), warble-fly infestation (Andrews, 1978), enzootic pneumonia (Goodwin, 1971a), dairy calf (Martin and Wiggins, 1973) and sheep (Howe, 1976; Purvis *et al.*, 1979) mortality, and bovine helminthiasis (Reid and Armour, 1978). The general principles of the measurement and evaluation of the financial effects of parasitic disease are described by Morris and Meek (1980).

# Cost-benefit analysis of disease control

The costs and benefits of disease control campaigns can be assessed using several methods, including **gross margin analysis**, **partial budgets** (Asby *et al.*, 1975) and **social cost-benefit analysis** (Pearce, 1971; Mishan, 1976; Sugden and Williams, 1978) which is a technique widely used for the appraisal of large-scale investment programmes. If it is necessary only to compare the effectiveness of two alternative control strategies, without fully assessing benefits and costs, then a **cost-effective** study is undertaken. The technique that has been applied widely to animal disease control evaluation is social cost-benefit analysis (CBA).

## *Principles of CBA*

Social cost-benefit analysis attempts to quantify the social advantages and disadvantages of a policy in terms of a common monetary unit. The building of a road will incur costs to society arising from the resources expended on construction and maintenance, the undesirable side-effects of pollution, increased noise level and spoiling of the landscape. The benefits include savings in travelling time, reduced congestion and decreased noise level in a town if the road is a bypass. Some of the costs or benefits (e.g. construction outlays—costs) are expressed easily in pecuniary values. Other costs or benefits (e.g. decreased noise level—a benefit), however, are much more difficult to translate into monetary terms; these are called **intangibles**. Only by using the common denominator of money is it possible to aggregate the gains and losses which ultimately interest society as the benefits and costs perceived in **real** terms, that is, as adding to or reducing people's sense of wellbeing. Consequently, it is important to quantify, in monetary units, all important factors as comprehensively as possible, and to make the problem areas explicit, although the value of intangibles is often assessed somewhat subjectively.

If a disease control programme were initiated, costs would include those of manpower, drugs, vaccines, quarantine buildings, compensation for slaughter, transportation and training programmes. The benefits would include increased productivity, decreased animal and (in the case of zoonotic diseases) human suffering, increased trade and the psychological wellbeing accompanying the decreased disease incidence. The prefix 'social' to CBA is often dropped from the name but is important. It emphasizes that CBA is used by an organization to maximize the **net benefits to society**, rather than maximizing its own purely private benefits (Pearce and Sturmey, 1966).

## 'Internal' and 'external' costs and benefits

**Internalities (private** costs and benefits) are those that accrue directly to an investment project. Costs and benefits accruing to others are termed **externalities**. It is the externalities that mainly are not reflected in the price mechanism (which therefore becomes inadequate as a guide to correct investment decisions from the point of view of society). For example, a farm mastitis control campaign includes dry-cow antibiotic therapy (a cost) and increased milk yield (a benefit), both of which are part of the farm's budget and therefore internal. However, antibiotic residues in milk may have undesirable side-effects on unknowing consumers. If they were aware of the risks they would be prepared to pay less for the milk (if, indeed, they would buy it at all). To protect consumers, and to 'internalize' the external effects, legislation limiting the use of antibiotics and affected milk may be necessary instead of reliance on a deficient price mechanism. Similarly, in a foot-and-mouth disease campaign in Britain, farmers' loss of slaughtered animals is an internal cost, whereas the inconvenience of restrictions on movement and access is an external cost.

## Discounting

Control campaigns may operate over several years. The value of a sum of money now is greater than the same sum of money at a later date because it could be invested now to produce a larger sum in the future as interest accrues. If the interest rate is 5% per annum, then £100 now is worth £105 compound in one year's time, £110.25 in 2 years, and so on. If costs and benefits, spread over several years, are to be compared then they must be adjusted to calculate their value now. The process of adjustment, which is the opposite of compounding, is called **discounting**. The formulae for its calculation are described by Gittinger (1972) and Little and Mirrlees (1974). The calculation uses a rate of discount that is usually defined by governments, for example, the World Bank Rate and, in Britain, the Treasury Rate. The latter is a target rate for public investments and is not the same as the Bank Rate. Cost-benefit analysis is performed in real terms which means that the rate of interest used in the calculations is adjusted to exclude the effects of price inflation.

## Shadow prices

The social value of a benefit may not always be the market price. For example, a litre of milk is valued at its market price by the farmer. However, in the European Economic Community, the value may be less because of a surplus of milk. A national disease control campaign that resulted in increased milk production therefore would use the value of the milk to the European Economic Community, termed a **shadow price**, in economic evaluation.

## Uncertainty

Any project is accompanied by uncertainty. The results of a control campaign cannot be known with certainty, but it is necessary to have an idea what the outcome might be. There are two approaches to dealing with uncertainty. First, if a model is constructed, the 'most probable outcome' can be defined; a sensitivity analysis (*see* Chapter 17) can then be conducted to determine whether changes in the model's parameters can produce major changes in the outcome. Alternatively, the likelihood of the various outcomes can be judged using probability theory (Reutlinger, 1970).

## Criteria for selecting a control campaign

Three important measures of economic efficiency, used as criteria for selecting a control campaign, are:

(1) Net present value (*NPV*);
(2) Benefit:cost ratio (*B/C*);
(3) Internal rate of return (*IRR*).

The **net present value** (*NPV*) is the value of the stream of discounted benefits less costs over $n$ time periods. It is given by:

$$NPV = \frac{B_0 - C_0}{(1 + r)^0} + \frac{B_1 \, C_1}{(1 + r)^1} + \cdots + \frac{B_n - C_n}{(1 + r)^n}$$

$$= \sum_{t=0}^{n} \frac{B_t - C_t}{(1 + r)^t}$$

where:

$C_t$ = value of costs incurred in time t,
$B_t$ = value of benefits gained in time t,
$r$ = discount rate,
$n$ = life of project.

A project is considered to be viable if the *NPV* is positive.

The **benefit:cost ratio** (*B/C*) is the ratio of the present value of benefits to that of costs. It is given by:

$$B/C = \sum_{t=0}^{n} \{B_t/(1+r)^t\}/\{C_t/(1+r)^t\}$$

$$= \sum_{t=0}^{n} \frac{B_t}{C_t}.$$

A project is viable if the ratio is greater than or equal to 1.

The **internal rate of return** (*IRR*) is the rate of discount that equates the present value of the costs with the present value of the benefits. It is given by solving for *r* such that:

$$NPV = \sum_{t=0}^{n} \frac{B_t - C_t}{(1 + r)^t} = 0.$$

If the internal rate of return of an investment project is greater than the actual interest rate, the project is economically worthwhile.

## An example of CBA

### Alternative policies for the prevention, control and eradication of infestation with *Chrysomyia bezziana* in Australia (Cason and Geering, 1980).

*C. bezziana*, the Old World screw-worm fly (SWF), causes serious economic losses in livestock in Africa, Asia and Papua New Guinea. Damage caused by burrowing larvae can result in a case fatality rate of up to 50% in young animals, and can cause loss of condition, occasional deaths and sterility (if genitalia are struck) in adults. The disease is not present in Australia, but if the fly entered Australia, potential losses have been estimated at around $100 million per annum. The most likely method of entry into Australia would be by movement of infested livestock across the Torres Strait islands from Papua New Guinea, although entry could also occur either by the direct flight of the flies or by transmission of the flies by migratory birds and aircraft.

Strategies to prevent the introduction and establishment of SWF in Australia include:

(1) improved quarantine surveillance, including training of local inhabitants and education programmes;
(2) better control of livestock in danger areas, possibly including total destocking of the Torres Strait islands—although this would probably be socially unacceptable to the islanders;
(3) the development of a SWF monitoring system, facilitated by a specific chemical bait (Swormlure);
(4) the construction of a clinic in the Torres Strait islands to neuter dogs and cats (potential hosts of SWF);
(5) eradication of SWF from Papua New Guinea.

The major strategy to control and eradicate an outbreak of infestation with SWF in Australia is ground control of the fly, consisting of restriction of movement of livestock, dipping and spraying with insecticides, the use of a sterile insect release method, by which sterile male flies compete with fertile male flies for each mating female, and the use of a screw-worm adult suppression system (SWASS), in which poisoned baits are released by aeroplane over infested areas. The quickest response to an outbreak of SWF infestation would be obtained if a sterile SWF facility were built in advance, but not opened until an outbreak occurred.

*Table 18.4* shows the benefit:cost ratios for the various strategies over a 20-year period, assuming

**Table 18.4 Cost-benefit analysis of strategies for the prevention, control and eradication of infestation with *Chrysomyia bezziana* in Australia. (The analysis is in present values over a 20-year period, and assumes that the methods prevent Australia-wide losses commencing year 1, year 10, year 20; discounted at 9%). (Modified from Cason and Geering, 1980)**

| Prevention method | Year infestation prevented | | | | | |
|---|---|---|---|---|---|---|
| | *1* | | *10* | | *20* | |
| | Benefit: $389m | | Benefit: $164m | | Benefit: $69m | |
| | Cost ($000) | Benefit:cost ratio | Cost ($000) | Benefit:cost ratio | Cost ($000) | Benefit:cost ratio |
| Strategic eradication from Papua New Guinea | 2 962 | 131 | 11 734 | 14 | 16 123 | 4 |
| Mothballed factory and maintenance colony | 1 394 | 279 | 1 670 | 98 | 1 809 | 38 |
| Ground control* | 2 523 | 154 | 1 065 | 154 | 449 | 155 |
| Destocking of Torres Strait islands | 657 | 592 | 776 | 212 | 836 | 83 |
| Improving quarantine | 124 | 3 137 | 417 | 394 | 563 | 123 |
| 'Swormlure' trapping and myiasis monitoring | 30 | 12 966 | 171 | 961 | 241 | 288 |
| Training | 26 | 14 961 | 69 | 2 383 | 91 | 763 |
| Extension | 13 | 29 923 | 83 | 1 980 | 119 | 583 |
| Torres Strait clinic | 7 | 55 571 | 40 | 4 110 | 56 | 1 239 |

*Includes the SWASS technique (*see* text).

that infestation occurred after 1, 10 or 20 years. In all cases the benefit:cost ratios are greater than 1, indicating that all techniques are economically justifiable.

In the example the benefits do not derive from increased production, but from decreasing the risk of infestation. Although the benefit:cost ratios are high, they have to be weighed against the probability of infestation occurring when a particular policy either is or is not adopted. These and other considerations are discussed by the authors of the study.

## Some problems associated with CBA

There are several general practical problems related to CBA. The technique assumes that the preferences and priorities of society are known; this may not always be true. The technique also applies the **current** social preferences, rather than future ones. Additionally, as indicated earlier, the costs and benefits of externalities and intangibles may be difficult to assess.

There are specific problems relating to disease control policy formulation (Grindle, 1980, 1986). Cost-benefit analysis is a relatively sophisticated technique but may be applied in situations—especially in the developing countries—where accurate basic data are lacking. For example, there may be inadequate information on livestock numbers, disease morbidity and the actual economic impact of disease. It may also be impossible to predict future market prices (e.g. of beef and milk) which need to be included in analyses. The sophistication of the economic techniques therefore needs to be balanced with the quality of the epidemiological data that are available. However, although CBA and other techniques of project evaluation are, at best, approximate (Gittinger, 1972), they play an essential role in economic evaluation. Despite its

limitations, CBA is a rigorous approach to project evaluation, and its application should help towards better informed decisions regarding the efficient use of scarce resources in disease control programmes.

## Further reading

ELLIS, P.R. and JAMES, A.D. (1979) The economics of animal health—(1) major disease control programmes. *Veterinary Record*, **105**, 504–506

ELLIS, P.R. and JAMES, A.D. (1979) The economics of animal health—(2) economics in farm practice. *Veterinary Record,* **105**, 523–526

ELLIS, P.R., SHAW, A.P.M. and STEPHENS, A.J. (Eds) (1976) *New Techniques in Veterinary Epidemiology and Economics*. Proceedings of a symposium, University of Reading, 12–15 July 1976

ERB, H. (1984) Economics for veterinary farm practice. *In Practice*, **6**, 33–37

GEERING, W.A., ROE, R.T. and CHAPMAN, L.A. (Eds) (1980) *Veterinary Epidemiology and Economics*. Proceedings of the Second International Symposium, Canberra, 7–11 May 1979. Australian Government Publishing Service, Canberra

HOWE, K.S. (1985) An economist's view of animal disease. In: Society for Veterinary Epidemiology and Preventive Medicine, Proceedings, Reading 27–29 March 1985. Ed. Thrusfield, M.V. Pp. 122–129

JAMES, A.D. and ELLIS, P.R. (1980) The evaluation of production and economic effects of disease. In: *Veterinary Epidemiology and Economics*. Eds Geering, W.A., Roe, R.T. and Chapman, L.A. Proceedings of the Second International Symposium, Canberra, 7–11 May 1979. Pp. 363–372. Australian Government Publishing Service, Canberra

KANEENE, J.B. and MATHER, E.C. (1982) *Cost Benefits of Food Animal Health*. Michigan State University and W.K. Kellogg Foundation, East Lansing

PEARCE, D.W. (1971) *Cost-Benefit Analysis*. The Macmillan Press Ltd, London

*PROCEEDINGS OF THE THIRD INTERNATIONAL SYMPOSIUM ON VETERINARY EPIDEMIOLOGY AND ECONOMICS* (1983) Held at Arlington, Virginia, 6–10 September 1982. Veterinary Medicine Publishing Company, Edwardsville

# 19

# Health and productivity schemes

## The development of health and productivity schemes

The traditional role of the veterinarian has been to attend individual sick animals when requested to do so by the owner: such attention has been called 'fire brigade' treatment. This approach was useful when most diseases, such as the classic epidemic infectious diseases, had a predominantly single cause and responded to a simple course of treatment. However, an appreciation during the 1960s of the multifactorial nature of many diseases, which coincided with intensification of animal industries in the developed countries, with a relative decrease in the value of individual animals, resulted in a change in attitude towards the management of diseases in livestock units (*see* Chapter 1). First, it became clear that diseases needed to be controlled by simultaneously manipulating all determinants: those associated with agent, host and environment. The veterinarian's objective should be to **prevent** rather than to treat disease. Secondly, it became necessary to consider disease in terms of its contribution to reduced performance (and therefore profitability) of a herd. Production, like disease, includes interaction between host, agent and environment. Thus, the number of piglets born alive can be reduced by, among other factors, early fetal deaths due to virus infections (agent) and by the genetic constitution of the sow and boar (host). Piglet mortality may be increased by deaths due to hypothermia (environment).

The first change stimulated the development of **preventive medicine programmes** in the early 1960s. The second change resulted in the evolution of comprehensive **herd health and productivity schemes**, encompassing preventive medicine and the assessment of productivity.

## Structure of health and productivity schemes

### Objectives

The goals of a health and productivity scheme are summarized by Blood (1976). They should:

(1) identify disease problems on a farm;
(2) rate the problems in order of importance, with reference to technical and economic criteria;
(3) initiate suitable control techniques and measure their success, not only technically but also with regard to the economic efficiency of the utilization of resources at the national and individual farm level, thereby indicating which technique should be increased and which should be reduced.

The scope of service offered by the veterinarian in a health and productivity scheme (Grunsell *et al.*, 1969) includes:

(1) the diagnosis and prevention of the major epidemic diseases;
(2) advice on environmental determinants (nutrition, housing and management);
(3) advice on production techniques and general policies of livestock farming.

This scope is broad and indicates that the veterinarian requires more than just a knowledge of the diagnosis and treatment of clinical disease. In many cases, the veterinarian may need to enlist further expert help from nutritionists, from building advisors, and from management specialists who have some knowledge of farm economics.

### Components

There are differences between the schemes applied to different species, but the principles are the same.

The main components of a health and productivity scheme are:

(1) the recording of a **farm profile** comprising details of animal numbers, stocking density, nutrition, usual management practices, disease status and current levels of production;
(2) identification of production shortfalls;
(3) monitoring of all aspects of production;
(4) identification of the major disease problems;
(5) routine prophylaxis against the major disease risks;
(6) definition of **production targets that are suitable for the system of management operating on the particular livestock units and for the aims of the farmer**;
(7) advice on management and husbandry, to achieve the predetermined targets;
(8) detection of unacceptable shortfalls in production (and therefore in profitability);
(9) correction of the shortfalls by eliminating the defects associated with host, agent and environment, or revising the production targets in the light of experience.

Regular visits to farms are an important part of health schemes. An **action list** is drawn up containing details of procedures (e.g. vaccination) to be followed at certain times of the year.

Health schemes require accurate records to be kept. Early schemes used longhand records, as do some modern ones (e.g. Blowey, 1983), but most contemporary systems store data on computers where the data can be analysed rapidly. The first computerized systems were run on mainframes and were organized by central advisory bureaux. Some current systems are network-based (e.g. FAHRMX, 1984; Bartlett *et al.*, 1985), therefore combining the benefits of local data storage and retrieval with the advantages of a centralized facility for data analysis. Some dairy health and productivity schemes are listed in *Table 11.3*; most are essentially microscale.

## Targets

The variables that are used to determine production targets are described below in relation to the different species. Targets have usually been defined as measures of position (e.g. mean age of dry sows) or as upper or lower limits (e.g. maximum calving interval or minimum first service pregnancy rate in dairy cattle). Measures of location do not indicate the dispersion of values in a herd and can be misleading; measures of dispersion, such as the standard deviation (when a variable is Normally distributed) or the semi-interquartile range, are more informative (*see* Chapter 12). Thus, if a farmer bred some cows very soon (less than 35 days) after calving, the measure of position would be reduced but the measure of dispersion would be increased.

This can eliminate the economic benefit that the owner thinks he is achieving because the economic benefit results from most cows calving with intervals close to 365 days (Morris, 1982); the benefit will not exist with a large dispersion.

Some variables that are used as production indices have frequency distributions that are skewed, in which case the mean may be far from the peak of the distribution. For example, the frequency distribution of calving to conception intervals is positively skewed; typically the median may be 10 days less than the mean. More appropriate measures of position and dispersion therefore would be the median and semi-interquartile range respectively. Logarithmic transformation of values (*see* Chapter 12) may be undertaken because this may convert skewed distributions to Normal ones. Morant (1984) discusses the appropriateness of measures in relation to dairy fertility, giving examples.

## Measuring shortfalls in production

Shortfalls in production are defined by an **action level** (also termed an **interference level**). This is the level at which the recorded production variable ceases to be acceptable in relation to its target level. Action levels are often identified by experience, based on financial criteria, and defined as levels beyond which there is unacceptable financial loss. When the measurement of location of a variable (the mean has commonly been used), recorded over a period of time, is beyond the action level, corrective measures are undertaken. This method does not consider the effects of random variation. These can be accommodated by defining the action levels as statistical parameters of the target level; the standard error is a suitable parameter for Normally distributed data. Suitable techniques for continuous data are the construction of cusums and Shewhart charts (*see* Chapter 12).

## Justification

A herd health and productivity scheme must be economically justifiable, that is, the cost of the scheme must be less than the revenue stemming from the increased productivity that it brings. The economic justification of these schemes is well documented (e.g. Williamson, 1980). Pharo *et al.* (1984) derived a benefit:cost ratio of approximately 3:1 for a computerized dairy herd health and productivity scheme in Britain over a 5-year period.

Details of schemes for the various species given below are presented only as introductory examples and therefore are not comprehensive descriptions of the systems. Radostits and Blood (1985) describe livestock health and productivity schemes thoroughly.

# Dairy health and productivity schemes

Dairy health and productivity schemes were developed in the 1950s and since then have received considerable attention. The main object of a dairy scheme is to improve productivity by maximizing milk yield and quality under the particular system of management on the farm. Optimum milk yield and quality are achieved by:

(1) efficient reproduction;
(2) decreasing important diseases (especially mastitis);
(3) optimum feeding.

## *Targets*

Some suggested targets for efficient reproduction for a dairy enterprise in the UK are listed in *Table 19.1*. De Kruif (1978) cites European targets, and Woods and Howard (1980) give North American ones. A target mean calving to conception interval of 85 days is often recommended. This facilitates an annual reproductive cycle because the cow's gestation period is approximately 280 days.

**Table 19.1 Suggested reproductive performance targets for a dairy herd in the UK. (From Esslemont *et al.*, 1985)**

| Index variable | Target | Range |
| --- | --- | --- |
| Period of lactation | 305 days | 300–320 days |
| Duration of pregnancy | 282 days | Varies somewhat with breed |
| Dry period | 60 days | 42–75 days |
| Calving interval | 365 days | 350–380 days |
| Calving to first service | Not less than 50 days, and not more than 60 days | |
| Calving to conception interval | 83 days | 69–98 days |
| Conception rate | 60% | |
| Heat detection efficiency | 80% | |
| Proportion of cows seen bulling and recorded as such by 60 days post-partum | 100% | |
| Herd calving index | 350–380 | |
| Proportion of animals involuntarily culled | <10% | |

## *Routine visits*

Regular farm visits are required to achieve reproductive targets. De Kruif (1980) recommends visits to cows:

(1) that have calved during the previous 3–6 weeks and have abnormal histories of parturition and of the early post-partum period;

(2) not seen in oestrus by 50–70 days post-partum;
(3) with abnormal discharges or irregular oestrous cycles;
(4) inseminated three or more times;
(5) served 35–60 days earlier (for pregnancy diagnosis).

A reproductive examination schedule is also described by Morrow (1980). Additionally, farmers are advised on the control of important diseases and on nutrition during routine visits.

## Decreasing important diseases

Mastitis is a major cause of loss of milk yield. A recommended control programme, recognizing the disease's various component causes (Kingwill *et al.*, 1970) includes:

(1) the dipping of teats in a suitable disinfectant immediately after milking;
(2) antibiotic therapy of chronic cases and of all cows at 'drying off';
(3) culling of recurrent cases;
(4) improved general husbandry, including milking machine maintenance.

Blood *et al.* (1983), Bramley *et al.* (1981) and Jarrett (1984) describe mastitis control in detail.

Pedal lameness is also an important cause of reduced production, especially when chronic. 'Lameness' is a disease definition based on presenting signs (*see* Chapter 9) which result from a range of lesions including hoof erosions, white line disease, sole trauma, sole ulceration, sandcrack, septic laminitis and interdigital hyperplasia. Component causes relate to host, agent and environment. Pododermatitis, for example, has a genetic component associated with sires (Peterse and Antonisse, 1981) and therefore might be controlled partially by sire selection. Laminitis appears to be related to diet (excess feeding of carbohydrate and protein: Nilsson, 1978) and to have a heritable component. Control of lameness therefore depends on identification of the major lesions and manipulation of their component causes. The survey illustrated in Chapter 14 (*see Figure 14.2*) was undertaken to identify the lesions associated with pedal lameness and their importance. Baggott (1982) describes hoof lameness in detail, and Edwards (1980) discusses its control.

## Optimum feeding

The correct nutritional balance is important in maintaining optimum milk yield, milk quality and fertility. The likelihood of deficiencies arising can be estimated by feed analysis. Blood analysis can be of value in diagnosing chronic deficiencies (e.g. chronic hypomagnesaemia and hypocuprosis).

A popular means of assessing the nutritional balance in dairy herds is the **metabolic profile** (Payne *et al.*, 1970). This involves estimating the levels of blood constituents that are important components of metabolism related to milk yield. Such constituents include minerals, protein metabolites, glucose, butyrates and free fatty acids.

Much has been learned since the initial use of metabolic profiles in dairy cattle. It has become apparent that planning of blood sampling according to feed changes and calving patterns is necessary, and that care must be taken when selecting cows 'typical' of the herd. Useful and sensible interpretation of biochemical results can only be carried out with access to background information on the cows' level of performance, stage of lactation and diet. With these caveats, some authors conclude that practical information can be obtained on some important aspects of the nutritional status of animals (Kelly and Whitaker, 1982; Whitaker *et al.*, 1983b). The usefulness of metabolic profiles is discussed by Lister and Gregory (1978) and, more recently, by MAFF/DAFS (1984).

Dairy health schemes are reviewed by Whitaker (1978) and described by Blood *et al.* (1978), Cannon *et al.* (1978), Morris *et al.* (1978a,b), Williamson *et al.* (1978), Lesch (1981), Noordhuizen (1984) and Esselmont *et al.* (1985).

# Pig health and productivity schemes

Intensively reared pigs are housed in large units, sometimes with over 100 sows in a herd (*see Table 1.5*).

There are four areas of concern:

(1) reproduction in the dry sow;
(2) production in the suckling sow;
(3) performance of the growing pig;
(4) performance of the boar.

Different constraints operate in each area. The dry sow's reproductive potential is governed by the service programme (the rate of reproduction), by the fertility of the sow (the sow's efficiency) and by disease. Productivity of the suckling sow is a function of the farrowing rate, the number of piglets born alive, piglet mortality, diseases of the sow, and the sucking piglets' growth rate. Performance of the growing pig is affected by the type of feed, feed costs, food conversion efficiency, disease and mortality. Boar performance, which affects the reproductive capacity of the sow, is affected by the age of the boar, the boar:sow ratio, frequency of mating, and the litter size and litter scatter attributable to the boar (litter scatter is the percentage of litters of eight or less).

**Table 19.2 Recommended variables to be recorded monthly in a pig health and productivity scheme. (From Douglas, 1984)**

*Stock numbers*
(1)  Boars
(2)  Sows and served gilts
(3)  Maidens
(4a)  Culls/deaths—sows
(4b)  Culls/deaths—boars

*Service area*
(5)  Number of 1st services
(6)  Number of 2nd services
(7)  Number of 3rd services

*Farrowing area*
(8)  Number of farrowings
(9)  Number of pigs born alive
(10)  Number of pigs born dead
(11)  Number of sows weaned
(12)  Number of pigs weaned
(13)  Number of pigs transferred to finishing area
(14a)  Deaths—sucking
(14b)  Deaths—weaning
(14c)  Deaths—finishing

*Finishing area*
(13)  Number of pigs in
(15)  Number of pigs sold (including number of gilts retained for breeding)

*Food (tonnes)*
(16)  Amount of sow food used
(17)  Amount of pre-weaning (creep) food used
(18)  Amount of post-weaning food used

*Table 19.2* lists the basic variables that should be recorded to produce and regularly update a farm profile.

## *Targets*

*Table 19.3* lists target and interference levels (the latter based on experience) for dry sows, suckling sows, growing pigs and boars in an intensively reared pig herd in NE England.

## *Routine visits*

A schedule for regular visits to a pig herd is recommended by Muirhead (1980). *Table 19.4* lists components of monthly visits to a herd of 150–300 sows. Smaller herds may be seen less frequently. Visits comprise a standard procedure and discussion of special topics. The standard procedure involves:

(1) pre-visit preparation, when previous reports, current investigations and clinical problems are studied;

**Table 19.3 Suggested targets and interference levels for an intensive pig unit in NE England. (From Muirhead, 1978b)**

| Index variable | Target | Interference level | Index variable | Target | Interference level |
|---|---|---|---|---|---|
| *(a) The dry sow* | | | Piglet mortality (%): | | |
| Average number of sows in herd | As determined | Fluctuation of 30% of target | Laid on | 5 | 7 |
| Average age | 24 months | 30 months | Congenital defects | 0.5 | 1.5 |
| Ratio of average number of maiden gilts:sows | 1:15 | | Low viability | 1.5 | 3 |
| | | | Starvation | 1 | 3 |
| | | | Scour | 0.5 | 2 |
| Service programme | As determined | >10% variation | Miscellaneous | 3 | 5 |
| | | | Pigs reared/sow/year | 21 | 19 |
| Weaning to service interval average | 7 days | 9 days | Sow feed (tonnes/year) | 1.1 | 1.2 |
| Normal repeat service (%) | 5 | 8 | *(c) The growing pig* | | |
| Abnormal repeat service (%) | 3 | 4 | Mortality (%) | 2.5 | 3.5 |
| Abortions (%) | 1 | 2.5 | Feed conversion from weaning: | | |
| Sows infertile not in pig (%) | <2 | 5 | Pork (60 kg) | 2.7 | 2.9 |
| Sow deaths (%) | 2 | 3 | Cutter (85 kg) | 2.9 | 3.2 |
| Sows culled due to disease (%) | <2 | 4 | Bacon (90 kg) | 2.9 | 3.2 |
| | | | Heavy (115 kg) | 3.6 | 3.8 |
| Farrowing rate (%) | 85–89 | 80 | Feed cost/kg liveweight gain | Variable with feed costs | Comparative figures |
| *Litters/sow/year | 2.25 | 2.0 | | | |
| *(b) The farrowing/suckling sow* | | | *(d) The boar* | | |
| | | | Average age | 20 months | 30 months |
| Number of piglets born alive/litter | 10.9 | 10 | Boar:sow ratio | 1:20 | 1:30 |
| | | | Matings/week | 4 | 5 |
| Number of piglets born dead (%) | 5 | 7 | Matings/sow | 2 | 3 |
| Number of mummified piglets (%) | 0.5 | 1 | Mating interval | 12 hours (variable) | — |
| | | | Boar litter scatter (%) | 15 | 25 |
| Number of piglets weaned/litter | 9.6 | 9 | Litter size | 9.8–10.8 | Obtained by boar comparison |
| Deaths until weaning (%) | 8–12 | 13 | Conception to first service (%) | >90 | 85 |
| **Litter scatter (%) | 10 | 18 | | | |

*Assuming 5-week weaning
**Litter of 8 or less (*see* text for definition)

**Table 19.4 A 12-monthly preventive medicine programme for a herd of 150–300 sows on monthly visits. (From Muirhead, 1980)**

| Visit No. | Special topics |
|---|---|
| (1) Standard procedure* | Herd security |
| (2) Standard procedure | Stock introduction; methods of gene movement; herd replacement policies; gilt selection requirements |
| (3) Standard procedure | Economic losses in the herd; feed costs and utilization |
| (4) Standard procedure | External/internal parasites; vermin control; vaccination programme |
| (5) Standard procedure | Fertility; boar management |
| (6) Standard procedure | Herd security check; farrowing sow diseases; parturition, mastitis, etc. |
| (7) Standard procedure | Piglet problems |
| (8) Standard procedure | Diseases, mortality and management of the weaned and fattening pigs |
| (9) Standard procedure | Housing utilization; alterations; associated diseases |
| (10) Standard procedure | Man management, disease and productivity |
| (11) Standard procedure | Slaughter house monitoring; pathological tests |
| (12) Standard procedure | 12-monthly appraisal and analysis |

*See text for details.

(2) a clinical examination of the reproductive and service areas, dry sows, the farrowing and weaning areas, and fattening pigs;
(3) a discussion with the farmer.

Comprehensive examination of a pig herd is described by Goodwin (1971b) and Muirhead (1978b). Routine preventive measures are described by Douglas (1984).

# Sheep health and productivity schemes

The major areas of concern in sheep health schemes, like schemes in other species, are reproductive efficiency, losses due to disease, and suboptimal production (which may be caused by subclinical disease).

Examples of health schemes include those developed in England (Hindson, 1982; Holland, 1984), W Australia (Bell, 1980), SW Australia (Morley *et al.*, 1983), New Zealand (McNeil *et al.*, 1984) and

**Table 19.5 An information sheet recording a farm profile and illustrating some recorded variables in a lowland sheep flock health programme. (From Holland, 1984)**

| INFORMATION SHEET |
|---|
| (1) RAMS Nos. Breed(s) |
|     – rams |
|     – ram lambs |
| (2) EWES Nos. Breed(s) |
|     – ewes |
|     – ewe lambs |
| (3) EWES TO TUP |
|     Nos. and date |
| (4) EWES LAMBED |
| (5) LAMBS BORN |
|     – alive |
|     –dead |
| (6) LAMB DEATHS BETWEEN BIRTH AND WEANING |
| (7) LAMBING COMMENCED – Date |
| (8) LAMBING COMPLETED – Date |
| (9) EWES HOUSED/HOUSED AT LAMBING/NOT HOUSED |
| (10) RATION |
|     (a) ewes |
|     (b) lamb creep |
|     (c) lamb fattener |
| (11) LAMB SALES |
|     (a) commenced |
|     (b) completed |
| (12) COMMENTS ON: |
|     (a) Results |
|     (b) Problem areas |
| (13) COMMENTS ON MASTITIS IN EWES |
|     (a) known cases this year |
|     (b) previous culling percentage |
| (14) CONDITION SCORING FULLY PRACTISED AND UNDERSTOOD? |

the Netherlands (Konig, 1985). The schemes are designed primarily for lowland flocks. The principles of such schemes are similar, although details vary depending on local management practices and disease problems.

Initially, a farm profile should be produced, comprising details of the breeds of rams and ewes, the size and stocking density of the flock, current feeding, breeding, pasture management and disease control. *Table 19.5* illustrates a simple sheet for recording a farm profile.

## *Targets*

Records of past performance of a flock enable the setting of suitable production targets. Examples of targets relating to a Scottish lowland flock are given in *Table 19.6*. In common with other health schemes, accurate records must be kept so that productivity can be assessed and corrective action taken if shortfalls are detected.

**Table 19.6 Performance targets for a Scottish lowland sheep flock (per 100 ewes put to the ram). (From Linklater and Speedy, 1980)**

| Index variable | Target |
|---|---|
| Barren ewes | 3% |
| Ewe deaths | 2% |
| Productive ewes | 95% |
| Total lambs born/ewe | 1.81 |
| Lambs born dead | 4% |
| Perinatal lamb mortality | 5% |
| Lambs surviving/ewe | 1.72 |
| Later lamb mortality | 2% |
| Lambs weaned or sold/ewe | 1.70 |
| Lamb growth rate to 1 August | 300 g/day |
| Target weight at 1 August | 41 kg |
| Proportion sold fat at 1 August (remainder sold fat by 30 September) | 50% |

## *Routine visits*

Advisory visits are made at important stages of sheep management. In Britain it is recommended (Holland, 1984) that visits should occur:

(1) in mid to late summer (i.e. before tupping);
(2) during the pregnancy of the ewe;
(3) at or around lambing;
(4) after lambing.

During the first visit, culling of ewes, based on examination of condition score, udders, mouths, feet and legs, should be advised. The genitals of rams should also be examined. Advice should be given on management of the breeding flock at tupping. The second visit (when the ewe is

212

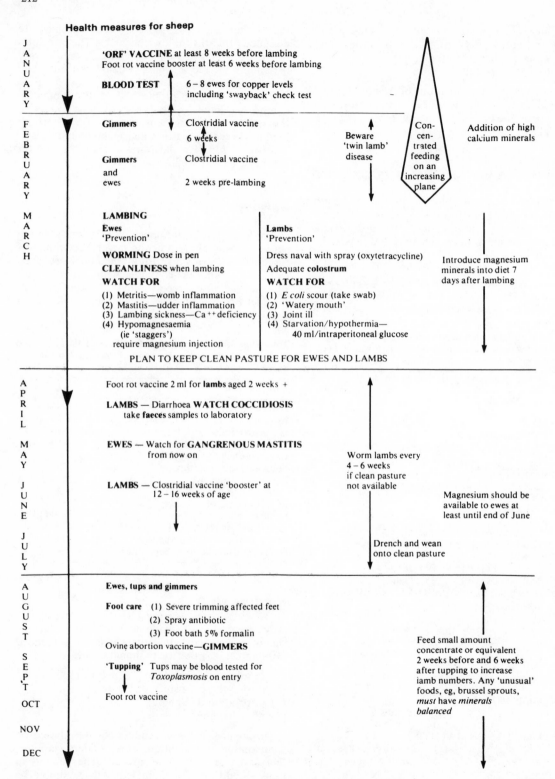

**Figure 19.1** An action list for a British health and productivity scheme for lowland sheep flocks. (From Hindson, 1982)

pregnant) is primarily concerned with nutritional advice. Nutrition of pregnant ewes is important (Russel, 1985) and metabolic profiles, based on butyrate examination, are valuable. The third visit deals with problems at birth, and is used as a further opportunity for offering advice on nutrition and management. The fourth visit is timed to provide advice on the growing lamb.

Specific disease problems should be identified during visits. In Britain, problem diseases can include orf, infectious abortion, mastitis, swayback, pregnancy toxaemia, mineral and trace element deficiencies, and ecto- and endoparasitism. Foot-rot (Egerton, 1981) is a major problem in many sheep-producing countries. Infection by *Clostridium* spp., however, is now controlled effectively by routine vaccination. *Figure 19.1* illustrates an action list for British lowland flocks incorporating control strategies for the important diseases.

# Beef health and productivity schemes

Beef cattle are managed less intensively than dairy cattle. There is also less contact between individual beef than dairy cattle; therefore fewer records are kept.

## *Targets*

Beef health and productivity schemes are designed to attain optimum reproductive efficiency and to reduce morbidity and mortality in the stock that are being fattened. Traditionally, the number of calves

**Table 19.7 Suggested reproductive performance and production variables for a beef enterprise in the USA. (From Rice, 1980a)**

| Index variable | Target |
|---|---|
| Average weaning weight | 500 lb |
| % Cows cycling during the first 21 days breeding | 90% |
| First service conception rate | 70% |
| % Cows pregnant | 95% |
| Calf survival: | |
| $\dfrac{\text{Live calves at 24 hours}}{\text{Number pregnant cows released}}$ | 95% |
| Nursing survival: | |
| $\dfrac{\text{Calves weaned}}{\text{Calves alive at 24 hours}}$ | 85% |
| % Calf crop weaned: | |
| $\dfrac{\text{Calves weaned}}{\text{Total cows exposed to breeding during the previous season}}$ | 85% |

reared is the sole measure of production. The production target of beef rearing is to produce one calf per cow per year. This objective is somewhat optimistic, requiring a breeding season restricted to 42–63 days, a 95% pregnancy rate, and a 100% reared calf crop during each year, none of which usually occurs.

*Table 19.7* lists some variables that are suggested as indices of reproduction and production, with target levels, for a North American feedlot enterprise.

## *Routine visits*

Routine visits should coincide with major events. Rice (1980b) suggests that the reproductive year should be divided into six periods:

(1) weaning;
(2) weaning to calving (90–120 days);
(3) calving (90 days);
(4) pre-breeding (30 days);
(5) breeding (60–90 days);
(6) post-breeding to pre-weaning.

Relevant management procedures and prophylaxis are carried out and advice is given during each period. During the weaning period, calves are identified, weighed, and vaccinated against blackleg, and their internal parasites are controlled; cows are examined for pregnancy, 'open', old and non-productive cows are culled and, if necessary, cows are vaccinated against leptospirosis and campylobacteriosis.

Beef health schemes are reviewed by Caldow (1984) and discussed in detail by Radostits (1983). Models of beef production systems in various developing countries are described by Levine and Hohenboken (1982) and of breeding systems in developed countries by Congleton and Goodwill (1980).

# Companion animal health schemes

Companion animal health schemes are concerned with disease prevention in the individual animal, rather than in a group (although several individuals may be involved in kennels and stables). Production is not relevant to companion animal schemes. (The track performance of racehorses and greyhounds is loosely described as 'production' but the animals are usually more commercial than companion.) Schemes involve:

(1) prophylaxis, such as vaccination;
(2) routine therapy, including dosing with anthelmintics;

**Table 19.8 A routine health programme (action list) for the prevention of helminth and microbial diseases in horses in the Netherlands. (Modified from Verberne and Mirck, 1976)**

*March* (all horses)
(1)  Parasitological faeces examination
(2)  Anthelmintic treatment
(3)  Immunization against influenza and tetanus (booster dose)

*June*
(1)  Parasitological faeces examination (foals)
(2)  Anthelmintic treatment (all horses)
(3)  Immunization of foals against tetanus (1st dose)

*August*
(1)  Anthelmintic treatment (all horses)
(2)  Immunization of foals against influenza (1st dose) and tetanus (2nd dose)

*October*
(1)  Parasitological faeces examination (all horses)
(2)  Anthelmintic treatment (all horses)
(3)  Immunization against influenza (foals) (2nd dose) and yearlings (2nd booster dose)

*December*
(1)  Anthelmintic treatment

(3)  advice on management relating to diet and housing;
(4)  routine examination of animals.

A preventive medicine scheme for commercial dog breeding kennels in the USA is given by Glickman (1980). It includes nutritional recommendations, vaccination, ecto- and endoparasite control, and the management of reproduction and common diseases. Systematic record keeping is advised, to provide a kennel profile, facilitating the detection of deviations from normal breeding performance and expected patterns of morbidity and mortality.

Fraser (1969) describes an equine schedule, including tetanus and influenza vaccination, haematological examination of foals to detect anaemia, dietary problems and helminth infestation, and routine attention to and advice on teeth and feet. Owen (1985) describes a similar equine schedule, including control of parasites, respiratory and genital tract infections, attention to feet, and nutritional advice. *Table 19.8* lists a Dutch equine action list for the prevention of helminth and microbial diseases. This programme starts in March because in the Netherlands most foals are born in April and May, and peak performance in showjumpers and racehorses is required between April and September. Under different circumstances, the programme would require modification.

## Further reading

EDDY, R.G. and DUCKER, M.J. (Eds) (1984) *Dairy Cow Fertility*. Proceedings of a joint British Veterinary Association and British Society of Animal Production conference, Bristol University, 28–29 June 1984. British Veterinary Association, London

ESSLEMONT, R.J., BAILIE, J.H. and COOPER, M.J. (1985) *Fertility Management in Dairy Cattle*. Collins Professional and Technical Books, London

PROCEEDINGS OF THE SYMPOSIUM ON COMPUTER APPLICATIONS IN VETERINARY MEDICINE, *13–15 OCTOBER 1982* (1983) College of Veterinary Medicine, Mississippi State University, Starkville

RADOSTITS, O.M. and BLOOD, D.C. (1985) *Herd Health: A Textbook of Health and Production Management of Agricultural Animals*. W.B. Saunders Company, Philadelphia

SECOND SYMPOSIUM ON COMPUTER APPLICATIONS IN VETERINARY MEDICINE (1985) Proceedings of the American Veterinary Computer Society, College of Veterinary Medicine, Mississippi State University, 23–25 May 1984

# 20

# The control of disease

The preceding chapters have outlined the scope of veterinary epidemiology. In reiteration: epidemiology is the study of disease and factors affecting its distribution in populations. This study involves the **description** and **analysis** of disease in groups of animals using three complementary techniques:

(1) observation and recording of the natural occurrence of disease and its determinants, and presentation of the recorded observations;
(2) statistical analysis of the observations;
(3) modelling.

These three techniques are used in conjunction with experimental, clinical and pathological investigations to:

(1) assess disease morbidity and mortality;
(2) elucidate the cause of disease;
(3) understand the ecology of disease (transmission, maintenance and nidality);
(4) investigate the efficiency of different techniques of disease control.

This final chapter outlines the ways in which the results of epidemiological investigations are applied to the control and eradication of disease.

## Disease control and eradication

### Definition of 'control' and 'eradication'

#### Control

Control is the reduction of the morbidity and mortality from disease. It can be achieved by **treating** diseased animals, which therefore reduces disease prevalence, and by **preventing** disease, which therefore reduces both incidence and prevalence. Veterinary medicine, like human medicine, developed as a healing art concerned with the treatment of sick individuals. This approach continues with the improvement of medical and surgical skills. However, prevention is an increasingly important part of disease control, being better than cure on humanitarian and, frequently, economic grounds.

#### Eradication

The term 'eradication' was first applied in the 19th century to the regional elimination of infectious diseases of animals, notably Texas fever from cattle in the USA, and pleuropneumonia, glanders and rabies from European animals. Since then the term has been used in four different senses.

First, it has been used to mean the extinction of an infectious agent (Cockburn, 1963); eradication has not been completed if a single infectious agent survives anywhere in nature. According to this definition, very few diseases have been eradicated; human smallpox is an example.

Secondly, eradication has been defined as the reduction of infectious disease prevalence in a specified area to a level at which transmission does not occur (Andrews and Langmuir, 1963). For instance, in local areas in northern Nigeria trypanosomiasis can be 'eradicated' by clearing the vector (the tsetse fly) from riverine areas.

Thirdly, eradication has been defined as the reduction of infectious disease prevalence to a level at which the disease ceases to be a major health problem, although some transmission may still take place (Maslakov, 1968). The term 'elimination' has been used to describe the reduction in the prevalence of either clinical disease or infection below that achieved by control, but without complete eradication of the pathogen (Payne, 1963).

Fourthly, and most commonly in veterinary medicine, eradication refers to the **regional** extinction of an infectious agent. For example, since the eradication of foot-and-mouth disease in the UK, no foot-and-mouth disease virus particles are believed to be present (apart from laboratory stocks).

## Strategies of control and eradication

### Doing nothing

In some cases the natural history of a disease is such that the incidence of the disease is reduced by doing nothing. This is not strictly a technique of control but illustrates that the incidence of disease may be reduced by natural changes in host/parasite relationships without the intervention of man. Thus, bluetongue does not occur in Cyprus in winter because the vector (*Culicoides* spp.) of the causal virus cannot survive then. Similarly, the incidence of trypanosomiasis in the dry savannah regions of Nigeria is reduced during the dry season when the tsetse fly is absent.

### Quarantine

Quarantine is the isolation of animals that are either infected or suspected of being so, or of non-infected animals that are at risk. Quarantine is an old method of disease control that is still very valuable. It is used to isolate animals when they are imported from countries where exotic diseases are endemic, for example, the compulsory quarantine of dogs, cats and zoo animals when they are imported to Britain to prevent the introduction of rabies. It is also used to isolate animals suspected of being infected, until infection is either confirmed or discounted, such as cows suspected of being infected with bovine brucellosis. Quarantine is commonly applied in human medicine during epidemics to isolate infected from susceptible individuals. The period of quarantine depends on the incubation period of the agent, the time taken for the infection to be confirmed and the time taken for an infected animal to become non-infectious (either with or without treatment).

### Slaughter

The productivity of animals is usually decreased when they are chronically diseased. If a disease is infectious, affected animals can be a source of infection to others. In such circumstances it may be economically and technically expedient to slaughter the affected animals. For example, clinical bovine

mastitis can produce a 15% drop in the milk yield of dairy cattle (Parsons, 1982); cows that have three of more bouts of mastitis per lactation therefore are often culled.

In eradication campaigns, infected or in-contact animals may be slaughtered to remove sources of infection. Thus, all cloven-hoofed animals in infected herds are slaughtered during foot-and-mouth disease epidemics in some countries.

### Vaccination

Vaccines can confer immunity to many bacteria and viruses, and to some helminths. They are used routinely to prevent disease, and may be used during epidemics to decrease the number of susceptible animals, thus assisting in terminating an epidemic. Vaccines may be **inactivated**, in which the antigenic organisms such as bacteria are killed, and viruses are denatured. Alternatively, they may be **live** and the organisms usually attenuated. Each type of vaccine has advantages and disadvantages. Inactivated vaccines are safer than live vaccines and can be produced more quickly when new agents are discovered. However, they cost more than live vaccines and stimulate mucosal and cell-mediated immunity less quickly and less effectively. On the other hand, there is a danger that the live immunizing agent might revert to a virulent form. Also, it may be difficult to differentiate between infections due to live vaccinal strains of agent and those due to natural 'field' strains.

Natural vaccination can occur when animals are exposed to a low level of challenge from agents in the environment. This mechanism has been enhanced in pigs by feeding faeces back to pregnant animals, a technique called 'feedback'. Immunity to pathogens, for example porcine transmissible gastroenteritis virus and parvovirus (Stein *et al.*, 1982), thus may be increased and passed passively to the piglets via colostrum after birth. Although this may be of value when no other means of control is available, there are dangers (Porter, 1979): some agents, such as enteropathogenic *Escherichia coli* can increase in virulence when passaged *in vivo*.

The use of vaccination as a control strategy is discussed in detail by Biggs (1982). The potential and application of vaccination for the control of several parasitic diseases, such as East Coast fever, haemonchosis and trypanosomiasis, are described by Urquhart (1980).

### Therapeutic and prophylactic chemotherapy

Antibiotics, anthelmintics, other drugs and hyperimmune serum are used (therapeutically) to treat diseases, and are administered (prophylactically) at times of high risk to prevent disease and thus to increase productivity. Examples include the addition of antibiotics to livestock feed to promote growth, and the postoperative use of antibiotics to prevent bacterial infections. These procedures can have undesirable consequences, notably the selection of strains of bacteria that are resistant to the antibiotic to which they have been exposed. Furthermore, resistance can be spread by transfer to other bacteria by conjugation and by transducing phages (*see* Chapter 5).

## Movement of hosts

Animals can be removed from 'high risk' areas where infections are endemic. This control strategy is implemented in tropical countries where hosts are seasonally migrated from areas in which biological vectors are active. The Fulani tribe in West Africa traditionally migrate, with their livestock, from the south to the north in the wet season to avoid the tsetse fly. Similarly, horses may be moved indoors at night to prevent infection with African horse sickness virus which is transmitted by night-flying vectors of the genus *Culicoides* (Chalmers, 1968).

## Mixed, alternate and sequential grazing

The level of infection with some nematodes can be reduced by mixed, alternate and sequential grazing (Brunsdon, 1980). The **mixed grazing** of susceptible animals with stock that are genetically or immunologically resistant to helminths reduces pasture contamination to an acceptable level. Thus, adult cattle (immune) can be grazed with calves (susceptible). Similarly, cattle (resistant to *Ostertagia circumcincta*) can be grazed with sheep (susceptible).

The **alternate grazing** of a pasture with different species of livestock again reduces pasture contamination. Thus, annual alternation of sheep and cattle in Norway has reduced to negligible levels the challenge to sheep from nematode species that overwinter (*Ostertagia* spp. and *Nematodirus* spp.: Helle, 1971).

The **sequential grazing** at different times of resistant and susceptible animals of the same species reduces pasture contamination. Thus, when clean grazing is not available in the late summer and autumn, trichostrongyle infections of calves (susceptible animals) can be reduced by transferring them to pastures that have been grazed by cows (resistant) (Burger, 1976).

## Control of biological vectors

Infectious diseases transmitted by biological vectors can be controlled by removing the vectors. Insect vectors can be killed with insecticides. The habitat of the vectors can be destroyed, for example by draining land to remove snails that are intermediate hosts of *Fasciola hepatica*. Alternatively, an animal that competes with the vector can be introduced into the habitat, for example the exclusion of the molluscan vectors of schistosomiasis by a snail that is not a vector (*see* Chapter 7). Some infections of definitive hosts may be prevented by the elimination of infective material found at post-mortem meat inspection of intermediate hosts, for instance the inspection of cattle to condemn meat containing *Cysticercus bovis* cysts.

## Control of mechanical vectors

Living organisms that mechanically transmit infectious agents can be controlled by destruction and disinfection. Biting fleas that transmit bacteria, for example, can be destroyed by insecticides. The veterinarian can also act as a mechanical vector and so must impose a strict procedure for personal disinfection when dealing with outbreaks of highly contagious infectious diseases such as foot-and-mouth disease.

## Fomite disinfection

Fomites (*see* Chapter 6) can be disinfected to prevent the transmission of infectious agents. Fomites include farm equipment, surgical instruments and sometimes drugs themselves, the last two being associated with iatrogenic transmission (*see* Chapter 6). Food is heat-treated (e.g. the pasteurization of milk) to destroy microbes and their heat-sensitive toxins, to prevent food-borne infection.

## Niche filling

The presence of one organism within a niche can prevent its occupation by another organism. This is epidemiological interference (*see* Chapter 7), and has been investigated experimentally in the poultry industry where suspensions of endogenous intestinal microbes have been fed to day-old chicks to prevent colonization of their digestive tract by virulent *Salmonella* spp. (Pivnick and Nurmi, 1982). This technique of control has the advantage over prophylactic antibiotic chemotherapy that antibiotic resistance is not encouraged. However, the technique has not been exploited widely and, like feedback, risks enhancement of virulence of the administered agents.

## Improvement in environment, husbandry and feeding

The diseases of intensively produced animals, particularly cattle and pigs, are major contemporary problems (e.g. Webster, 1982) which can be controlled only when epidemiological investigations have identified the determinants associated with inadequate management. Thus, the increase in Britain of bovine mastitis associated with *E. coli* and *Streptococcus uberis* ('environmental mastitis') has paralleled the increase in the number of cows that are housed loosely in cubicles. Poor hygiene has been incriminated as the most important environmental cause (Francis *et al.*, 1979). Recommendations to reduce this disease (Sumner, quoted by Webster, 1982) therefore include:

(1) adjustment of head rails to minimize soiling of cubicles;
(2) removal of faeces and soiled litter twice daily;
(3) addition of clean litter daily;
(4) scraping cubicle passages at least twice daily.

## Genetic improvement

Many diseases of both agricultural and companion animals (Foley *et al.*, 1979) have a variable heritable component. The disease may be determined predominantly genetically, as in canine cyclic neutropenia (the gray collie syndrome: Cheville, 1975) which is carried by a simple autosomal recessive lethal gene. Alternatively, the disease may be determined by several factors, only one of which is genetic, as in canine hip dysplasia (Riser, 1974) whose determinants also include growth rate, body type, and pelvic muscle mass. The incidence of such diseases can be reduced by early detection, for example, by radiography in the case of hip dysplasia, followed by voluntary agreement of owners of affected animals not to breed from the animals.

A valuable aid to the identification of genetic diseases is **genetic screening** (Jolly *et al.*, 1981) to identify diseased animals by screening either the total population at risk or the part that is mainly responsible for the maintenance of a particular disease. The latter technique is commonly applied in veterinary medicine because animal populations tend to be very large, and most animals of 'superior' genetic potential are concentrated in pedigree 'nuclei' that are used for breeding. Human populations are screened to detect hereditary dietary deficiencies (e.g. aminoacidurias, so facilitating dietary control), and to identify serious genetic diseases prenatally so that elective abortion can be considered. In veterinary medicine the main value of screening is the reduction in defective gene frequency by identifying and removing normal and partially expressed carriers. The relatively short generation time of domestic animals, and artificial breeding techniques, help towards this objective.

Defects can be identified by clinical examination of animals (e.g. canine progressive retinal atrophy: Black, 1972). However, the main benefit of screening is in the detection of heterozygotes where disease is either subclinical or transmitted by healthy carriers. Techniques include test matings, cytogenetic studies (e.g. bovine Robertsonian translocations: Gustavsson, 1969) and biochemical analyses (e.g. bovine mannosidosis: Jolly *et al.*, 1973).

The requirements for a genetic screening programme are listed by Jolly *et al.* (1981):

(1) the disease must occur in a defined population sufficiently frequently to make the disease of economic or social importance; the defined population may be a family, a herd, or a breed of animal within certain geographical boundaries;
(2) a simple, relatively inexpensive test, capable of identifying heterozygotes with a high degree of accuracy, should be available; as most tests in biological systems do not have a sensitivity and specificity of 100%, there should be provision for follow-up testing, either with a more specific supplementary test or by replication of the original method;
(3) control by culling of heterozygotes should neither have a deleterious effect on the overall genetic make-up of the population nor deplete breeding stock to an uneconomic or disadvantageous level;
(4) the logistics of the programme should be acceptable to the breeders and be preceded by adequate educational and public relations programmes;
(5) the logistics of the programme should satisfy the breeders but not encroach on other necessary disease prevention programmes; where possible, the programme should be integrated with other disease control schemes to simplify specimen collection;
(6) there should be provision for adequate genetic counselling and either breed society or kennel club rules or legislation to ensure that control is instigated on the basis of information provided by the screening tests.

*Table 20.1* illustrates the economic benefit of a screening programme for bovine mannosidosis. This disease causes a lethal nervous syndrome in Angus and Murray Gray cattle. It is inherited recessively; carriers can be detected biochemically because their blood $\alpha$-mannosidase levels are approximately half of the normal. The cost-benefit analysis relates to New Zealand, where the prevalence of heterozygotes before the programme was 10%, and approximately one million Angus and Murray Gray calves are born each year, with a total estimated loss due to the disease of $281 000. Different values for the prevalence, number and value of susceptible cattle, cost of screening test and discount rate affect the results of such an analysis and therefore the economic viability of the control programme.

Other genetic diseases to which screening can be applied are bovine protoporphyria and canine

**Table 20.1 Cost-benefit analysis of a genetic screening programme for bovine mannosidosis in New Zealand, at different levels of heterozygote prevalence. (From Jolly and Townsley, 1980)**

| *Time horizon* | *Costs and benefits 10% discount rate* | *Prevalence of heterozygotes* | | | |
|---|---|---|---|---|---|
| | | *10%* | *7.5%* | *5.0%* | *2.5%* |
| Incurred first 8 years | Cumulative costs | $500 000 | $500 000 | $500 000 | $500 000 |
| | Discounted costs | $333 433 | $333 433 | $333 433 | $333 433 |
| 20 years | Cumulative benefits | $3 471 600 | $1 910 800 | $874 300 | $211 100 |
| | Discounted benefits | $963 838 | $530 850 | $243 588 | $58 576 |
| | Benefit:cost ratio | 2.89 | 1.59 | 0.73 | 0.18 |
| Infinity | Discounted benefits | $1 381 527 | $760 951 | $348 951 | $83 994 |
| | Benefit:cost ratio | 4.14 | 2.28 | 1.04 | 0.25 |
| Break even time | Undiscounted benefits and costs | 9 years | 11 years | 15 years | >20 years |

inherited bleeding and eye defects (Jolly *et al.*, 1980).

The incidence of some infectious diseases can be reduced by selective breeding. For example, certain cattle are known to be tolerant to trypanosomiasis (so-called 'trypanotolerant' cattle: Murray *et al.*, 1979). Other infectious diseases for which genetic resistance has been reported include foot-and-mouth disease and tuberculosis in cattle, jaagziekte and scrapie in sheep, brucellosis and leptospirosis in pigs, and Newcastle disease, infectious bronchitis, Marek's disease and coccidiosis in poultry (Payne, 1982).

## Minimal disease methods

Disease can be reduced in intensively reared livestock by disinfecting infected premises and by treating infected animals or removing them from the animal unit. Uninfected animals can be produced by caesarean section and by hatching uninfected eggs from poultry. These combined techniques are termed **minimal disease** methods. They have been applied commercially only in pig and poultry units. Successes include the eradication of enzootic pneumonia from some pig herds in the UK.

Techniques of control and eradication have developed gradually. Until the germ theory of infectious disease was adequately supported in the 19th century, only those people who believed in contagion could attempt to control infectious disease. Thus, Lancisi controlled rinderpest in Italy by a slaughter policy (*see* Chapter 1). Those who accepted the miasmatic theory of cause occasionally succeeded in controlling disease by applying basic sanitary principles such as disinfection and fumigation.

**Table 20.2 Some eradicable diseases in the UK and chosen methods of eradication. (Adapted from Sellers, 1982)**

| *Method of eradication* | *Cattle* | *Sheep* | *Pigs* | *Poultry* |
|---|---|---|---|---|
| Slaughter of infected and in-contact animals | Exotic infections, e.g. foot-and-mouth disease | Exotic infections, e.g. foot-and-mouth disease | Exotic infections, e.g. foot-and-mouth disease | Exotic infections, e.g. Newcastle disease, fowl plague |
| Identify infected animal and either destroy or treat or vaccinate | Tuberculosis, brucellosis, warble fly infection, leptospirosis, enzootic bovine leucosis, Johne's disease, infectious bovine rhinotracheitis (stud bulls) | Sheep scab, Johne's disease | Tuberculosis | Pullorum disease, fowl typhoid, egg drop syndrome, fowl pox, duck hepatitis |
| Improvement of environment and management, and treatment | Streptococcal mastitis, coliform mastitis | Foot-rot, liver fluke | Streptococcal meningitis, mange | Chronic respiratory disease, *Mycoplasma meleagridis* infection |
| Minimal disease methods | | Maedi-visna | Enzootic pneumonia, atrophic rhinitis | |

A combination of the various techniques that have been described is applied to the control and eradication of disease. An example is the use of vaccination, followed by mass testing of animals and slaughter of infected animals to control contagious bovine pleuropneumonia in Nigeria (David-West, 1980). The choice of technique involves assessing, technically and economically, the most efficient strategy for a particular disease and system of management (Sellers, 1982).

*Table 20.2* lists some eradicable diseases in the UK and the methods chosen for eradication. Slaughter and quarantine campaigns against widespread epidemics and exotic diseases are usually conducted at the national level by government veterinary services. These campaigns are frequently supported by legislation.

Vaccination, treatment, alteration in environment and minimal disease techniques are generally carried out at the local level, and are often concerned with individual or herd problems, such as distemper in dogs (vaccination), and helminthiasis in herds of cattle and flocks of sheep (treatment and management practices). Vaccination may sometimes be carried out as part of a national government policy, for example, against bovine brucellosis.

## Important factors in control and eradication programmes

Before either a control or an eradication campaign can be undertaken, several factors must be considered. These include:

(1) the level of knowledge about the cause of the disease and, if infectious, also about its transmission and maintenance, including host range and the nature of the host/parasite relationship;
(2) veterinary infrastructure;
(3) diagnostic feasibility;
(4) availability of replacement stock;
(5) producers' and society's views;
(6) the disease's public health significance;
(7) the existence of suitable legislation with provision for compensation;
(8) the possible ecological consequences;
(9) economic costs and the availability of funds for the programme.

### Knowledge of the cause, maintenance and transmission of disease

A complete knowledge of the natural history of a disease, although not always necessary to control or eradicate it (recall Lancisi's eradication of rinderpest), is necessary to develop the **most effective** means of control. When the various disease determinants have been defined, often by epidemiological studies, a suitable control strategy can be selected, for example improving ventilation to reduce respiratory disease in intensively reared pigs. If a disease is infectious then a knowledge of its method of transmission, including the life-cycle and habitat of any vectors, assists in control. Thus, identification of *Limnea truncatula* as the molluscan intermediate host of *F. hepatica* has helped to identify land drainage as a possible control strategy for fascioliasis because the snail requires a moist habitat. A knowledge of the host range of an infectious agent and the host/parasite relationship (considered separately below) is also desirable.

### Host range

An infectious agent that infects or can be transmitted by only one species of host is easier to control than an agent with a wide host range. The global eradication of human smallpox was possible because the virus infected only humans; control, by quarantine and vaccination, therefore needed to be directed towards only humans. Similarly, the British bovine brucellosis eradication programme required control of infection only in cattle because only cattle can transmit *Brucella abortus* significantly. On the contrary, the current obstacle to the control of bovine tuberculosis in England, by intradermal testing of cattle and slaughter of reactors, is the presence of transmissible infection in badgers (Little *et al.*, 1982). Agents that are transmitted by arthropod vectors may be particularly difficult to control because of the problems of controlling infection in the arthropod.

### Nature of the host/parasite relationship

Exogenous agents (*see* Chapter 5) have been (*see* Table 1.1) and still are the causes of the major animal plagues. Control is relatively straightforward and eradication is possible. Infected animals can be identified relatively easily using clinical and laboratory diagnosis, and can be removed by slaughter or quarantine.

The endogenous agents, by definition, are ubiquitous and their eradication is therefore impracticable because it would require elimination of the agent from most animals, including healthy ones in which no disease is present. Many infections of intensively reared animals are endogenous. Diseases in which endogenous agents are incriminated are best controlled by alteration of other determinants, for example by improving hygiene to prevent mastitis involving *E. coli*.

## Veterinary infrastructure

Veterinary services must be capable of implementing control and eradication campaigns. There are three main requirements:

(1) a mobile field service, comprising adequately trained veterinarians and veterinary auxiliaries;
(2) adequate diagnostic facilities;
(3) adequate research facilities.

The first two requirements are important when controlling the infectious diseases such as the classic animal plagues whose causes are understood. The third requirement must be fulfilled to improve the techniques of controlling the diseases whose causes are not known, and is also needed to elucidate the causes of new and emerging diseases, such as those of intensive animal production, so that the most appropriate control strategies can be selected.

Most developed countries possess the first two requirements, mainly because their veterinary services evolved at the beginning of this century to deal with the major plagues that were common then, such as foot-and-mouth disease, pleuropneumonia and rinderpest. The developing countries often lack the first two requirements. These countries have over half of the world's livestock units (*see Table 1.2*), but contain only 20% of the world's veterinary force. Disease control programmes in these countries should therefore include two stages (Mussman *et al.*, 1980):

(1) a short-term programme that includes the development of diagnostic and field services, training of personnel to deal with the major exotic diseases, and associated control techniques, such as prevention of entry of diseases across borders;
(2) a long-term programme, similar to those present in some developed countries, that includes disease reporting systems, facilities for field surveys, and economic and epidemiological modelling.

## Diagnostic feasibility

Control and eradication can be carried out successfully only if a disease can be recognized. The main techniques of recognition are by:

(1) clinical signs;
(2) pathological changes;
(3) isolation of causal agents;
(4) demonstration of an immune, allergic or biochemical response;
(5) epidemiological identification of changes of a variable in a population.

Clinical signs may be observed either in the individual sick animal or in its offspring (e.g. congenital abnormalities). The value of signs varies because they can be either pathognomonic or indicative of several lesions and causes (*see Figure 9.1*).

Identification of pathological changes may substantiate clinical impressions and may be of value when clinical signs are absent, but again the changes may have several causes.

Isolation of causal agents is the most valuable means of identification of disease, but agents may be missed in a specimen (i.e. there may be false negatives).

Identification of an immune reaction is frequently used in control programmes. Each serological test has its own inherent sensitivity and specificity (*see* Chapter 16) whose acceptability for the control programme must be considered. Note that the predictive value of a test depends on the prevalence of the disease: the predictive value of a positive result decreases as control reduces prevalence because the proportion of false positives increases (*see Table 16.11*).

Criteria must be defined for interpreting the results of tests that are used during control and eradication campaigns because biological responses show natural variation (*see* Chapter 12). *Table 20.3*, for example, shows the criteria employed to interpret the comparative intradermal tuberculin test, which was used to identify **reactors** (cattle assumed to be infected by *Mycobacterium tuberculosis*) in the British tuberculosis eradication scheme. Note that the criteria and interpretation can vary, depending on circumstances. In this example, if there is a recent history of confirmed bovine tuberculosis on a farm, then a more severe interpretation is used than if the farm had been free from the disease for some time, thus decreasing the number of false negatives (*see Figure 16.1*).

Epidemiological diagnosis includes the detection of changes in disease or production trends in populations, for example by constructing Shewhart charts and cusums (*see* Chapter 12).

## Availability of replacement stock

If a control or an eradication campaign involves the slaughter of many animals, sufficient replacement stock should be available in the livestock industry to minimize disruption to production. This consideration has not been critical hitherto, although it has been cited as a potential problem if a slaughter campaign were used to control or eradicate bovine tuberculosis in developing countries (FAO/WHO, 1967).

## Producers' opinions and cooperation

The opinions of animal producers can affect the success of control and eradication campaigns. In Mexico in the 1940s a slaughter campaign to

**Table 20.3 Interpretation of the comparative intradermal test for bovine tuberculosis and subsequent action in Great Britain**

| Test result | Action following standard interpretation (applied to herds with no recent history of tuberculosis, or no evidence of infection at post-mortem examination of previous reactors) | Action following severe interpretation (applied to herds with recent tuberculosis problems, or herds with one or more reactors at the current test in which tuberculosis is confirmed on post-mortem examination |
|---|---|---|
| B (−ve) A (+ve or −ve)<br>B (+ve) > 2 mm < A (+ve) | Retain animal | Retain animal |
| B (+ve) = 1 or 2 mm < A (+ve)<br>B (+ve) = A (+ve) | Retain animal | Retest animal |
| B (+ve) = 1 or 2 mm > A (+ve) | Retest animal | Retest animal |
| B (+ve) = 3 or 4 mm > A (+ve) | Retest animal | Remove animal |
| B (+ve) 1 – 4 mm > A (−ve) | Retest animal | Remove animal |
| B (+ve) > 4 mm > A (+ve or −ve) | Remove animal | Remove animal |

B = reaction to bovine tuberculin; A = reaction to avian tuberculin.
A positive reaction is an increase in skin thickness at the site of tuberculin inoculation of 2 mm or more, **or** the presence of oedema at the site.

eradicate foot-and-mouth disease had to be abandoned because local farmers strongly disagreed with the technique. Producers' opinions and the degree of their cooperation are influenced by their understanding of the control campaign; an important preliminary step is a detailed explanation of its rationale to farmers. In developed countries, pamphlets and audiovisual presentations are useful, such as posters at ports of entry warning of the risk of bringing rabies into the UK. In developing countries, especially where illiteracy is widespread, these techniques may not be satisfactory and may need to be replaced or supplemented by more direct contact with farmers (Chain, 1980).

## Public opinion

The opinion of society may be an important consideration in devising a control or eradication scheme. Bovine brucellosis and canine distemper have a similar natural history. Both are transmitted by a single host species: cattle in the case of brucellosis, dogs in the case of distemper (ferrets and mink are excluded because their contribution is minor). In situations where bovine brucellosis can be eradicated on economically justifiable grounds, a vaccination and slaughter campaign is socially acceptable in most countries (excepting Hindu countries for religious reasons). A slaughter campaign to control distemper, even though technically feasible, would not be acceptable in many Western countries because of social attitudes towards dogs. In other countries, slaughter of dogs may be acceptable to the public, for example to improve environmental hygiene in China (*The Times*, 1983). Again, education of the public plays an important part in influencing attitudes. The virtual eradication

of echinococcosis from Iceland over the last century has been achieved by explaining to the public the dangers of keeping dogs unhygienically (Beard, 1973), beginning with the publication, in the 19th century, of a pamphlet that outlined precautions against infection (Krabbe, 1864).

A knowledge of social and cultural anthropology may also be valuable. In the border region of New Guinea, oestrus postponement drugs have been injected into village bitches to regulate the dog population in relation to the control of diseases, such as rabies, that might enter the country from Indonesia. Treated dogs were tagged with brightly coloured discs. However, villagers removed the discs to wear for personal adornment. Thus, treated bitches subsequently could not be identified.

## Public health considerations

Over 70% of the known pathogens are infectious to both man and other animals. Many of these—the zoonoses—are naturally transmissible between man and animals. The control of zoonotic diseases is the main concern of veterinary public health authorities.

The public health significance of a disease may be a major factor in determining the need for control, usually when human infection is either fatal, for example rabies (and, in the past, glanders), or when the infection can be clinically severe, such as occupationally acquired leptospirosis in farmers and abattoir workers.

In many cases, however, prevention of human infection is secondary to control of the infection in animals. Routine prophylactic administration of anthelmintics to dogs, for instance, is practised primarily to prevent clinical and subclinical disease in dogs, although animal owners are sometimes made aware of the potential risk of human infection (e.g. Woodruff, 1976). The control of infectious disease in livestock is usually undertaken because of the financial impact of diseases; a decrease in the incidence of human infection is an added bonus, for example when controlling bovine brucellosis.

## The requirement for legislation and compensation

Control and eradication programmes are more effective when supported by **legislation**, sometimes accompanied by penalties when the legislation is contravened. For example, in the UK, Ireland, Australia, New Zealand, Papua New Guinea and other areas in which rabies is absent, there is legislation forbidding the entry, without quarantine, of animals from countries in which the disease is present. Severe fines are imposed (and the imported animals sometimes destroyed) if the legislation is ignored.

The benefits of disease control in agriculture are frequently realized by the consumer; thus, tuberculosis eradication results in uninfected milk. The culling of an infected cow, however, represents a financial loss to the farmer. An essential part of many control programmes therefore is the **compensation** of producers for the loss of infected animals as a result of the programme. In other cases, bonuses can be offered to increase cooperation of owners, for example awarding a bonus to farmers whose cows' bulk milk cell count (which is an indirect measure of bovine mastitis) is below a defined level; farmers whose cows' bulk cell count is above a higher defined level are penalized.

## Ecological consequences

It has been argued that control and, particularly, eradication of an infectious agent may disturb the 'balance of nature' in an ecosystem (*see* Yekutiel, 1980, for a detailed discussion). The elimination of an infectious agent may free a niche that could be occupied by a more virulent organism.

The use of insecticides to destroy arthropod vectors could kill other animals in the arthropods' ecosystem. These considerations have, so far, been only theoretical in relation to animal disease control, although the use of insecticides to control insect pests has resulted in the death of birds and other animals that have ingested the insecticides (Carson, 1963).

## Financial support

Control and eradication campaigns require financial support. The control of companion animal diseases readily draws financial support from owners; canine, equine and feline vaccination programmes are examples.

Livestock disease control campaigns are usually funded either totally or partially by the government, or by non-governmental sources (Parsons, 1982). Total government support is often given to the control of exotic infectious diseases of major economic importance. Diagnostic tests, vaccines, disinfection, compensation, quarantine facilities and veterinary staff are funded by the government. Examples of such diseases are foot-and-mouth disease and swine vesicular disease. There may be partial government support, for example when a control scheme initially is voluntary (funded by the producer) and then becomes compulsory (funded by the government). An example is the British bovine brucellosis scheme which initially was financed by farmers, with incentives and compensation awarded for inclusion in the scheme, and which then became compulsory. Alternatively, costs may be shared by government and the livestock industry. For example, in Britain sheep scab is controlled by dipping; the dips are provided by farmers; veterinary supervision is funded by the government.

State financial support may also be provided indirectly, for example through the State laboratory diagnostic services and participation in herd health schemes. Non-governmental financial support is supplied indirectly by the pharmaceutical industry in the development of therapeutic and prophylactic drugs and vaccines. In Israel, a part of farm insurance premiums is directed towards disease control. In West Germany, levies on farm products are used to support control programmes. The extent of government support is reflected by current political and economic attitudes. Support may be reduced in circumstances when the government becomes less 'paternalistic' and when it supports private enterprise rather than state control.

In all cases of financial support, the cost of control has to be weighed against the cost of disease.

# Veterinary medicine towards the end of this century

Chapter 1 described how veterinary medicine coped with various challenges during its development. This final chapter ends with some thoughts on the direction of the veterinary profession in the near future. The topic is discussed in greater detail by Henderson (1982) and Hugh-Jones (1983).

## *Livestock medicine*

Multifactorial diseases are the major problems in intensive livestock enterprises. Investigation of their cause does not involve the study of a simple infectious agent, but of several determinants associated with host, agent and environment. Sophisticated environmental monitoring devices that log variables, such as cough rates, are now available and can be linked directly to computers for analysis. The environment too is recognized as important, not only because of its role in the cause of disease but also because of its significance to animal welfare.

Modelling of livestock units, using variables associated with disease and production, is likely to be developed. Models can predict disease morbidity, for example the prevalence of pneumonia in pig herds, using management and environmental variables as risk indicators (Morrison and Morris, 1985). They also facilitate definition of the most suitable index variables and action levels, and indicate methods of assessing the economic impact of disease.

A prerequisite for an economic assessment of disease is accurate morbidity data. Computerized recording systems provide a powerful means of collecting and analysing data. They will be more valuable when many data bases can be analysed communally; networks provide the technological means of linking such data.

Similarly, in developing countries, there is a need for an improvement in the 'quality' of data. The epidemic infectious diseases still pose problems. Eradication campaigns have sometimes been unsuccessful because of recurrence; rinderpest in Africa, cited in Chapter 1, is an example. There is a need to improve the planning of the terminal stages of some eradication campaigns in these countries.

Techniques of identification of infectious diseases are becoming more sensitive and refined. Smaller quantities of antigen can be detected, and subtle differences between strains can be identified using ELISA tests, monoclonal antibodies, and oligonucleotide fingerprinting (McMillan and Hanson, 1983).

New techniques are producing safer vaccines. For example, subunit vaccines comprise only virus capsid antigens and lack nucleic acid, and therefore cannot be pathogenic. Vaccines against helminths (e.g. *Dictyocaulus viviparus*) are few but they have a considerable advantage over the current anthelmintics, because of the latter's associated risk of resistance and short period of action. The breeding of resistant stock, however, may be more useful because techniques such as embryo cloning, superovulation and nuclear transplantation can accelerate this otherwise slow process.

Financial support is needed for research, therefore the interest shown by grant-awarding organizations will determine which techniques are investigated (Henderson, 1980).

## Companion animal medicine

Companion animals are of considerable value to their owners. The quality of individual patient care

will continue to improve, involving better surgical techniques and medical therapy. The aim of medical epidemiologists is to ensure that each person enjoys a long healthy life with morbidity confined to a short period before death. This goal can be shared by veterinarians, and its achievement requires research on improved preventive techniques, such as vaccination, and on the determinants associated with chronic and refractory diseases, such as canine heart disease and dermatoses. This research is currently hampered by a lack of basic demographic and morbidity data from a wide cross-section of the companion animal population. However, the increasing availability of inexpensive microcomputers to veterinary practitioners and the expansion of computer networks should facilitate the gathering of these data.

Epidemiology plays a central role in the continuing development and improvement of livestock and companion animal veterinary medicine. Its contemporary objectives are similar to those of ancient Greek medicine, described by Hippocrates in the 'Second Constitution' of Book 1 of his *Epidemics*, as to:

'Declare the past, diagnose the present, foretell the future'

(Jones, 1923)

## Further reading

BIGGS, P.M. (1985) Infectious disease and its control. *Philosophical Transactions of the Royal Society of London, Series B*, **310**, 259–274

BRANDER, G.C. and ELLIS, P.R. (1977) *The Control of Disease*. Baillière Tindall, London

DAVIES, G. (1985) Art, science and mathematics: new approaches to animal health problems in the agricultural industry. *Veterinary Record*, **117**, 263–267

FOOD AND AGRICULTURE ORGANIZATION OF THE UNITED NATIONS (1984) *Ticks and Tick-borne Disease Control. Vol. 1, Tick Control. Vol. 2, Tick-borne Disease Control*. FAO, Rome

REPORT OF A BRITISH VETERINARY ASSOCIATION TRUST PROJECT ON THE FUTURE OF ANIMAL HEALTH CONTROL (1982) *The Control of Infectious Diseases in Farm Animals*. British Veterinary Association, London

SCHWABE, C.W. (1980) Animal disease control. Part II. Newer methods, with possibility for their application in the Sudan. *Sudan Journal of Veterinary Science and Animal Husbandry*, **21**, 55–64

YEKUTIEL, P. (1980) *Eradication of Infectious Disease—A Critical Study*. Contributions to Epidemiology and Biostatistics Vol. 2. Karger, Basel

# General reading

CAMPBELL, R.S.F. (Ed.) (1983) *A Course Manual in Veterinary Epidemiology*. Australian Universities' International Development Program, Canberra

ELLIS, P.R., SHAW, A.P.M. and STEPHENS, A.J. (1976) *New Techniques in Veterinary Epidemiology and Economics*. Proceedings of a Symposium held at the University of Reading, 12–15 July 1976

*EPIDEMIOLOGY IN ANIMAL HEALTH* (1983) Proceedings of a symposium held at the British Veterinary Association's Centenary Congress, Reading, 22–25 September 1982. Society for Veterinary Epidemiology and Preventive Medicine

GEERING, W.A., ROE, R.T. and CHAPMAN, L.A. (Eds) (1980) *Veterinary Epidemiology and Economics*. Proceedings of the Second International Symposium, Canberra, 7–11 May 1979. Australian Government Publishing Service, Canberra

HALPIN, B. (1975) *Patterns of Animal Disease*. Baillière Tindall, London

LEECH, F.B. and SELLERS, K.C. (1979) *Statistical Epidemiology in Veterinary Science*. Charles Griffin and Company Ltd, London and High Wycombe

*PROCEEDINGS OF THE THIRD INTERNATIONAL SYMPOSIUM ON VETERINARY EPIDEMIOLOGY AND ECONOMICS* (1983) Arlington, Virginia, 6–10 September 1982

*PROCEEDINGS OF THE FOURTH INTERNATIONAL SYMPOSIUM ON VETERINARY EPIDEMIOLOGY AND ECONOMICS* (1986) Singapore, 18–22 November 1985. Singapore Veterinary Association

SCHWABE, C.W., RIEMANN, H.P. and FRANTI, C.E. (1977) *Epidemiology in Veterinary Practice*. Lea and Febiger, Philadelphia

SCHWABE, C.W. (1984) *Veterinary Medicine and Human Health*. 3rd edn. Williams and Wilkins, Baltimore and London

THRUSFIELD, M.V. (Ed.) (1983) Society for Veterinary Epidemiology and Preventive Medicine, Proceedings, Southampton, 12–13 April 1983

THRUSFIELD, M.V. (Ed.) (1984) Society for Veterinary Epidemiology and Preventive Medicine, Proceedings, Edinburgh, 10–11 April 1984

THRUSFIELD, M.V. (Ed.) (1985) Society for Veterinary Epidemiology and Preventive Medicine, Proceedings, Reading, 27–29 March 1985

THRUSFIELD, M.V. (Ed.) (1986) Society for Veterinary Epidemiology and Preventive Medicine, Proceedings, Edinburgh, 2–4 April 1986

General reading

# Appendices

Appendices III, IV, V and X are taken from Tables III, IV, VII and V, respectively, in *Statistical Tables for Biological, Agricultural and Medical Research*, 6th edition (1974), edited by Fisher, R.A. and Yates, F. and published by Longman Group Limited (previously published by Oliver and Boyd Limited, Edinburgh), and are reproduced with the permission of the authors and publishers.

# Appendix I

# Glossary of terms

This glossary provides brief definitions of some common epidemiological terms that are used in this book. A more comprehensive guide is given in *A Dictionary of Epidemiology* (edited by J.M. Last, Oxford University Press, New York, 1983), from which some of the definitions below are derived.

**Accuracy:** the degree to which an individual measurement represents the true value of the attribute that is being measured: the greater the accuracy, the greater the degree.

**Antibody:** a protein produced by an animal's immunological system in response to exposure to a foreign substance (an antigen; q.v.). Sometimes antibodies are produced against the individual's own proteins, causing autoimmune disease. Antibodies display specificity (q.v.) to particular antigens.

**Antigen:** a substance (usually a protein) that induces a specific immune response (e.g. circulating antibody production).

**Association:** the relationship between two variables (*see* Appendix II). The association is 'positive' when the variables occur together more frequently than is expected by chance; the association is 'negative' when they occur less frequently than is expected by chance.

**Bias:** systematic (as opposed to random) departure from true values.

**Binomial distribution:** a probability distribution relating to two mutually exclusive and exhaustive outcomes (e.g. the birth of either male or female animals), where successive outcomes (e.g. births) are independent and occur with constant probability.

**Carrier:**

(1) an animal that is infected with an infectious agent without displaying clinical signs, and that can be a source of infection to other animals;

(2) (genetic) an animal that is heterozygous for a normal and an abnormal gene, the latter of which is not expressed but may be detected by tests.

**Case-control study:** an observational study (q.v.) in which a group of diseased animals (cases) is compared with a group of non-diseased animals (controls) with respect to exposure to an hypothesized cause.

**Cohort study:** an observational study (q.v.) in which a group of animals exposed to an hypothesized cause is compared with a group not so exposed, with respect to development of a disease.

**Commensals:** microbes found on the skin or within the body that do not usually cause disease (cf. pathogens).

**Confidence interval:** a range of values within which the value of a parameter (*see* Appendix II) lies with a specified level of confidence.

**Confounding:** the inseparability from a given data set of the effects of two possible causes of an observed result, because both occur together.

**Continuous variable:** a variable (*see* Appendix II) that may take any value in an interval; the interval may be finite or infinite.

**Cost-benefit analysis:** *see* Social cost-benefit analysis.

**Cross-sectional study:**

(1) an observational study (q.v.) in which animals are classified according to presence or absence of disease, and presence or absence of exposure to an hypothesized causal factor, at a particular point in time;

(2) an observational study (q.v.) in which a simple random sample of a population is selected, and the sample's members are classified according to presence or absence of disease, and presence or absence of exposure (either current or previous), to an hypothesized cause.

**Cross-sectional survey:** a survey (q.v.) undertaken at a particular point in time.

**Data base:** a structured collection of data.

**Determinant:** a factor that affects the health of a population.

**Discrete variable:** a variable (*see* Appendix II) for which there is a definite distance from one value of the variable to the next possible value (e.g. numbers of cases of disease: 1, 2, 3 ... where the distance is 1).

**Endemic:** an adjective describing:
(1) the predictable level of occurrence of disease, infection, antibody etc.
(2) the usual presence of disease, infection, antibody etc.

**Endogenous:**
(1) normally from within an animal;
(2) (characteristic) an innate characteristic of an animal (e.g. breed).

**Epidemic:** an occurrence of disease in excess of its anticipated frequency (also used adjectivally).

**Epidemic curve:** a graph plotting the number of new cases against time of onset of disease; thus, an epidemic curve plots incidence.

**Epidemiology (veterinary):** the investigation of disease, other health-related events, and production in animal populations and the making of inferences from the investigation in an attempt to improve the health and productivity of the populations.

**Exogenous:**
(1) normally from outside an animal;
(2) (characteristic) a characteristic, that is not innate, to which an animal is exposed (e.g. climate, toxic substances and microbes).

**Experimental study:** a study (q.v.) in which the investigator can allocate animals to different categories; thus, the conditions of the study are controlled by the investigator.

**Extrinsic factor:** *see* Exogenous (2).

**Extrinsic incubation period:** the time between the entry of an infectious agent into an arthropod vector and the time at which the arthropod becomes infectious.

**Fomites (singular: fomes):** inanimate communicators of infection (cf. vector).

**Health and productivity schemes:** systems for recording disease and productivity in groups of animals (usually herds and flocks), their aim being to improve health and productivity of the groups.

**Horizontal (lateral) transmission:** transmission of an infection from an individual to any other individual in a population, but excluding vertical transmission (q.v.).

**Hypothesis:** a proposition that can be tested formally; after which the hypothesis may be either 'supported' or 'rejected'.

**Inapparent infection:** an infection that does not produce clinical signs.

**Incidence:** the number of new cases that occur over a specified period of time. It is expressed usually in relation to the population at risk and the time during which the population is observed.

**Interaction:**
(1) **(biological)** the interdependent operation of two or more causes to produce an effect;
(2) **(statistical)** in an epidemiological context, a quantitative interdependence between two or more factors, such that the frequency of disease when two or more factors are present is either in excess of that expected from the combined effects of each factor (positive interaction) or less than the combined effect (negative interaction).

**Intrinsic factor:** *see* Endogenous (2).

**Longitudinal study:**
(1) a cohort study (q.v.);
(2) a general description of both cohort and case-control studies (q.v.), so called because these studies investigate exposure to an hypothesized cause and development of disease (the effect) when cause and effect are separated temporally.

**Longitudinal survey:** a survey (q.v.) that records events over a period of time.

**Misclassification:** the incorrect allocation of individuals or features to categories to which they do not belong (e.g. the classification of a diseased animal as non-diseased).

**Model:** a representation of a physical process; in epidemiology models are usually mathematical and attempt to analyse and predict processes quantitatively.

**Monitoring:** the routine collection of information on disease, productivity and other characteristics possibly related to them in a population.

**Morbidity:** the amount of disease in a population (commonly defined in terms of incidence or prevalence; q.v.).

**Mortality:** a measure of the number of deaths in a population.

**Multifactorial disease:** a disease that depends on the presence of several factors for its induction. Most diseases are multifactorial, although some may have one major component cause (e.g. foot-and-mouth disease virus in the cause of foot-and-mouth disease), in which case they are commonly termed 'unifactorial'.

**Necessary cause:** a cause that must always be present for a disease to occur (e.g. *Mycobacterium tuberculosis* is the necessary cause of tuberculosis).

**Nidality:** the characteristic of an infectious agent to occur in distinct nidi (q.v.) associated with particular geographic, climatic and ecological conditions.

**Nidus (plural: nidi):** a focus of infection.

**Normal distribution:** a probability distribution relating to continuous data and characterized by a symmetric, bell-shaped distribution with 'tails' extending to infinity.

**Observational study:** an epidemiological study (q.v.) in which the investigator has no freedom, or does not exercise his freedom, to allocate animals to different categories: disease is studied as it occurs 'naturally'.

**Odds ratio:** usually defined as the ratio of (the number of diseased animals exposed to a factor multiplied by the number of non-diseased animals not exposed to the factor) to (the number of non-diseased animals exposed to the factor multiplied by the number of diseased animals not exposed to the factor). It is a measure of association commonly used in observational studies.

**Outbreak:** an identified occurrence of disease involving one or more animals. The term generally implies that several animals are affected. Livestock in developed countries are usually kept as separated populations and so 'outbreak' can be applied unambiguously to an occurrence of disease on an individual farm. However, in developing countries, animal populations frequently are contiguous and so it may be difficult to define the limits of one outbreak. *Office International des Epizooties* has suggested that the occurrence of disease within a 50 km$^2$ area constitutes an outbreak, even though the disease may be found in several places in that area.

**Pandemic:** a geographically widespread (sometimes global) epidemic (also used adjectivally).

**Parameter:** *see* Appendix II.

**Pathogen:** an organism that produces disease.

**Pathogenicity:** the ability of an infectious agent to cause disease.

**Point (common) source epidemic:** an epidemic resulting from exposure of animals to a single common cause.

**Poisson distribution:** a probability distribution relating to the distribution of events, independently, either throughout space (an area) or over time.

**Population at risk:** the population that is naturally susceptible to a disease.

**Precision:**
(1) the reciprocal of the variance of an estimate;
(2) the quality of being lucidly and clearly defined.

**Prevalence:** the number of occurrences of disease, infection, antibody presence, and so on in a population, usually relating to a particular point in time; it is commonly expressed as the proportion of the population at risk.

**Predictive value:**
(1) of a positive test result: the probability that an animal with a 'positive' test is a true 'positive';
(2) of a negative test result: the probability that an animal with a 'negative' test result is a true 'negative'.

**Proportion:** a ratio (q.v.) in which the numerator is part of the denominator.

**Prospective study:** a cohort study.

**Rate:** a ratio (q.v.) that indicates the change in one quantity with respect to one or more others; the latter usually include 'time'. Thus incidence rate is the number of new cases of disease per defined size of population at risk per defined time period (e.g. 10 cases per 1000 animals per year).

**Ratio:** a value obtained by dividing one quantity (the numerator) by another (the denominator), for example, the number of males born per female birth. Proportions and rates are ratios.

**Refinement:** the quality of being sharply defined. Thus, a refined serological test will detect subtle antigenic differences between microbes, whereas a less refined test will only identify major antigenic groups.

**Relative risk:** the ratio of disease incidence in individuals exposed to an hypothesized cause, to the incidence in those not so exposed. It is a measure of association commonly used in observational studies.

**Reliability:** the degree of stability exhibited when a measurement is repeated under identical conditions; reliability therefore may be demonstrated by repeating a measurement.

**Reservoir:** an animate or inanimate object on or in which an infectious agent usually lives, and which therefore is often a source of infection by the agent.

**Retrospective study:**
(1) a case-control study (so-called because the study **looks back** from effect to cause);
(2) any study that collects and utilizes historical data.

**Sample:** a selected part of a population.

**Screening:** the presumptive identification of an unrecognized disease or defect using tests or other procedures that can be applied rapidly to a population or a selected subset.

**Sensitivity** (of a test):
(1) the proportion of diseased animals that are detected by a test;
(2) the ability of a test to detect amounts of antigen, enzyme, and so on; a sensitive test will detect small amounts.

**Social cost-benefit analysis:** an economic technique used in epidemiology to assess the costs of disease and impaired productivity in relation to the benefits that accrue from their control.

**Specificity:**
(1) (of a test) the proportion of non-diseased animals that are detected by a test;
(2) degree of refinement; the greater the specificity, the greater the degree.

**Sporadic:** an adjective describing the irregular, unpredictable occurrence of disease or infection.

**Study:** an investigation that involves the testing of a causal hypothesis. A study may be either experimental (q.v.) or observational (q.v.).

**Sufficient cause:** the complex of component causes that induces a disease. Several different sufficient causes may induce the same disease.

**Surveillance:** an intensive form of monitoring (q.v.),

designed so that appropriate action can be taken to improve the health status of a population, and therefore frequently used in disease control campaigns.

**Survey:** an investigation involving the collection of information and in which a causal hypothesis usually is not tested (cf. study). It may suggest aspects worthy of study.

**Synergism:** a positive statistical interaction (q.v.) where a causal pathway can be inferred (other authors may use the term differently).

**Threshold level:**

(1) the spatial density of susceptible animals required to initiate an epidemic;

(2) the minimum concentration of an infectious agent in a vertebrate host's circulation that allows successful transmission to an arthropod vector.

**Validity:** a term with a variety of meanings; in this book it is the degree to which a diagnostic test or survey produces, **on average**, an accurate result. It is therefore a **long-run** property of the test or survey.

**Variable:** *see* Appendix II.

**Vector:** a living organism (frequently an arthropod) that communicates an infectious agent from an infected to a susceptible animal.

**Vertical transmission:** transmission of an infection from one individual to its offspring.

**Virulence:** the disease-evoking power of an infectious agent in a particular host.

**Zoonosis:** an infection shared in nature by man and other vertebrates.

# Appendix II

# Basic mathematical notation and terms

## Variables

There are properties of members of a population that vary between the members, for example, weights of cows or breed of pig. The values (sometimes known as **variates**) are donated by Roman letters which usually take the lower case, $x$, $y$, $z$ etc. The letters often have **subscripts** (small-sized numbers to the right of and slightly below the letter), for example:

the weights $x_1$, $x_2$, $x_3$, of three calves
$x_1 = 230$ kg, $x_2 = 221$ kg, $x_3 = 155$ kg.

## Constants

There are two types of constant:

(1) **Universal constants** have a single value, for example, $\pi = 3.141...$
(2) **Parameters** are constants that are fixed for a particular study, but which may change from one study to another. Greek letters, $\lambda$, $\mu$ and so on, usually denote parameters. For example, the infectivity rate of a particular parasite could be denoted by $\lambda$, where $\lambda$ may change from one isolate to another.

## Summation notation: $\Sigma$

$\Sigma$ is used to denote the sum of a set of data. For example:

$$\sum_{i=1}^{6} x_i = x_1 + x_2 + x_3 + x_4 + x_5 + x_6.$$

This means 'the sum of all the values of $x$ from $x_1$ to $x_6$ inclusive'. This notation is of value if, for instance, one wanted to add $x_3$, $x_4$ and $x_5$ from the series of values, in which case one would write:

$$\sum_{i=3}^{5} x_i$$

In biological calculations it is usually necessary to add **all** of the values of $x$ from $x_1$ to the last value of $x$, omitting none of the values in the series. It is therefore sufficient to write $\Sigma x$, in which case it is assumed that all of the $x$ values in the series are being added.

This system of notation can also be applied to powers. For example, $\Sigma x^2$ means 'square all the individual values of $x$ in the series and then add these square values together':

$x_1 = 2$, $x_2 = 3$, $x_3 = 2$,

then $\Sigma x^2 = x_1^2 + x_2^2 + x_3^2 = 4 + 9 + 4 = 17$.

$(\Sigma x)^2$ means 'add together all the values of $x$ in the series and then square the result'. For example:

$x_1 = 2$, $x_2 = 3$, $x_3 = 2$,
then $(\Sigma x)^2 = (x_1 + x_2 + x_3)^2 = (2 + 3 + 2)^2 = 49$.

## Order of calculation

Multiplication and division are conducted before addition and subtraction. Thus:

$6 \times 3 + 1$
$= 18 + 1$
$= 19$.

Brackets are used to indicate the order of calculation, when calculations would otherwise be ambiguous. Three types of bracket are commonly used: parentheses (), braces {}, and square brackets [], usually, but not always, in that order.

Thus: 3 [ 3 + { 6(4+2) } ]

is calculated as 4 + 2 = 6
then 6 × 6 = 36
then 3 + 36 = 39
then 3 × 39 = 117.

## *Magnitude notation*

> = greater than (e.g. 6 > 5)
< = less than (e.g. 5 < 6)
≥ = greater than or equal to
≤ = less than or equal to

A line through any of these symbols means 'not', for example ≯ means 'not greater than'.

## *Factorial notation: x!*

$x!$ is used to denote the successive multiplication of all positive integers (whole numbers) between $x$ and 1. For example:

6! = 6 × 5 × 4 × 3 × 2 × 1 = 720
2! = 2 × 1 = 2
1! = 1.

Note, however, that 0! is an exception because it equals 1, **not** 0.

## *Modulus notation: $|x|$*

Vertical lines on each side of a numerical quantity, $x$, mean that the positive sign of the value of $x$ should be used. For example, $|-2|$ and $|2|$ are both read as +2. Similarly $|-6 +1|$ will simplify to $|-5|$ which is read as +5.

# Appendix III

## Student's *t*-distribution

| Degrees of freedom | Probability | | | | | | | | | | | | |
|---|---|---|---|---|---|---|---|---|---|---|---|---|---|
| | .9 | .8 | .7 | .6 | .5 | .4 | .3 | .2 | .1 | .05 | .02 | .01 | .001 |
| 1 | .158 | .325 | .510 | .727 | 1.000 | 1.376 | 1.963 | 3.078 | 6.314 | 12.706 | 31.821 | 63.657 | 636.619 |
| 2 | .142 | .289 | .445 | .617 | .816 | 1.061 | 1.386 | 1.886 | 2.920 | 4.303 | 6.965 | 9.925 | 31.598 |
| 3 | .137 | .277 | .424 | .584 | .765 | .978 | 1.250 | 1.638 | 2.353 | 3.182 | 4.541 | 5.841 | 12.924 |
| 4 | .134 | .271 | .414 | .569 | .741 | .941 | 1.190 | 1.533 | 2.132 | 2.776 | 3.747 | 4.604 | 8.610 |
| 5 | .132 | .267 | .408 | .559 | .727 | .920 | 1.156 | 1.476 | 2.015 | 2.571 | 3.365 | 4.032 | 6.869 |
| 6 | .131 | .265 | .404 | .553 | .718 | .906 | 1.134 | 1.440 | 1.943 | 2.447 | 3.143 | 3.707 | 5.959 |
| 7 | .130 | .263 | .402 | .549 | .711 | .896 | 1.119 | 1.415 | 1.895 | 2.365 | 2.998 | 3.499 | 5.408 |
| 8 | .130 | .262 | .399 | .546 | .706 | .889 | 1.108 | 1.397 | 1.860 | 2.306 | 2.896 | 3.355 | 5.041 |
| 9 | .129 | .261 | .398 | .543 | .703 | .883 | 1.100 | 1.383 | 1.833 | 2.262 | 2.821 | 3.250 | 4.781 |
| 10 | .129 | .260 | .397 | .542 | .700 | .879 | 1.093 | 1.372 | 1.812 | 2.228 | 2.764 | 3.169 | 4.587 |
| 11 | .129 | .260 | .396 | .540 | .697 | .876 | 1.088 | 1.363 | 1.796 | 2.201 | 2.718 | 3.106 | 4.437 |
| 12 | .128 | .259 | .395 | .539 | .695 | .873 | 1.083 | 1.356 | 1.782 | 2.179 | 2.681 | 3.055 | 4.318 |
| 13 | .128 | .259 | .394 | .538 | .694 | .870 | 1.079 | 1.350 | 1.771 | 2.160 | 2.650 | 3.012 | 4.221 |
| 14 | .128 | .258 | .393 | .537 | .692 | .868 | 1.076 | 1.345 | 1.761 | 2.145 | 2.624 | 2.977 | 4.140 |
| 15 | .128 | .258 | .393 | .536 | .691 | .866 | 1.074 | 1.341 | 1.753 | 2.131 | 2.602 | 2.947 | 4.073 |
| 16 | .128 | .258 | .392 | .535 | .690 | .865 | 1.071 | 1.337 | 1.746 | 2.120 | 2.583 | 2.921 | 4.015 |
| 17 | .128 | .257 | .392 | .534 | .689 | .863 | 1.069 | 1.333 | 1.740 | 2.110 | 2.567 | 2.898 | 3.965 |
| 18 | .127 | .257 | .392 | .534 | .688 | .862 | 1.067 | 1.330 | 1.734 | 2.101 | 2.552 | 2.878 | 3.922 |
| 19 | .127 | .257 | .391 | .533 | .688 | .861 | 1.066 | 1.328 | 1.729 | 2.093 | 2.539 | 2.861 | 3.883 |
| 20 | .127 | .257 | .391 | .533 | .687 | .860 | 1.064 | 1.325 | 1.725 | 2.086 | 2.528 | 2.845 | 3.850 |
| 21 | .127 | .257 | .391 | .532 | .686 | .859 | 1.063 | 1.323 | 1.721 | 2.080 | 2.518 | 2.831 | 3.819 |
| 22 | .127 | .256 | .390 | .532 | .686 | .858 | 1.061 | 1.321 | 1.717 | 2.074 | 2.508 | 2.819 | 3.792 |
| 23 | .127 | .256 | .390 | .532 | .685 | .858 | 1.060 | 1.319 | 1.714 | 2.069 | 2.500 | 2.807 | 3.767 |
| 24 | .127 | .256 | .390 | .531 | .685 | .857 | 1.059 | 1.318 | 1.711 | 2.064 | 2.492 | 2.797 | 3.745 |
| 25 | .127 | .256 | .390 | .531 | .684 | .856 | 1.058 | 1.316 | 1.708 | 2.060 | 2.485 | 2.787 | 3.725 |
| 26 | .127 | .256 | .390 | .531 | .684 | .856 | 1.058 | 1.315 | 1.706 | 2.056 | 2.479 | 2.779 | 3.707 |
| 27 | .127 | .256 | .389 | .531 | .684 | .855 | 1.057 | 1.314 | 1.703 | 2.052 | 2.473 | 2.771 | 3.690 |
| 28 | .127 | .256 | .389 | .530 | .683 | .855 | 1.056 | 1.313 | 1.701 | 2.048 | 2.467 | 2.763 | 3.674 |
| 29 | .127 | .256 | .389 | .530 | .683 | .854 | 1.055 | 1.311 | 1.699 | 2.045 | 2.462 | 2.756 | 3.659 |
| 30 | .127 | .256 | .389 | .530 | .683 | .854 | 1.055 | 1.310 | 1.697 | 2.042 | 2.457 | 2.750 | 3.646 |
| 40 | .126 | .255 | .388 | .529 | .681 | .851 | 1.050 | 1.303 | 1.684 | 2.021 | 2.423 | 2.704 | 3.551 |
| 60 | .126 | .254 | .387 | .527 | .679 | .848 | 1.046 | 1.296 | 1.671 | 2.000 | 2.390 | 2.660 | 3.460 |
| 120 | .126 | .254 | .386 | .526 | .677 | .845 | 1.041 | 1.289 | 1.658 | 1.980 | 2.358 | 2.617 | 3.373 |
| ∞ | .126 | .253 | .385 | .524 | .674 | .842 | 1.036 | 1.282 | 1.645 | 1.960 | 2.326 | 2.576 | 3.291 |

The table gives the percentage points most frequently required for significance tests and confidence limits based on Student's *t*-distribution. Thus the probability of observing a value of *t*, with 10 degrees of freedom, greater in **absolute value** than 3.169 (i.e. $<-3.169$ or $>+3.169$) is exactly 0.01 or 1 per cent.

# Appendix IV

# The $\chi^2$-distribution

| Degrees of freedom | Value of P | | | | |
|---|---|---|---|---|---|
| | 0.99 | 0.95 | 0.05 | 0.01 | 0.001 |
| 1 | 0.000157 | 0.00393 | 3.841 | 6.635 | 10.83 |
| 2 | 0.0201 | 0.103 | 5.991 | 9.210 | 13.82 |
| 3 | 0.115 | 0.352 | 7.815 | 11.34 | 16.27 |
| 4 | 0.297 | 0.711 | 9.488 | 13.28 | 18.47 |
| 5 | 0.554 | 1.145 | 11.07 | 15.09 | 20.51 |
| 6 | 0.872 | 1.635 | 12.59 | 16.81 | 22.46 |
| 7 | 1.239 | 2.167 | 14.07 | 18.48 | 24.32 |
| 8 | 1.646 | 2.733 | 15.51 | 20.09 | 26.13 |
| 9 | 2.088 | 3.325 | 16.92 | 21.67 | 27.88 |
| 10 | 2.558 | 3.940 | 18.31 | 23.21 | 29.59 |
| 11 | 3.053 | 4.575 | 19.68 | 24.72 | 31.26 |
| 12 | 3.571 | 5.226 | 21.03 | 26.22 | 32.91 |
| 13 | 4.107 | 5.892 | 22.36 | 27.69 | 34.53 |
| 14 | 4.660 | 6.571 | 23.68 | 29.14 | 36.12 |
| 15 | 5.229 | 7.261 | 25.00 | 30.58 | 37.70 |
| 16 | 5.812 | 7.962 | 26.30 | 32.00 | 39.25 |
| 17 | 6.408 | 8.672 | 27.59 | 33.41 | 40.79 |
| 18 | 7.015 | 9.390 | 28.87 | 34.81 | 42.31 |
| 19 | 7.633 | 10.12 | 30.14 | 36.19 | 43.82 |
| 20 | 8.260 | 10.85 | 31.41 | 37.57 | 45.31 |
| 21 | 8.897 | 11.59 | 32.67 | 38.93 | 46.80 |
| 22 | 9.542 | 12.34 | 33.92 | 40.29 | 48.27 |
| 23 | 10.20 | 13.09 | 35.17 | 41.64 | 49.73 |
| 24 | 10.86 | 13.85 | 36.42 | 42.98 | 51.18 |
| 25 | 11.52 | 14.61 | 37.65 | 44.31 | 52.62 |
| 26 | 12.20 | 15.38 | 38.89 | 45.64 | 54.05 |
| 27 | 12.88 | 16.15 | 40.11 | 46.96 | 55.48 |
| 28 | 13.56 | 16.93 | 41.34 | 48.28 | 56.89 |
| 29 | 14.26 | 17.71 | 42.56 | 49.59 | 58.30 |
| 30 | 14.95 | 18.49 | 43.77 | 50.89 | 59.70 |

The table gives the percentage points most frequently required for significance tests based on $\chi^2$. Thus the probability of observing a $\chi^2$ with 5 degrees of freedom **greater** in value than 11.07 is 0.05 or 5 per cent. Again, the probability of observing a $\chi^2$ with 5 degrees of freedom **smaller** in value than 0.554 is $1 - 0.99 = 0.01$ or 1 per cent.

# Appendix V

# The correlation coefficient

| Degrees of freedom | Value of P | | | | |
|---|---|---|---|---|---|
| | 0.10 | 0.05 | 0.02 | 0.01 | 0.001 |
| 1 | 0.9877 | 0.99692 | 0.99951 | 0.99988 | 0.9999988 |
| 2 | 0.9000 | 0.9500 | 0.9800 | 0.9900 | 0.9990 |
| 3 | 0.805 | 0.878 | 0.9343 | 0.9587 | 0.9911 |
| 4 | 0.729 | 0.811 | 0.882 | 0.9172 | 0.9741 |
| 5 | 0.669 | 0.754 | 0.833 | 0.875 | 0.9509 |
| 6 | 0.621 | 0.707 | 0.789 | 0.834 | 0.9249 |
| 7 | 0.582 | 0.666 | 0.750 | 0.798 | 0.898 |
| 8 | 0.549 | 0.632 | 0.715 | 0.765 | 0.872 |
| 9 | 0.521 | 0.602 | 0.685 | 0.735 | 0.847 |
| 10 | 0.497 | 0.576 | 0.658 | 0.708 | 0.823 |
| 11 | 0.476 | 0.553 | 0.634 | 0.684 | 0.801 |
| 12 | 0.457 | 0.532 | 0.612 | 0.661 | 0.780 |
| 13 | 0.441 | 0.514 | 0.592 | 0.641 | 0.760 |
| 14 | 0.426 | 0.497 | 0.574 | 0.623 | 0.742 |
| 15 | 0.412 | 0.482 | 0.558 | 0.606 | 0.725 |
| 16 | 0.400 | 0.468 | 0.543 | 0.590 | 0.708 |
| 17 | 0.389 | 0.456 | 0.529 | 0.575 | 0.693 |
| 18 | 0.378 | 0.444 | 0.516 | 0.561 | 0.679 |
| 19 | 0.369 | 0.433 | 0.503 | 0.549 | 0.665 |
| 20 | 0.360 | 0.423 | 0.492 | 0.537 | 0.652 |
| 25 | 0.323 | 0.381 | 0.445 | 0.487 | 0.597 |
| 30 | 0.296 | 0.349 | 0.409 | 0.449 | 0.554 |
| 35 | 0.275 | 0.325 | 0.381 | 0.418 | 0.519 |
| 40 | 0.257 | 0.304 | 0.358 | 0.393 | 0.490 |
| 45 | 0.243 | 0.288 | 0.338 | 0.372 | 0.465 |
| 50 | 0.231 | 0.273 | 0.322 | 0.354 | 0.443 |
| 60 | 0.211 | 0.250 | 0.295 | 0.325 | 0.408 |
| 70 | 0.195 | 0.232 | 0.274 | 0.302 | 0.380 |
| 80 | 0.183 | 0.217 | 0.257 | 0.283 | 0.357 |
| 90 | 0.173 | 0.205 | 0.242 | 0.267 | 0.338 |
| 100 | 0.164 | 0.195 | 0.230 | 0.254 | 0.321 |

The table gives percentage points for the distribution of the estimated correlation coefficient $r$ when the true value $\varrho$ is zero. Thus when there are 10 degrees of freedom (i.e. in samples of 12) the probability of observing an $r$ greater in **absolute value** than 0.576 (i.e. $< -0.576$ or $> +0.576$) is 0.05 or 5 per cent.

# Appendix VI

# Technique of selecting a simple random sample

**Example:** An investigator requires a random sample of 10 animals from a population of 88.

Construct a sampling frame of all animals and label them consecutively from 1 to 88. The random numbers in this table are arranged in groups of 5 columns for visual convenience (other tables may have different numbers of columns grouped together).

(1) Select two columns arbitrarily, to correspond to tens and units—use columns 11 and 12, for visual convenience.
(2) Select a row arbitrarily—say row 1 for visual convenience: number 32.

(3) Move down the columns: 32, 50, 81, 89, 47, 89, 12, 38, 76, 76, 65, 24, 23, 72. All numbers greater than 88 are ignored. The first 10 numbers are then: 32, 50, 81, 47, 12, 38, 76, 76, 65, 24.
(4) Number 76 has been selected twice. The second 76 should be rejected* and the next available number chosen: 23.

The sample size of 10 is then made up of animals labelled: 32, 50, 81, 47, 12, 38, 76, 65, 24, 23.

If the table is used repeatedly, then the row and column starting point should be changed.

---

*Rejection of numbers that occur more than once is performed if animals are not returned to the selection pool, after having been selected once: sampling 'without replacement'. If animals are returned to the pool after being selected once, so that they can be selected again—sampling 'with replacement'—then a number corresponding to an animal can be selected more than once (number 76 in this example).

## Table of random numbers*

```
72137 73850 32733 35321 80647 39713 61060 57865 88049 20557 43375 50914 83628 73935 72502 48174 62551 96122 22375 96488
04254 60099 50584 10961 57642 19101 30613 01549 96531 83936 45842 78222 83481 44933 12839 20750 47116 58973 99018 22769
48083 50731 81250 57995 41467 29834 80059 22945 72193 36077 82577 16210 76092 87730 90049 02115 37096 20505 91937 69776
16602 26772 89693 92558 38394 84119 68486 17622 78267 31568 58297 88922 50436 86135 42726 54307 29170 13045 65527
29910 55480 47184 79775 09779 04314 08718 17643 63252 00232 98059 07255 90786 95246 15280 61692 45137 17539 31799 64780

77708 83761 89238 86521 82711 79266 47763 26173 36183 65869 64355 91271 49295 98354 28005 69792 01480 15557 50726 35862
90715 65115 12870 89922 24696 44062 94896 97561 96490 35454 51623 98381 11055 32951 28363 16451 67912 66404 76254 75495
79666 48119 38525 82189 34921 49838 47558 92343 47408 99542 44247 12762 54488 74321 36224 95619 16238 25374 13653 25345
53294 49761 76235 55814 29900 03796 73326 94291 10739 36087 32326 52225 72447 77804 57045 27552 72387 34001 83792 66764
44422 78305 76369 20601 39701 80769 17322 78280 42376 64899 62390 68375 42921 28545 33167 85710 11035 40171 04840 69848

12601 54432 65017 91131 50515 97477 80691 31834 32401 11994 97820 06653 27477 61364 22681 02280 53815 47479 44017 37563
65664 73669 24910 25458 23699 86413 19985 49355 24358 02915 81553 92012 50435 73814 96290 86827 81430 45597 82296 28947
18363 66515 23098 22384 87756 63896 63646 50963 99099 62895 09202 48494 95974 33534 94657 71126 11770 16092 03942 90111
00491 53688 72033 68063 86104 90576 04119 65531 30304 39202 82110 82210 03669 03281 11613 36336 98297 48100 71594 52667
02878 83197 94318 47901 85252 91124 32939 75043 40325 53252 18175 09457 83810 46392 02705 85591 33192 65127 80852 42030

79920 22780 43100 83886 26378 66010 00020 80666 66861 17820 50756 80608 35695 72641 26306 76298 32532 22644 96853 18610
97556 54260 42361 12741 56996 48177 85725 36668 45531 85245 12710 60264 74650 92126 08152 32147 17457 56298 48964 64733
79435 52143 12322 12254 04314 98550 58315 78036 24355 85822 44424 88508 66190 74060 93206 92840 04833 81146 64060 62975
93903 78220 09178 33676 58996 78675 11648 96220 54127 24804 24720 66501 74157 42246 41688 72835 87258 89384 11251 34329
04758 50961 90230 72006 24268 77817 10524 60304 79352 31942 85419 93017 28087 78323 77109 56832 78400 24190 37978 85863

53841 28758 93442 42983 25254 96336 16570 89358 36619 12838 10933 99964 13468 17211 48046 51122 92668 96750 11139 06275
07626 78473 17708 59059 33584 52451 11575 55992 83228 38546 49559 71671 53603 24491 57570 90789 32932 67449 05115 45941
40645 27008 16341 05870 42604 79286 08720 13175 89573 38051 39391 92039 71664 40219 97707 93975 66981 19556 24605 52169
82666 14127 94390 07069 39152 10357 94612 56748 75428 28101 38543 54214 48928 32818 51963 87353 15094 29529 87305 01361
60147 99378 58310 34655 48242 58656 30544 01860 08322 70476 44242 54227 28598 64422 29361 20359 48577 05971 92373 22765

61557 43927 11643 65522 76713 95782 34956 67384 47654 64999 11468 74149 81386 94127 67342 38010 92522 57728 39432 27914
71522 16545 68464 62540 76143 06328 94718 58404 84099 73641 52165 54336 89196 40042 37889 06003 58033 59082 49988 62152
05366 66273 49518 25413 20346 22719 18255 47685 78475 67421 83093 77038 55399 67893 89597 85630 08050 35757 49479 63531
72668 62720 08971 97908 15905 86615 97559 68107 10649 30976 66455 90790 08450 50120 17795 55604 51222 17900 55553 02980
51497 78491 83680 08319 51223 19735 72708 82599 28127 29660 30790 65154 19582 20942 81439 83917 90452 64753 99645 19799

66170 68781 91423 86645 02925 51327 41022 76893 29200 82747 97297 74420 18783 93471 89055 56413 77817 10655 52915 68198
23361 60672 52451 03774 06365 94880 70978 57385 70532 46978 87390 53319 90155 03154 20301 47831 86786 11284 49160 79852
53608 59661 70966 24937 56559 98856 19207 41684 20288 19783 82215 35810 39852 43795 21530 96315 55657 76473 08217 46810
24079 01177 02666 35515 24819 73382 50172 23114 28745 12224 35844 63265 26451 06986 08707 99251 06260 74779 96285 31998
50495 87947 20592 91917 59595 55083 43112 94833 72864 58785 53473 06308 56778 30474 57277 23425 27092 47759 18422 56074

93550 48308 20282 92711 74402 51335 64031 41740 69680 69373 73674 97914 77989 47280 71804 74587 70563 77813 50242 60398
16269 03381 09798 89487 33632 47073 92357 38870 73784 95662 83923 90790 49474 11901 30322 80254 96008 17019 17892 76813
32868 72831 15570 90166 01599 09471 79945 42580 86605 97758 08206 54199 41327 01170 21745 71318 09978 35440 26128 10545
80722 21328 19977 82161 29385 62151 48030 05125 70866 72154 86385 35490 57482 32921 33795 43155 30413 48384 85430 51828
07362 87389 00559 98456 70498 40173 80016 81500 48061 25583 74101 87573 01556 89183 64830 16779 35724 82103 61658 20296

83452 92994 85019 57720 36951 03383 34265 65728 89776 04006 06089 84076 12445 47416 83620 59151 97420 23689 74515 55211
51168 41624 94768 53124 55920 04777 82534 76335 21108 42302 79496 21054 80132 67719 72662 58360 57384 65406 63918 17046
83805 28803 63272 65480 08764 16379 72055 61146 82780 89411 53131 57879 39099 42715 24830 60045 23250 39847 46616 17817
59782 50488 77081 10186 86577 28581 26999 96294 20431 30114 23035 30380 76272 60343 57573 42492 47962 21439 54664 97968
09627 26695 79373 09119 79765 99918 01628 47335 17893 53176 07436 14799 78197 48601 97557 83918 20530 61565 69344 71964

20160 50603 71684 34875 60617 77991 66322 27390 73834 73494 21527 93579 20049 85666 25102 64733 93872 72698 87520 43340
04375 15463 49139 17369 71179 74472 96239 18521 67354 41385 58939 36222 43935 36272 47817 90287 91434 86453 84477 03559
67163 48629 25607 27003 09721 70206 10497 83617 39176 45062 63903 33862 14903 38096 60027 41702 78189 28598 12707 91106
49380 42273 93835 33621 60848 67721 69712 33438 85908 58620 50646 47857 96024 58568 67614 44370 40276 85964 71604 05691
56013 02278 53110 33235 62949 53799 51375 42451 76889 68090 80657 91046 95340 70209 23825 46031 45306 64476 31460 61553

46596 51960 02957 56574 18672 02994 39960 02489 53079 72789 22562 39359 38220 13972 86115 17196 24569 26820 66299 50962
52928 66296 15570 31407 54988 78749 16135 82797 31296 93268 10104 95616 82618 85756 51156 74037 12501 94162 42006 99213
09403 50848 71088 31308 35677 49046 10870 72107 11550 61175 33345 56717 07896 74085 59886 03051 78702 13402 74318 20992
30328 72163 66728 81091 52307 78952 60261 11207 73065 48286 57057 49472 55241 84360 13960 95736 46372 46726 19080 72417
78707 57821 28410 64908 30432 38760 36880 02564 96978 62332 77321 92228 53849 26578 39954 86726 91039 13884 25376 60187

73597 94657 72927 46459 61325 50908 25601 30838 78786 65197 65283 18169 72967 53031 47906 99501 27753 69946 66875 31598
07446 66408 19958 65159 11338 39231 72802 70630 87336 16385 32784 38073 87910 89260 66444 15979 83469 76952 50065 89540
47870 55448 14158 83451 58729 42430 42234 04905 83274 22459 75032 93544 10482 34277 40177 01081 57788 08612 39886 33050
84269 35324 35508 49481 56478 30246 41771 61398 98154 61644 12405 45037 68034 98561 46747 30655 41878 93610 51745 97527
52704 71441 50581 65679 37597 17182 60733 11765 09293 70076 40751 95846 80277 92450 60888 18689 45966 25837 70906 62841

19020 09999 08316 32781 89773 52148 09111 64205 77930 32391 69076 13649 59896 78185 60268 03650 36814 88460 34049 19544
19442 94873 36976 30366 65815 68895 27222 17378 59359 00055 66780 54939 78369 04163 77673 73342 78915 20537 06156 92480
39523 74227 51895 39733 29426 76685 93548 87546 17536 12240 52277 32277 23015 54261 95020 77705 81682 96907 37411 90717
01201 85057 93409 81200 21176 85162 18960 40702 79038 68639 52527 62992 55171 85448 12455 75992 08790 88992 69756 46722
51725 60273 84903 84374 31438 26959 83719 67123 98030 83821 58095 62204 69319 00672 96037 78680 98734 92743

91045 72642 42684 32419 12825 58785 84563 62071 17799 96994 41635 52830 19700 98193 37600 70617 58959 45486 58338 12464
54896 95603 17290 91508 95605 82514 32257 15699 02654 83110 44278 95523 12666 87597 23190 26243 36690 75829 71060 91605
92324 88115 77848 38006 45600 02181 79261 49705 31491 25318 52586 72294 66685 05344 71633 68536 18786 28575 08455 93825
88397 78035 06366 37342 62070 74459 62026 13032 14048 16304 11959 78684 72590 47283 45445 35611 98354 53680 45747 87442
52118 65337 13461 18438 16099 57330 05018 92605 10316 07351 78020 86361 30286 06434 50220 09070 44848 09990 77753 49227

37202 05623 23595 79677 59772 37141 63390 48093 02366 05407 08325 52046 87494 95585 25547 53500 45047 08406 66984 71128
71637 80269 83299 89743 94628 26784 17792 09214 53781 90102 25774 92525 32301 25923 76556 13274 39776 97027 56919 88547
35790 19603 31212 34419 34728 47391 93272 09887 34196 98251 62453 37703 70711 37921 54989 17828 60976 57662 61757 71249
99087 72525 34402 50115 09825 54728 37514 24437 01316 04770 06534 17768 36086 05468 41631 95632 78154 38634 47463 99728
09768 36608 49108 92337 79809 81934 06370 18703 90858 55130 40869 88243 37403 42231 17073 49097 54147 03656 14735 78351

83816 00718 94663 39629 27812 28250 44983 33834 54280 67850 96025 96117 00768 14821 69029 25453 48798 15486 73835 51776
00806 20667 81224 24296 39967 60239 89494 34431 44890 59897 79682 20308 82510 53609 13258 89631 80497 49167 81559 47202
65733 03902 29140 05414 62087 65727 54430 52632 94126 95597 48338 67645 44676 14730 22642 21919 21050 87791 76192 56686
60671 23190 47433 86979 45281 69750 96999 42104 34377 63309 82181 00278 28209 95625 59043 48564 87355 27209 09827
45326 86280 74876 51858 03263 10215 87947 09427 32380 43636 58578 07761 28456 46570 11623 50417 37763 30136 58254 71090

54419 65493 88741 89069 10789 00973 30238 46126 85306 37114 22718 50584 02291 56575 24075 43889 40909 18741 86154 20843
72845 68939 06483 40835 16564 75047 22938 13073 32066 43098 75738 94910 15403 80151 73322 18370 90586 46115 87375 79147
01828 48113 60005 87083 90000 22346 89182 27750 63314 87302 49472 24885 79506 60638 07132 00908 92035 75518 30878 14979
89871 81320 05251 25930 37320 11895 16187 03303 40287 52435 23926 92544 54099 31497 03063 22864 72620 74169 25311 80669
74883 93005 77888 64673 19302 54669 21526 07401 30925 46148 20138 33874 56715 38424 38273 11361 15203 64912 62494 31231

25493 56247 46907 25634 84761 76421 42907 27146 37012 43361 03173 97911 71313 44256 66609 42504 76799 46790 28464
28278 93841 13134 25129 65536 19838 21479 48265 01674 47274 56350 37512 14883 96673 62298 33948 32456 28675 04242 20735
44834 89816 52509 85192 32114 83770 90076 70233 25043 16686 54737 57403 21008 20803 69645 37970 06573 49516 09035
23329 74767 85661 54449 76606 02131 93202 25355 93941 84434 22384 13240 93617 51549 28532 57150 77261 62643 74966 08777
33176 16108 98143 27652 76918 41000 46059 72208 90475 10341 39703 83224 37858 61657 04184 15597 29448 01922 05709 77900

44597 28074 92908 22392 38034 83739 32876 98604 75652 95680 51386 48724 76069 94867 93519 20306 31712 96238 57864 86267
81456 81110 94771 13664 07478 80992 58485 18882 13238 59865 55644 05528 94935 58972 43340 94718 97397 92197 51257 73187
91503 59589 22803 18122 17790 00236 93750 20468 92189 66781 06210 18208 13973 57905 66878 55721 67437 61709 88182 92769
63651 64109 13207 68346 42140 00052 04099 48767 23355 42505 34539 51129 48580 93386 62209 29754 77409 48146 50411 50511
30709 25869 68851 65221 69392 35106 36393 27129 17326 86452 69952 68433 72332 62502 76323 38379 07293 76788 84281 58581

50664 89487 41973 98456 51147 51327 26590 94684 58103 96936 71276 30275 22753 46046 67196 65135 54879 71903 23541 92400
80089 83750 36605 85343 26090 28447 33179 09680 39039 61170 50381 43130 88108 64709 15916 68718 58375 66747 19880 76129
19293 91304 37043 82077 42231 31534 54358 52939 26655 72687 26616 09608 92273 74533 64986 49667 78039 61030 46122 54941
97754 28401 62533 98641 48553 35996 08033 91811 70471 81538 20017 11963 81103 37642 41866 96777 08667 74544 92903 58427
47923 38366 81939 61526 27691 13988 21630 00957 10599 91260 72832 89364 14158 71740 91289 61204 91185 23485 18424 65084
```

*Extracted from *Documenta Geigy Scientific Tables*, 7th edition, Basle, 1970. Courtesy Ciba-Geigy Limited, Basle, Switzerland.

# Appendix VII

## Sample sizes

This Appendix comprises sample sizes required to attain a desired confidence interval around expected prevalence values of 5%, 10%, 20%, 30%, 40% and 50% (From WHO, 1973). For example, if the expected prevalence is 30%, consult *Figure 4*. A sample-size of 200 will produce a 95% confidence interval of 24% to 36%. A sample size of 800 will produce a 95% confidence interval of 27% to 33%.

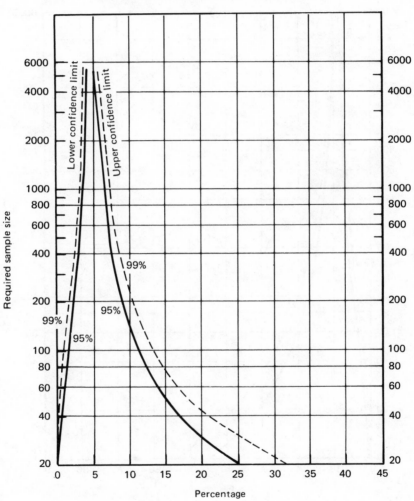

Figure 1

242

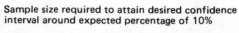

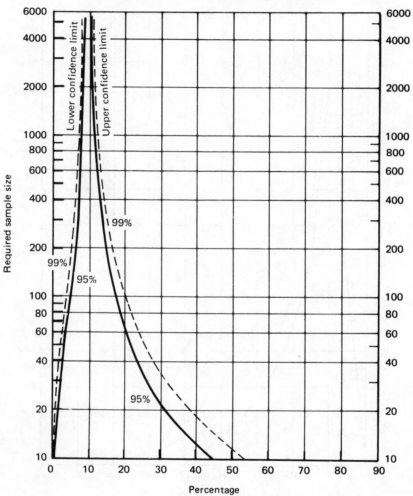

Figure 2

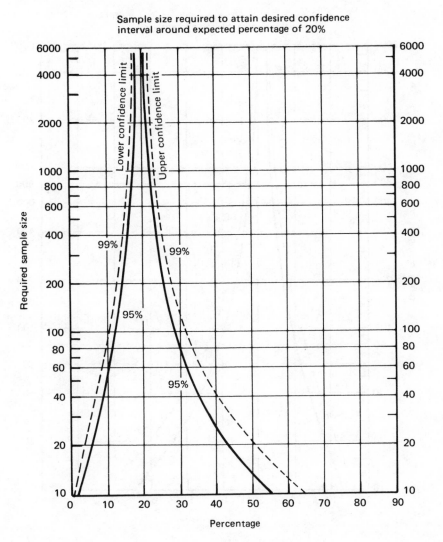

Figure 3

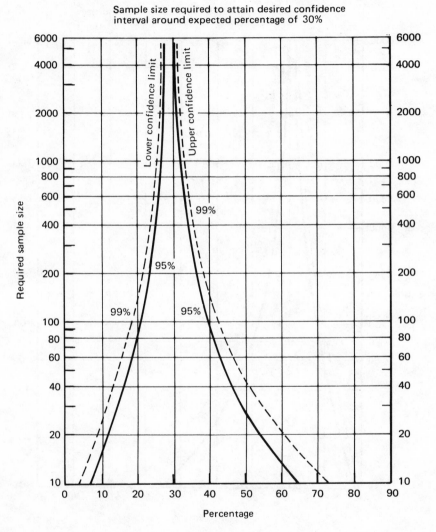

**Figure 4**

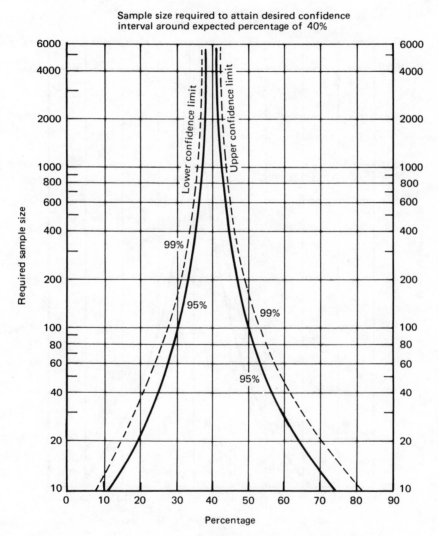

**Figure 5**

246

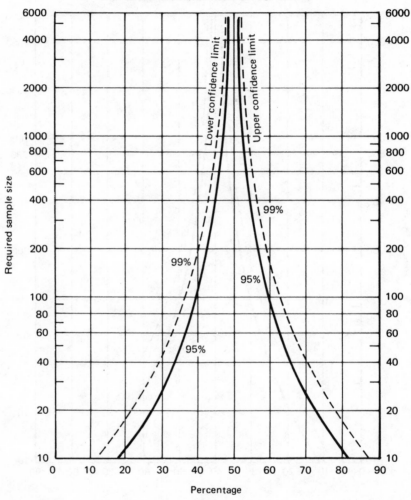

Sample size required to attain desired confidence
interval around expected percentage of 50%

Figure 6

# Appendix VIII

# The probability of detecting a small number of cases in a population

(Modified from Cannon and Roe, 1982)

These tables give the probability of detecting at least one case for different sampling fractions and numbers of cases in the population.

**Example:** A 40% sample from a herd of 20 animals would have a 97.6% chance of including at least one positive if six were present in the herd.

### 20% Sampling

| Population size | Number sampled | Number of positives in the population | | | | | | | |
|---|---|---|---|---|---|---|---|---|---|
| | | 1 | 2 | 3 | 4 | 5 | 6 | 7 | 8 |
| 10 | 2 | 0.200 | 0.378 | 0.533 | 0.667 | 0.778 | 0.867 | 0.933 | 0.978 |
| 20 | 4 | 0.200 | 0.368 | 0.509 | 0.624 | 0.718 | 0.793 | 0.852 | 0.898 |
| 30 | 6 | 0.200 | 0.366 | 0.501 | 0.612 | 0.702 | 0.773 | 0.830 | 0.874 |
| 40 | 8 | 0.200 | 0.364 | 0.498 | 0.607 | 0.694 | 0.764 | 0.819 | 0.863 |
| 50 | 10 | 0.200 | 0.363 | 0.498 | 0.603 | 0.689 | 0.758 | 0.813 | 0.857 |
| 60 | 12 | 0.200 | 0.363 | 0.495 | 0.601 | 0.686 | 0.755 | 0.809 | 0.853 |
| 70 | 14 | 0.200 | 0.362 | 0.494 | 0.599 | 0.684 | 0.752 | 0.807 | 0.850 |
| 80 | 16 | 0.200 | 0.362 | 0.493 | 0.598 | 0.683 | 0.751 | 0.804 | 0.847 |
| 90 | 18 | 0.200 | 0.362 | 0.492 | 0.597 | 0.682 | 0.749 | 0.803 | 0.846 |
| 100 | 20 | 0.200 | 0.362 | 0.492 | 0.597 | 0.681 | 0.748 | 0.802 | 0.844 |
| ∞ | ∞ | 0.200 | 0.360 | 0.486 | 0.590 | 0.672 | 0.738 | 0.790 | 0.832 |

### 30% Sampling

| Population size | Number sampled | Number of positives in the population | | | | | | | |
|---|---|---|---|---|---|---|---|---|---|
| | | 1 | 2 | 3 | 4 | 5 | 6 | 7 | 8 |
| 10 | 3 | 0.300 | 0.533 | 0.708 | 0.833 | 0.917 | 0.967 | 0.992 | 1.000 |
| 20 | 6 | 0.300 | 0.521 | 0.681 | 0.793 | 0.871 | 0.923 | 0.956 | 0.976 |
| 30 | 9 | 0.300 | 0.517 | 0.672 | 0.782 | 0.857 | 0.909 | 0.943 | 0.965 |
| 40 | 12 | 0.300 | 0.515 | 0.668 | 0.776 | 0.851 | 0.902 | 0.936 | 0.960 |
| 50 | 15 | 0.300 | 0.514 | 0.666 | 0.773 | 0.847 | 0.898 | 0.933 | 0.956 |
| 60 | 18 | 0.300 | 0.514 | 0.665 | 0.770 | 0.844 | 0.895 | 0.930 | 0.954 |
| 70 | 21 | 0.300 | 0.513 | 0.663 | 0.769 | 0.842 | 0.893 | 0.928 | 0.952 |
| 80 | 24 | 0.300 | 0.513 | 0.663 | 0.768 | 0.841 | 0.892 | 0.927 | 0.951 |
| 90 | 27 | 0.300 | 0.512 | 0.662 | 0.767 | 0.840 | 0.891 | 0.926 | 0.950 |
| 100 | 30 | 0.300 | 0.512 | 0.661 | 0.766 | 0.839 | 0.890 | 0.925 | 0.949 |
| ∞ | ∞ | 0.300 | 0.510 | 0.657 | 0.760 | 0.832 | 0.882 | 0.918 | 0.942 |

**40% Sampling**

| Population size | Number sampled | Number of positives in the population | | | | | | | |
|---|---|---|---|---|---|---|---|---|---|
| | | *1* | *2* | *3* | *4* | *5* | *6* | *7* | *8* |
| 10 | 4 | 0.400 | 0.667 | 0.833 | 0.929 | 0.976 | 0.995 | 1.000 | 1.000 |
| 20 | 8 | 0.400 | 0.653 | 0.807 | 0.898 | 0.949 | 0.976 | 0.990 | 0.996 |
| 30 | 12 | 0.400 | 0.648 | 0.799 | 0.888 | 0.940 | 0.969 | 0.984 | 0.993 |
| 40 | 16 | 0.400 | 0.646 | 0.795 | 0.884 | 0.935 | 0.965 | 0.981 | 0.990 |
| 50 | 20 | 0.400 | 0.645 | 0.793 | 0.881 | 0.933 | 0.963 | 0.980 | 0.989 |
| 60 | 24 | 0.400 | 0.644 | 0.791 | 0.879 | 0.931 | 0.961 | 0.978 | 0.988 |
| 70 | 28 | 0.400 | 0.643 | 0.790 | 0.878 | 0.930 | 0.960 | 0.977 | 0.987 |
| 80 | 32 | 0.400 | 0.643 | 0.789 | 0.877 | 0.929 | 0.959 | 0.977 | 0.987 |
| 90 | 36 | 0.400 | 0.643 | 0.789 | 0.876 | 0.928 | 0.959 | 0.976 | 0.987 |
| 100 | 40 | 0.400 | 0.642 | 0.788 | 0.876 | 0.927 | 0.958 | 0.976 | 0.986 |
| ∞ | ∞ | 0.400 | 0.640 | 0.784 | 0.870 | 0.922 | 0.953 | 0.972 | 0.983 |

**50% Sampling**

| Population size | Number sampled | Number of positives in the population | | | | | | | |
|---|---|---|---|---|---|---|---|---|---|
| | | *1* | *2* | *3* | *4* | *5* | *6* | *7* | *8* |
| 10 | 5 | 0.500 | 0.778 | 0.917 | 0.976 | 0.996 | 1.000 | 1.000 | 1.000 |
| 20 | 10 | 0.500 | 0.763 | 0.895 | 0.957 | 0.984 | 0.995 | 0.998 | 0.994 |
| 30 | 15 | 0.500 | 0.759 | 0.888 | 0.950 | 0.979 | 0.992 | 0.997 | 0.999 |
| 40 | 20 | 0.500 | 0.756 | 0.885 | 0.947 | 0.976 | 0.990 | 0.996 | 0.998 |
| 50 | 25 | 0.500 | 0.755 | 0.883 | 0.945 | 0.975 | 0.989 | 0.995 | 0.998 |
| 60 | 30 | 0.500 | 0.754 | 0.881 | 0.944 | 0.974 | 0.988 | 0.995 | 0.998 |
| 70 | 35 | 0.500 | 0.754 | 0.880 | 0.943 | 0.973 | 0.988 | 0.994 | 0.998 |
| 80 | 40 | 0.500 | 0.753 | 0.880 | 0.942 | 0.973 | 0.987 | 0.994 | 0.997 |
| 90 | 45 | 0.500 | 0.753 | 0.879 | 0.942 | 0.972 | 0.987 | 0.994 | 0.997 |
| 100 | 50 | 0.500 | 0.753 | 0.879 | 0.941 | 0.972 | 0.987 | 0.994 | 0.997 |
| ∞ | ∞ | 0.500 | 0.750 | 0.875 | 0.937 | 0.969 | 0.984 | 0.992 | 0.996 |

**60% Sampling**

| Population size | Number sampled | Number of positives in the population | | | | | | | |
|---|---|---|---|---|---|---|---|---|---|
| | | *1* | *2* | *3* | *4* | *5* | *6* | *7* | *8* |
| 10 | 6 | 0.600 | 0.867 | 0.967 | 0.994 | 1.000 | 1.000 | 1.000 | 1.000 |
| 20 | 12 | 0.600 | 0.853 | 0.951 | 0.986 | 0.994 | 0.997 | 1.000 | 1.000 |
| 30 | 18 | 0.600 | 0.848 | 0.946 | 0.982 | 0.994 | 0.997 | 1.000 | 1.000 |
| 40 | 24 | 0.600 | 0.846 | 0.943 | 0.980 | 0.993 | 0.997 | 0.999 | 1.000 |
| 50 | 30 | 0.600 | 0.845 | 0.942 | 0.979 | 0.993 | 0.997 | 0.999 | 1.000 |
| 60 | 36 | 0.600 | 0.844 | 0.941 | 0.978 | 0.992 | 0.997 | 0.999 | 1.000 |
| 70 | 42 | 0.600 | 0.843 | 0.940 | 0.978 | 0.992 | 0.997 | 0.999 | 1.000 |
| 80 | 48 | 0.600 | 0.843 | 0.940 | 0.977 | 0.992 | 0.997 | 0.999 | 1.000 |
| 90 | 54 | 0.600 | 0.843 | 0.939 | 0.977 | 0.991 | 0.997 | 0.999 | 1.000 |
| 100 | 60 | 0.600 | 0.842 | 0.939 | 0.977 | 0.991 | 0.997 | 0.999 | 1.000 |
| ∞ | ∞ | 0.600 | 0.840 | 0.936 | 0.974 | 0.990 | 0.996 | 0.998 | 1.000 |

# Appendix IX

## The probability of failure to detect cases in a population

(From Cannon and Roe, 1982)

The table gives the probability of failure to detect diseased animals from an 'infinite' population with the specified proportion of positives in the population.

**Example:** Tests of a series of random samples of 25 animals from a large population in which 10% of animals are positive would fail to detect any positives in 7.2% of such sample groups.

| Prevalence | Number of animals in sample tested | | | | | | | | | |
|---|---|---|---|---|---|---|---|---|---|---|
| | 5 | 10 | 25 | 50 | 75 | 100 | 200 | 250 | 500 | 1000 |
| 1% | 0.951 | 0.904 | 0.778 | 0.605 | 0.471 | 0.366 | 0.134 | 0.081 | 0.007 | 0.000 |
| 2% | 0.904 | 0.817 | 0.603 | 0.364 | 0.220 | 0.133 | 0.018 | 0.006 | 0.000 | |
| 3% | 0.859 | 0.737 | 0.467 | 0.218 | 0.102 | 0.048 | 0.002 | 0.000 | | |
| 4% | 0.815 | 0.665 | 0.360 | 0.130 | 0.047 | 0.017 | 0.000 | | | |
| 5% | 0.774 | 0.599 | 0.277 | 0.077 | 0.021 | 0.006 | 0.000 | | | |
| 6% | 0.734 | 0.539 | 0.213 | 0.045 | 0.010 | 0.002 | 0.000 | | | |
| 7% | 0.696 | 0.484 | 0.163 | 0.027 | 0.004 | 0.001 | 0.000 | | | |
| 8% | 0.659 | 0.434 | 0.124 | 0.015 | 0.002 | 0.000 | | | | |
| 9% | 0.624 | 0.389 | 0.095 | 0.009 | 0.001 | 0.000 | | | | |
| 10% | 0.590 | 0.349 | 0.072 | 0.005 | 0.000 | | | | | |
| 12% | 0.528 | 0.279 | 0.041 | 0.002 | 0.000 | | | | | |
| 14% | 0.470 | 0.221 | 0.023 | 0.001 | 0.000 | | | | | |
| 16% | 0.418 | 0.175 | 0.013 | 0.000 | | | | | | |
| 18% | 0.371 | 0.137 | 0.007 | 0.000 | | | | | | |
| 20% | 0.328 | 0.107 | 0.004 | 0.000 | | | | | | |
| 24% | 0.254 | 0.064 | 0.001 | 0.000 | | | | | | |
| 28% | 0.193 | 0.037 | 0.000 | | | | | | | |
| 32% | 0.145 | 0.021 | 0.000 | | | | | | | |
| 36% | 0.107 | 0.012 | 0.000 | | | | | | | |
| 40% | 0.078 | 0.006 | 0.000 | | | | | | | |
| 50% | 0.031 | 0.001 | 0.000 | | | | | | | |
| 60% | 0.010 | 0.000 | | | | | | | | |

# Appendix X

# The variance-ratio ($F$) distribution

**5 per cent points**

| $f_2$ | | | | | | | | $f_1$ | | | | | | | |
|---|---|---|---|---|---|---|---|---|---|---|---|---|---|---|---|
| | 1 | 2 | 3 | 4 | 5 | 6 | 7 | 8 | 9 | 10 | 12 | 15 | 20 | 30 | ∞ |
| 1 | 161.4 | 199.5 | 215.7 | 224.6 | 230.2 | 234.0 | 236.8 | 238.9 | 240.5 | 241.9 | 143.9 | 245.9 | 248.0 | 250.1 | 254.3 |
| 2 | 18.51 | 19.00 | 19.16 | 19.25 | 19.30 | 19.33 | 19.35 | 19.37 | 19.38 | 19.40 | 19.41 | 19.43 | 19.45 | 19.46 | 19.50 |
| 3 | 10.13 | 9.55 | 9.28 | 9.12 | 9.01 | 8.94 | 8.89 | 8.85 | 8.81 | 8.79 | 8.74 | 8.70 | 8.66 | 8.62 | 8.53 |
| 4 | 7.71 | 6.94 | 6.59 | 6.39 | 6.26 | 6.16 | 6.09 | 6.04 | 6.00 | 5.96 | 5.91 | 5.86 | 5.80 | 5.75 | 5.63 |
| 5 | 6.61 | 5.79 | 5.41 | 5.19 | 5.05 | 4.95 | 4.88 | 4.82 | 4.77 | 4.74 | 4.68 | 4.62 | 4.56 | 4.50 | 4.36 |
| 6 | 5.99 | 5.14 | 4.76 | 4.53 | 4.39 | 4.28 | 4.21 | 4.15 | 4.10 | 4.06 | 4.00 | 3.94 | 3.87 | 3.81 | 3.67 |
| 7 | 5.59 | 4.74 | 4.35 | 4.12 | 3.97 | 3.87 | 3.79 | 3.73 | 3.68 | 3.64 | 3.57 | 3.51 | 3.44 | 3.38 | 3.23 |
| 8 | 5.32 | 4.45 | 4.07 | 3.84 | 3.69 | 3.58 | 3.50 | 3.44 | 3.39 | 3.35 | 3.28 | 3.22 | 3.15 | 3.08 | 2.93 |
| 9 | 5.12 | 4.26 | 3.86 | 3.63 | 3.48 | 3.37 | 3.29 | 3.23 | 3.18 | 3.14 | 3.07 | 3.01 | 2.94 | 2.86 | 2.71 |
| 10 | 4.96 | 4.10 | 3.71 | 3.48 | 3.33 | 3.22 | 3.14 | 3.07 | 3.02 | 2.98 | 2.91 | 2.85 | 2.77 | 2.70 | 2.54 |
| 11 | 4.84 | 3.98 | 3.59 | 3.36 | 3.20 | 3.09 | 3.01 | 2.95 | 2.90 | 2.85 | 2.79 | 2.72 | 2.65 | 2.57 | 2.40 |
| 12 | 4.75 | 3.89 | 3.49 | 3.26 | 3.11 | 3.00 | 2.91 | 2.85 | 2.80 | 2.75 | 2.69 | 2.62 | 2.54 | 2.47 | 2.30 |
| 13 | 4.67 | 3.81 | 3.41 | 3.18 | 3.03 | 2.92 | 2.83 | 2.77 | 2.71 | 2.67 | 2.60 | 2.53 | 2.46 | 2.38 | 2.21 |
| 14 | 4.60 | 3.74 | 3.34 | 3.11 | 2.96 | 2.85 | 2.76 | 2.70 | 2.65 | 2.60 | 2.53 | 2.46 | 2.39 | 2.31 | 2.13 |
| 15 | 4.54 | 3.68 | 3.29 | 3.06 | 2.90 | 2.79 | 2.71 | 2.64 | 2.59 | 2.54 | 2.48 | 2.40 | 2.33 | 2.25 | 2.07 |
| 16 | 4.49 | 3.63 | 3.24 | 3.01 | 2.85 | 2.74 | 2.66 | 2.59 | 2.54 | 2.49 | 2.42 | 2.35 | 2.28 | 2.19 | 2.01 |
| 17 | 4.45 | 3.59 | 3.20 | 2.96 | 2.81 | 2.70 | 2.61 | 2.55 | 2.49 | 2.45 | 2.38 | 2.31 | 2.23 | 2.15 | 1.96 |
| 18 | 4.41 | 3.55 | 3.16 | 2.93 | 2.77 | 2.66 | 2.58 | 2.51 | 2.46 | 2.41 | 2.34 | 2.27 | 2.19 | 2.11 | 1.92 |
| 19 | 4.38 | 3.52 | 3.13 | 2.90 | 2.74 | 2.63 | 2.54 | 2.48 | 2.42 | 2.38 | 2.31 | 2.23 | 2.16 | 2.07 | 1.88 |
| 20 | 4.35 | 3.49 | 3.10 | 2.87 | 2.71 | 2.60 | 2.51 | 2.45 | 2.39 | 2.35 | 2.28 | 2.20 | 2.12 | 2.04 | 1.84 |
| 21 | 4.32 | 3.47 | 3.07 | 2.84 | 2.68 | 2.57 | 2.49 | 2.42 | 2.37 | 2.32 | 2.25 | 2.18 | 2.10 | 2.01 | 1.81 |
| 22 | 4.30 | 3.44 | 3.05 | 2.82 | 2.66 | 2.55 | 2.46 | 2.40 | 2.34 | 2.30 | 2.23 | 2.15 | 2.07 | 1.98 | 1.78 |
| 23 | 4.28 | 3.42 | 3.03 | 2.80 | 2.64 | 2.53 | 2.44 | 2.37 | 2.32 | 2.27 | 2.20 | 2.13 | 2.05 | 1.96 | 1.76 |
| 24 | 4.26 | 3.40 | 3.01 | 2.78 | 2.62 | 2.51 | 2.42 | 2.36 | 2.30 | 2.25 | 2.18 | 2.11 | 2.03 | 1.94 | 1.73 |
| 25 | 4.24 | 3.39 | 2.99 | 2.76 | 2.60 | 2.49 | 2.40 | 2.34 | 2.28 | 2.24 | 2.16 | 2.09 | 2.01 | 1.92 | 1.71 |
| 26 | 4.23 | 3.37 | 2.98 | 2.74 | 2.59 | 2.47 | 2.39 | 2.32 | 2.27 | 2.22 | 2.15 | 2.07 | 1.99 | 1.90 | 1.69 |
| 27 | 4.21 | 3.35 | 2.96 | 2.73 | 2.57 | 2.46 | 2.37 | 2.31 | 2.25 | 2.20 | 2.13 | 2.06 | 1.97 | 1.88 | 1.67 |
| 28 | 4.20 | 3.34 | 2.95 | 2.71 | 2.56 | 2.45 | 2.36 | 2.29 | 2.24 | 2.19 | 2.12 | 2.04 | 1.96 | 1.87 | 1.65 |
| 29 | 4.18 | 3.33 | 2.93 | 2.70 | 2.55 | 2.43 | 2.35 | 2.28 | 2.22 | 2.18 | 2.10 | 2.03 | 1.94 | 1.85 | 1.64 |
| 30 | 4.17 | 3.32 | 2.92 | 2.69 | 2.53 | 2.42 | 2.33 | 2.27 | 2.21 | 2.16 | 2.09 | 2.01 | 1.93 | 1.84 | 1.62 |
| 40 | 4.08 | 3.23 | 2.84 | 2.61 | 2.45 | 2.34 | 2.25 | 2.18 | 1.12 | 2.08 | 2.00 | 1.92 | 1.84 | 1.74 | 1.51 |
| 60 | 4.00 | 3.15 | 2.76 | 2.53 | 2.37 | 2.25 | 2.17 | 2.10 | 2.04 | 1.99 | 1.92 | 1.84 | 1.75 | 1.65 | 1.39 |
| 120 | 3.92 | 3.07 | 2.68 | 2.45 | 2.29 | 2.17 | 2.09 | 2.02 | 1.96 | 1.91 | 1.83 | 1.75 | 1.66 | 1.55 | 1.25 |
| ∞ | 3.84 | 3.00 | 2.60 | 2.37 | 2.21 | 2.10 | 2.01 | 1.94 | 1.88 | 1.83 | 1.75 | 1.67 | 1.57 | 1.46 | 1.00 |

The table gives the 5 per cent points of the distribution of the variance-ratio, $F = s_1^2/s_2^2$, where the numerator and denominator have $f_1$ and $f_2$ degrees of freedom respectively. Thus if $f_1 = 7$ and $f_2 = 15$, the probability that the observed value of $F$ is **greater** than 2.71 is exactly 0.05 or 5 per cent.

**1 per cent points**

| $f_2$ | $f_1$ | | | | | | | | | | | | | | |
|---|---|---|---|---|---|---|---|---|---|---|---|---|---|---|---|
| | *1* | *2* | *3* | *4* | *5* | *6* | *7* | *8* | *9* | *10* | *12* | *15* | *20* | *30* | *∞* |
| 1 | 4052 | 4999 | 5403 | 5625 | 5764 | 5859 | 5928 | 5982 | 6022 | 6056 | 6106 | 6157 | 6209 | 6261 | 6366 |
| 2 | 98.50 | 99.00 | 99.17 | 99.25 | 99.30 | 99.33 | 99.36 | 99.37 | 99.39 | 99.40 | 99.42 | 99.43 | 99.45 | 99.47 | 99.50 |
| 3 | 34.12 | 30.82 | 29.46 | 28.71 | 28.24 | 27.91 | 27.67 | 27.49 | 27.35 | 27.23 | 27.05 | 26.87 | 26.69 | 26.50 | 26.13 |
| 4 | 21.20 | 18.00 | 16.69 | 15.98 | 15.52 | 15.21 | 14.98 | 14.80 | 14.66 | 14.55 | 14.37 | 14.20 | 14.02 | 13.84 | 13.46 |
| 5 | 16.26 | 13.27 | 12.06 | 11.39 | 10.97 | 10.67 | 10.46 | 10.29 | 10.16 | 10.05 | 9.89 | 9.72 | 9.55 | 9.38 | 9.02 |
| 6 | 13.75 | 10.92 | 9.78 | 9.15 | 8.75 | 8.47 | 8.26 | 8.10 | 7.98 | 7.87 | 7.72 | 7.56 | 7.40 | 7.23 | 6.88 |
| 7 | 12.25 | 9.55 | 8.45 | 7.85 | 7.46 | 7.19 | 6.99 | 6.84 | 6.72 | 6.62 | 6.47 | 6.31 | 6.16 | 5.99 | 5.65 |
| 8 | 11.26 | 8.65 | 7.59 | 7.01 | 6.63 | 6.37 | 6.18 | 6.03 | 5.91 | 5.81 | 5.67 | 5.52 | 5.36 | 5.20 | 4.86 |
| 9 | 10.56 | 8.02 | 6.99 | 6.42 | 6.06 | 5.80 | 5.61 | 5.47 | 5.35 | 5.26 | 5.11 | 4.96 | 4.81 | 4.65 | 4.31 |
| 10 | 10.04 | 7.56 | 6.55 | 5.99 | 5.64 | 5.39 | 5.20 | 5.06 | 4.94 | 4.85 | 4.71 | 4.56 | 4.41 | 4.25 | 3.91 |
| 11 | 9.65 | 7.21 | 6.22 | 5.67 | 5.32 | 5.07 | 4.89 | 4.74 | 4.63 | 4.54 | 4.40 | 4.25 | 4.10 | 3.94 | 3.60 |
| 12 | 9.33 | 6.93 | 5.95 | 5.41 | 5.06 | 4.82 | 4.64 | 4.50 | 4.39 | 4.30 | 4.16 | 4.01 | 3.86 | 3.70 | 3.36 |
| 13 | 9.07 | 6.70 | 5.74 | 5.21 | 4.86 | 4.62 | 4.44 | 4.30 | 4.19 | 4.10 | 3.96 | 3.82 | 3.66 | 3.51 | 3.17 |
| 14 | 8.86 | 6.51 | 5.56 | 5.04 | 4.69 | 4.46 | 4.28 | 4.14 | 4.03 | 3.94 | 3.80 | 3.66 | 3.51 | 3.35 | 3.00 |
| 15 | 8.68 | 6.36 | 5.42 | 4.89 | 4.56 | 4.32 | 4.14 | 4.00 | 3.89 | 3.80 | 3.67 | 3.52 | 3.37 | 3.21 | 2.87 |
| 16 | 8.53 | 6.23 | 5.29 | 4.77 | 4.44 | 4.20 | 4.03 | 3.89 | 3.78 | 3.69 | 3.55 | 3.41 | 3.26 | 3.10 | 2.75 |
| 17 | 8.40 | 6.11 | 5.18 | 4.67 | 4.34 | 4.10 | 3.93 | 3.79 | 3.68 | 3.59 | 3.46 | 3.31 | 3.16 | 3.00 | 2.65 |
| 18 | 8.29 | 6.01 | 5.09 | 4.58 | 4.25 | 4.01 | 3.84 | 3.71 | 3.60 | 3.51 | 3.37 | 3.23 | 3.08 | 2.92 | 2.57 |
| 19 | 8.18 | 5.93 | 5.01 | 4.50 | 4.17 | 3.94 | 3.77 | 3.63 | 3.52 | 3.43 | 3.30 | 3.15 | 3.00 | 2.84 | 2.49 |
| 20 | 8.10 | 5.85 | 4.94 | 4.43 | 4.10 | 3.87 | 3.70 | 3.56 | 3.46 | 3.37 | 3.23 | 3.09 | 2.94 | 2.78 | 2.42 |
| 21 | 8.02 | 5.78 | 4.87 | 4.37 | 4.04 | 3.81 | 3.64 | 3.51 | 3.40 | 3.31 | 3.17 | 3.03 | 2.88 | 2.72 | 2.36 |
| 22 | 7.95 | 5.72 | 4.82 | 4.31 | 3.99 | 3.76 | 3.59 | 3.45 | 3.35 | 3.26 | 3.12 | 2.98 | 2.83 | 2.67 | 2.31 |
| 23 | 7.88 | 5.66 | 4.76 | 4.26 | 3.94 | 3.71 | 3.54 | 3.41 | 3.30 | 3.21 | 3.07 | 2.93 | 2.78 | 2.62 | 2.26 |
| 24 | 7.82 | 5.61 | 4.72 | 4.22 | 3.90 | 3.67 | 3.50 | 3.36 | 3.26 | 3.17 | 3.03 | 2.89 | 2.74 | 2.58 | 2.21 |
| 25 | 7.77 | 5.57 | 4.68 | 4.18 | 3.85 | 3.63 | 3.46 | 3.32 | 3.22 | 3.13 | 2.99 | 2.85 | 2.70 | 2.54 | 2.17 |
| 26 | 7.72 | 5.53 | 4.64 | 4.14 | 3.82 | 3.59 | 3.42 | 3.29 | 3.18 | 3.09 | 2.96 | 2.81 | 2.66 | 2.50 | 2.13 |
| 27 | 7.68 | 5.49 | 4.60 | 4.11 | 3.78 | 3.56 | 3.39 | 3.26 | 3.15 | 3.06 | 2.93 | 2.78 | 2.63 | 2.47 | 2.10 |
| 28 | 7.64 | 5.45 | 4.57 | 4.07 | 3.75 | 3.53 | 3.36 | 3.23 | 3.12 | 3.03 | 2.90 | 2.75 | 2.60 | 2.44 | 2.06 |
| 29 | 7.60 | 5.42 | 4.54 | 4.04 | 3.73 | 3.50 | 3.33 | 3.20 | 3.09 | 3.00 | 2.87 | 2.73 | 2.57 | 2.41 | 2.03 |
| 30 | 7.56 | 5.39 | 4.51 | 4.02 | 3.70 | 3.47 | 3.30 | 3.17 | 3.07 | 2.98 | 2.84 | 2.70 | 2.55 | 2.39 | 2.01 |
| 40 | 7.31 | 5.18 | 4.31 | 3.83 | 3.51 | 3.29 | 3.12 | 2.99 | 2.89 | 2.80 | 2.66 | 2.52 | 2.37 | 2.20 | 1.80 |
| 60 | 7.08 | 4.98 | 4.13 | 3.65 | 3.34 | 3.12 | 2.95 | 2.82 | 2.72 | 2.63 | 2.50 | 2.35 | 2.20 | 2.03 | 1.60 |
| 120 | 6.85 | 4.79 | 3.95 | 3.48 | 3.17 | 2.96 | 2.79 | 2.66 | 2.56 | 2.47 | 2.34 | 2.19 | 2.03 | 1.86 | 1.38 |
| ∞ | 6.63 | 4.61 | 3.78 | 3.32 | 3.02 | 2.80 | 2.64 | 2.51 | 2.41 | 2.32 | 2.18 | 2.04 | 1.88 | 1.70 | 1.00 |

The table gives the 1 per cent points of the distribution of the variance-ratio, $F = s_1^2/s_2^2$, where the numerator and denominator have $f_1$ and $f_2$ degrees of freedom respectively. Thus if $f_1 = 7$ and $f_2 = 15$, the probability that the observed value of $F$ is **greater** than 4.14 is exactly 0.01 or 1 per cent.

# References

AALUND, O., WILLEBERG, P., MANDRUP, M. and RIEMANN, H. (1976) Lung lesions at slaughter: association to factors in the pig herd. *Nordisk Veterinaermedicin*, **28**, 481–486

ALEXANDER, M. (1971) *Microbial Ecology*. John Wiley and Sons Inc., New York

ALGERS, B. and HENNICHS, K. (1985) The effects of exposure to 400 kv transmission lines on the fertility of cows. A retrospective cohort study. *Preventive Veterinary Medicine*, **3**, 351–361

ALGERS, B., EKESBO, I. and STROMBERG, S. (1978) The impact of continuous noise on animal health. *Acta Veterinaria Scandinavica*, **19**, Suppl. 67, 1–26

ANDERSON, D.E., LUSH, J.L. and CHAMBERS, C. (1957) Studies on bovine ocular squamous carcinoma ('cancer eye'). II. Relationships between eyelid pigmentation and occurrence of cancer eye lesions. *Journal of Animal Science*, **16**, 739–746

ANDERSON, H., HENRICSON, B., LUNDQUIST, P.-G., WENDENBERG, E. and WESALL, J. (1968) Genetic hearing impairment in the Dalmatian dog. *Acta-otolaryngologica*, Suppl., **232**, 1–34

ANDERSON, R.S. (1983) Trends in pet populations. In: Society for Veterinary Epidemiology and Preventive Medicine, Proceedings, Southampton, 12–13 April 1983. Ed. Thrusfield, M.V. Pp. 94–97

ANDREWS, A.H. (1978) Warble fly: the life-cycle, distribution, economic losses and control. *Veterinary Record*, **103**, 348–353

ANDREWS J.M. and LANGMUIR, A.D. (1963) The philosophy of disease eradication. *American Journal of Public Health*, **53**, 1–6

ANON (1984) Tattoos to help keep track of pets. *Veterinary Practice*, **16**, (20), 8

ARCHIBALD, A.L. and IMLAH, P. (1985) The halothane sensitivity locus and its linkage relationships. *Animal Blood Groups and Biochemical Genetics*, **16**, 253–263

ARMENIAN, H.K. and LILIENFELD, A.M. (1974) The distribution of incubation periods of neoplastic disease. *American Journal of Epidemiology*, **99**, 92–100

ASBY, C.G., GRIFFIN, T.K., ELLIS, P.R. and KINGWILL, R.G. (1975) The Benefits and Costs of a System of Mastitis Control in Individual Herds. Study No. 17. University of Reading

AUDY, J.R. (1958) The localisation of disease with special reference to the zoonoses. *Transactions of the Royal Society of Tropical Medicine and Hygiene*, **52**, 308–328

AUDY, J.R. (1960) *Relation of Foci of Zoonoses to Interspersed or Mosaic Vegetation*. Papers of the First WHO course on natural foci of infections, USSR

AUDY, J.R. (1961) The ecology of scrub typhus. In: *Studies in Disease Ecology*. Ed. May, J.M. Pp. 389–432. Hafner Publishing Company, New York

AUDY, J.R. (1962) *Behavioral and Sociocultural Aspects of Natural Foci of Infections*. Papers of the Second WHO course on natural foci of infections, Leningrad

BABUDIERI, B. (1958) Animal reservoirs of leptospirosis. *Annals of the New York Academy of Science*, **70**, 393–413

BAGGOTT, D. (1982) Hoof lameness in dairy cattle. *In Practice*, **4**, 133–141

BAILEY, N.T.J. (1975) *The Mathematical Theory of Infectious Diseases*, 2nd edn. Charles Griffin and Company, London and High Wycombe

BAILEY, N.T.J. (1981) *Statistical Methods in Biology*, 2nd edn. Hodder and Stoughton, London

BAKER, M. (1974) *Folklore and Customs of Rural England*. David and Charles, Newton Abbot

BAKER, R.J. and NELDER, J.A. (1978) *The GLIM System Release 3 Generalised Linear Interactive Modelling*. The Royal Statistical Society, London. Available from the Numerical Algorithms Group, 7, Banbury Road, Oxford, OX2 6NN

BANG, F.B. (1975) Epidemiological interference. *International Journal of Epidemiology*, **4**, 337–342

BARGER, I.A., DASH, K.M. and SOUTHCOTT, W.H. (1978) Epidemiology and control of liver fluke in sheep. In: *The Epidemiology and Control of Gastrointestinal Parasites of Sheep in Australia*. Eds Donald, A.D., Southcott, W.H. and Dineen, J.K. Pp. 65–74. Division of Animal Health, Commonwealth Scientific and Industrial Research Organisation, Australia

BARNARD, G.A. (1959) Control charts for stochastic processes. *Journal of the Royal Statistical Society, Series B*, **21**, (2), 239–271

BARRON, B.A. (1977) The effects of misclassification on the estimation of relative risk. *Biometrics*, **33**, 414–418

BARTLETT, M.S. (1957) Measles periodicity and community size. *Journal of the Royal Statistical Society, Series A*, **120**, 48–70

BARTLETT, P.C., KANEENE, J., GIBSON, C.D., ERICKSON, R. and MATHER, E.C. (1982) Development of a computerised dairy management and disease surveillance system: FAHRMX. In: Proceedings of the First Symposium on Computer Applications in Veterinary Medicine. College of Veterinary Medicine, Mississippi State University, 13–15 October 1982. Pp. 21–29

BARTLETT, P.C., KIRK, J.H., MATHER, E.C., GIBSON, C. and KANEENE, J.B. (1985) FAHRMX: a computerized dairy herd health management network. *The Compendium on Continuing Education for the Practising Veterinarian*, **7**, S124–S133

BASSON, P.A. and HOFMEYER, J.M. (1973) Mortalities associated with wildlife capture operations. In: *The Capture and Care of Wild Animals*. Pp. 151–160. Ed. Young, E. Human and Rousseau, Cape Town and Pretoria

BATES, D.J., CORKISH, J.D. and DAVIES, G. (1984) The financial consequences of an outbreak of abortion in a dairy herd. In: Society for Veterinary Epidemiology and Preventive Medicine, Proceedings, Edinburgh, 10–11 July 1984. Ed. Thrusfield, M.V. Pp. 104–112

BEARD, T.C. (1983) The elimination of echinococcosis from Iceland. *Bulletin of the World Health Organization*, **48**, 653–660

BECKER, F.F. (1981) Recent concepts of initiation and promotion in carcinogenesis. *American Journal of Pathology*, **105**, 3–9

BEECH, M.W.H. (1911) *The Suk, their Language and Folklore*. Clarendon Press, Oxford

BEHBEHANI, K. and HASSOUNAH, O. (1976) The role of native and domestic animals in the dissemination of *Echinococcus* infection among dogs in the State of Kuwait. *Journal of Helminthology*, **50**, 275–280

BELL, K.J. (1980) A study of productivity in sheep flocks. The application and evaluation of health and productivity programmes in south-west Australia. In: Proceedings of the 10th Seminar of the Sheep and Beef Cattle Society of the New Zealand Veterinary Association. Lincoln College, Canterbury, 11–12 July 1980. Pp. 108–114

BENDER, A.P., BENDER, G.P., DORN, C.R. and SCHNEIDER, R. (1982) Association between canine benign and malignant neoplasms. *Preventive Veterinary Medicine*, **1**, 77–87

BENDER, A.P., POLICELLO, G.E., DORN, C.R. and ROBINSON, R.A. (1983) Cautions about the estimation of summary relative risk from veterinary epidemiologic studies. In: Proceedings of the Third International Symposium on Veterinary Epidemiology and Economics. Arlington, Virginia, 6–10 September 1982. Pp. 60–67. Veterinary Medicine Publishing Company, Edwardsville

BERGSMA, D.R. and BROWN, K.S. (1971) White fur, blue eyes, and deafness in the domestic cat. *Journal of Heredity*, **62**, 171–185

BEYNON, V.H. (1964) *The Cost of Disease*. Pig Industry Development Authority Report. Pig Health and Profits Conference, Buxton

BIBIKOVA, V.A. (1977) Contemporary views on the interrelationships between fleas and the pathogens of human and animal diseases. *Annual Review of Entomology*, **22**, 23–32

BIELFELT, S.W., REDMAN, H.C. and McCLELLAN, R.O. (1971) Sire- and sex-related differences in rates of epileptiform seizures in a purebred beagle dog colony. *American Journal of Veterinary Research*, **32**, 2039–2048

BIGGS, P.M. (1982) Vaccination. In: *The Control of Infectious Diseases in Farm Animals*. British Veterinary Association Trust Project on the future of animal health control, London. Pp. 21–27

BLACK, A. (1972) Progressive retinal atrophy: a review of the genetics and an appraisal of the eradication scheme. *Journal of Small Animal Practice*, **13**, 295–314

BLACK, F.L. (1975) Infectious diseases in primitive societies. *Science*, **187**, 515–518

BLACKMORE, D.K. (1963) The incidence and aetiology of thyroid dysplasia in budgerigars (*Melopsittacus undulatus*). *Veterinary Record*, **75**, 1068–1072

BLACKMORE, D.K. (1964) A survey of disease in British wild foxes (*Vulpes vulpes*). *Veterinary Record*, **76**, 527–533

BLACKMORE, D.K. (1983) Practical problems associated with the slaughter of stock. In: *Stunning of Animals for Slaughter*. Ed. Eikelenboom, G. Pp. 167–178. Martin Nijhoff Publishers, The Hague

BLACKMORE, D.K. and HATHAWAY, S.C. (1980) The nidality of zoonoses. In: *Veterinary Epidemiology and Economics*. Proceedings of the Second International Symposium, Canberra, 7–11 May 1979. Eds Geering, W.A., Roe, R.T. and Chapman, L.A. Pp. 207–213. Australian Government Publishing Service, Canberra

BLACKMORE, D.K. and SCHOLLUM, L.M. (1983) The serological investigation of occupational exposure to leptospirosis. In: Proceedings of the Third International Symposium on Veterinary Epidemiology and Economics. Arlington, Virginia, 6–10 September 1982. Pp. 544–551. Veterinary Medical Publishing Company, Edwardsville

BLACKMORE, D.K., HILL, A. and JACKSON, O.F. (1971) The incidence of mycoplasma in pet and colony maintained cats. *Journal of Small Animal Practice*, **12**, 207–216

BLAJAN, L. (1982) National and international reporting services. In: *Epidemiology in Animal Health*. Proceedings of a symposium held at the British Veterinary Association's Centenary Congress, Reading, 22–25 September 1982. Pp. 90–98. Society for Veterinary Epidemiology and Preventive Medicine

BLAMIRE, R.V., CROWLEY, A.J. and GOODHAND, R.H. (1970) A review of some animal diseases encountered at meat inspection 1960–1968. *Veterinary Record*, **87**, 234–238

BLAMIRE, R.V., GOODHAND, R.H. and TAYLOR, K.C. (1980) A review of some animal diseases encountered at meat inspections in England and Wales, 1969 to 1978. *Veterinary Record*, **106**, 195–199

BLOOD, D.C. (1976) The principles of herd health programmes. In: Proceedings Number 28. Refresher course for veterinarians on mastitis. Pp. 47–64. The University of Sydney Post-graduate Committee on Veterinary Science in association with the Australian Veterinary Association and the Veterinary Clinic Centre, University of Melbourne

BLOOD, D.C., MORRIS, R.S., WILLIAMSON, N.B., CANNON, C.M. and CANNON, R.M. (1978) A health program for commercial dairy herds. 1. Objectives and methods. *Australian Veterinary Journal*, **54**, 207–215

BLOOD, D.C., RADOSTITS, O.M. and HENDERSON, J.A. (1983) *Veterinary Medicine*, 6th edn. Baillière Tindall, London

BLOT, W.J. and DAY, N.E. (1979) Synergism and interaction: are they equivalent? *American Journal of Epidemiology*, **110**, 99–100

BLOWEY, R.W. (1983) Data recording and analysis in dairy herds. In: Society for Veterinary Epidemiology and Preventive Medicine, Proceedings, Southampton, 12–13 April 1983. Ed Thrusfield, M.V. Pp. 19–28

BOOTH, A.J., STAGDALE, L. and GREGOR, J.A. (1984) Salmon poisoning disease in dogs in Southern Vancouver Island. *Canadian Veterinary Journal*, **25**, 2–6

BOOTH, J.M. and WARREN, M.E. (1984) The use of a computerized herd fertility monitor. In: Society for Veterinary Epidemiology and Preventive Medicine, Proceedings, Edinburgh, 10–11 July 1984. Ed. Thrusfield, M.V. Pp. 166–173

BORG, K. and HUGOSON, G. (1980) Wildlife as an indicator of environmental disturbances. In: *Veterinary Epidemiology and Economics*. Proceedings of the Second International Symposium, Canberra, 7–11 May, 1979. Eds Geering,W.A., Roe, R.T. and Chapman, L.A. Pp. 250–253.Australian Government Publishing Service,Canberra

BOSTOCK, D.E. and CURTIS, R. (1984) Comparison of canine oropharyngeal malignancy in various geographical locations. *Veterinary Record*, **114**, 341–342

BOYCOTT, J.A. (1971) *Natural History of Infectious Disease*. Studies in Biology No. 26. Edward Arnold, London

BRAMLEY, A.J., DODD, F.H. and GRIFFIN, T.K. (Eds) (1981) *Mastitis Control and Herd Management*. The proceedings of a course organized by the National Institute for Research in Dairying, 22–24 September 1980. National Institute for Research in Dairying/Hannah Research Institute. Technical Bulletin 4

BRAVERMAN, Y., UNGAR-WARON, H., FRITH, K., ADLER, H., DANIELI, Y., BAKER, K.P. and QUINN, P.J. (1983) Epidemiological and immunological studies of sweet itch in horses in Israel. *Veterinary Record*, **112**, 521–524

BROADBENT, D.W. (1979) Field collection of animal disease data in developing countries. *World Animal Review*, **29**, 38–42

BRODEY, R.S. (1970) Canine and feline neoplasia. *Advances in Veterinary Science and Comparative Medicine*, **14**, 309–354

BRODEY, R.S., MCDONOUGH, S.F., FRYE, F.L. and HARDY, W.D. (1970) Epidemiology of feline leukemia (lymphosarcoma). In: Proceedings of the 4th International Symposium on Comparative Leukaemia Research, Cherry Hill, New Jersey. Ed. Dutcher, R.M. *Bibliotheca Haematologica*, **36**, 333–342

BROOKSBY, J.B. (1972) Epizootiology of foot-and-mouth disease in developing countries. *World Animal Review*, **1**, 10–13

BROTHWELL, D. and SANDISON, A.T. (Eds) (1967) *Diseases in Antiquity*. Charles C. Thomas, Springfield

BROWNLEE, J. (1915) Historical note on Farr's theory of the epidemic. *British Medical Journal*, ii, 250–252

BRUNSDON, R.V. (1980) Principles of helminth control. *Veterinary Parasitology*, **6**, 185–215

BRYANT, T.N. and SMITH, J.E. (1981) *Report on Analysis of Biochemical, Haematological, Serological and Microbiological Data from Healthy Racehorses Using Principal Components Analysis and Other Methods. I. Recognition and Analysis of Horse Conditions*. Department of Microbiology, University of Surrey, Guildford (obtainable from The Equine Research Station, Newmarket, Suffolk, UK)

BRYSON, R.W. (1982) Kikuyu poisoning and the army worm. *Journal of the South African Veterinary Association*, **53**, 161–165

BUCHANAN, J.W. (1977) Chronic valvular disease (endocardiosis) in dogs. *Advances in Veterinary Science*, **21**, 75–106

BUESCHER, E.L., SCHERER, W.F., McCLURE, H.E., MOYER, J.T., ROSENBERG, M.Z., YOSHII, M. *et al*. (1959) Ecologic studies of Japanese Encephalitis virus in Japan. IV. Avian infection. *American Journal of Tropical Medicine and Hygiene*, **8**, 678–688

BURGDORFER, W. (1960) Colorado Tick Fever: II The behaviour of Colorado Tick Fever virus in rodents. *Journal of Infectious Diseases*, **107**, 384–388

BURGER, H.J. (1976) Trichostrongyle infestation in autumn on pastures grazed exclusively by cows or by calves. *Veterinary Parasitology*, **1**, 359–366

BURNET, M. and WHITE, D.O. (1972) *Natural History of Infectious Disease*, 4th edn. Cambridge University Press, London

BURRIDGE, M.J. and McCARTHY, S.M. (1979) The Florida veterinary clinical data retrieval system. In: Proceedings of an International Syposium on Animal Health and Disease Data Banks, 4–6 December 1978, Washington, D.C. Pp. 155–161. United States Department of Agriculture. Miscellaneous Publication No. 1381

BURRIDGE, M.J., SCHWABE, C.W. and PULLUM, T.W. (1977) Path analysis: application in an epidemiological study of echinococcosis in New Zealand. *Journal of Hygiene, Cambridge*, **78**, 135–149

CALDOW, G.L. (1984) The potential for veterinary involvement in the reproductive management of beef suckler herds. MSc thesis. University of Edinburgh

CANNON, R.M. and ROE, R.T. (1982) *Livestock Disease Surveys: A Field Manual for Veterinarians*. Australian Government Publishing Service, Canberra

CANNON, R.M., MORRIS, R.S., WILLIAMSON, N.B., CANNON, C.M. and BLOOD, D.C. (1978) A health program for commercial dairy herds. 2. Data processing. *Australian Veterinary Journal*, **54**, 216–230

CARMICHAEL, L.E. and BINN, L.N. (1981) New enteric viruses in the dog. *Advances in Veterinary Science and Comparative Medicine*, **25**, 1–37

CARSON, R.L. (1963) *Silent Spring*. Hamish Hamilton, London

CASLEY, J.D. and LURY, D.A. (1981) *Data Collection in Developing Countries*. Clarendon Press, Oxford

CASON, R. and GEERING, W.A. (1980) An economic evaluation of possible Australian policies to meet the threat of an exotic pest—the screw-worm fly, *Chrysomyia bezziana*. In: *Veterinary Epidemiology and Economics*. Proceedings of the Second International Symposium, Canberra, 7–11 May 1979. Eds Geering, W.A., Roe, R.T. and Chapman, L.A. Pp. 463–470. Australian Government Publishing Service, Canberra

CHAIN, P. (1980) Public participation and communications in Latin American disease control programs. In: *Veterinary Epidemiology and Economics*. Proceedings of the Second International Symposium, Canberra, 7–11 May 1979. Eds Geering, W.A., Roe, R.T. and Chapman, L.A. Pp. 335–340. Australian Government Publishing Service, Canberra

CHALMERS, A.W. (1968) African horse sickness. *Equine Veterinary Journal*, **1**, 83–86

CHAMBERLAIN, A.T. and CRIPPS, P.J. (1986) The derivation of prognostic indicators in the downer cow syndrome: an epidemiological approach to a multifactorial condition. In: Society for Veterinary Epidemiology and Preventive

Medicine, Proceedings, Edinburgh, 2–4 April 1986. Ed. Thrusfield, M.V. Pp. 142–159

CHAPMAN, R.N. (1928) The quantitative analysis of environmental factors. *Ecology*, **9**, 111–122

CHAPMAN, R.N. (1931) *Animal Ecology with Special Reference to Insects*. McGraw Hill, New York

CHATFIELD, C. and COLLINS, A.J. (1980) *Introduction to Multivariate Analysis*. Chapman and Hall, London

CHEVILLE, N.F. (1975) The gray collie syndrome (cyclic neutropenia). *Journal of the American Animal Hospitals Association*, **11**, 350–352

CHRISTIAN, M.K., BAKER, J.P. and GARDNER, T.W. (1973) Observations on disease during the first two years of operation of a large pig fattening unit. Part II. Costs. *Veterinary Record*, **93**, 153–155

CHRISTIANSEN, K.H. (1980) Laboratory management and disease surveillance information system. In: *Veterinary Epidemiology and Economics*. Proceedings of the Second International Symposium, Canberra, 7–11 May 1979. Eds Geering, W.A., Roe, R.T. and Chapman, L.A. Pp. 59–64. Australian Government Publishing Service, Canberra

CLIFF, A.D. and ORD, J.K. (1981) *Spatial Processes. Models and Applications*. Pion Limited, London

COCHRAN, W.G. (1977) *Sampling Techniques*. John Wiley and Sons, London

COCKBURN, A. (1963) *The Evolution and Eradication of Infectious Diseases*. Johns Hopkins Press, Baltimore

COHEN, D., BOOTH, S. and SUSSMAN, O. (1959) An epidemiological study of canine lymphoma and its public health significance. *American Journal of Veterinary Research*, **20**, 1026–1031

COHEN, D., BRODEY, R.S. and CHEN, S.M. (1964) Epidemiologic aspects of oral and pharyngeal neoplasms of the dog. *American Journal of Veterinary Research*, **25**, 1776–1779

COLE, P. and MacMAHON, B. (1971) Attributable risk percent in case-control studies. *British Journal of Preventive and Social Medicine*, **25**, 242–244

COLINVAUX, P.A. (1973) *Introduction to Ecology*. John Wiley and Sons, New York

CONGLETON, W.R. and GOODWILL, R.E. (1980) Simulated comparisons of breeding plans for beef production. Part 1: A dynamic model to evaluate the mating plan on herd age structure and productivity. *Agricultural Systems*, **5**, 207–219

COOMBS, M.M. (1980) Chemical carcinogenesis: a view at the end of the first half-century. *Journal of Pathology*, **130**, 117–146

COPELAND, K.T., CHECKOWAY, H., McMICHAEL, A.J. and HOLBROOK, R.H. (1977) Bias due to misclassification in the estimation of relative risk. *American Journal of Epidemiology*, **105**, 408–495

CORDES, D.O., LIMER, K.L. and McENTEE, K. (1981) Data management for the International Registry of Reproductive Pathology using SNOMED coding and computerization. *Veterinary Pathology*, **18**, 342–350

CORIA, M.F. and McCLURKIN, A.W. (1978) Specific immune tolerance in an apparently healthy bull persistently infected with bovine viral diarrhoea. *Journal of the American Veterinary Medical Association*, **172**, 449–451

COTCHIN, E. (1984) Veterinary oncology: a survey. *Journal of Pathology*, **142**, 101–127

COX, D.R. (1970) *Analysis of Binary Data*. Methuen, London

CROSSMAN, P.J. (1978) Gastric torsion in sows. *The Pig Veterinary Society Proceedings*, **2**, 47–49

CSIZA, C.K., SCOTT, F.W., LAHUNTA, A. DE and GILLESPIE, J.H. (1971) Feline viruses. XIV. Transplacental infections in spontaneous panleukopenia of cats. *Cornell Veterinarian*, **61**, 423–439

CUTHBERTSON, J.C. (1983) Sheep disease surveillance based on condemnations at three Scottish abattoirs. *Veterinary Record*, **112**, 219–221

DANIELS, P.W., ROBERTS, G. and JOHNSON, R.H. (1986) The aetiology of squamous cell carcinoma of sheep—epidemiological observations. In: Proceedings of the 4th International Conference on Veterinary Epidemiology and Economics. 18–22 November 1985, Singapore. Singapore Veterinary Association. In press

DANT, C.M. and BLACKMORE, D.J. (1981) Equine clinical data requirements. In: *A Computerised Veterinary Clinical Data Base*. Proceedings of a symposium, Edinburgh, 30 September 1981. Ed. Thrusfield, M.V. Pp. 10–16. Department of Animal Health, Royal (Dick) School of Veterinary Studies, Edinburgh

DARKE, P.G.G. (1982) The value of clinical case records in small animal cases. In: *Epidemiology in Animal Health*. Proceedings of a symposium held at the British Veterinary Association's Centenary Congress, Reading, 22–25 September 1982. Pp. 103–106. Society for Veterinary Epidemiology and Preventive Medicine

DARKE, P.G.G., THRUSFIELD, M.V. and AITKEN, C.G.G. (1985) Association between tail injuries and docking in dogs. *Veterinary Record*, **116**, 409

DAS, K.M. and TASHJIAN, R.J. (1965) Chronic mitral valve disease in the dog. *Veterinary Medicine/Small Animal Clinician*, **60**, 1209–1216

DAVID, F.N. and BARTON, D.E. (1966) Two space-time interaction tests for epidemicity. *British Journal of Preventive and Social Medicine*, **20**, 44–48

DAVID-WEST, K.B. (1980) Planning and implementation of contagious bovine pleuropneumonia control programs in Nigeria. In: *Veterinary Epidemiology and Economics*. Proceedings of the Second International Symposium, Canberra, 7–11 May 1979. Eds Geering, W.A., Roe, R.T. and Chapman, L.A. Pp. 575–580. Australian Government Publishing Service, Canberra

DAVIES, E.B. and WATKINSON, J.H. (1966) Uptake of native and applied selenium by pasture species. I. Uptake of Se by browntop, ryegrass, cocksfoot, and white clover from Atiamuri sand. *New Zealand Journal of Agricultural Research*, **9**, 317–327

DAVIES, F.G. (1975) Observations on the epidemiology of Rift Valley fever in Kenya. *Journal of Hygiene, Cambridge*, **75**, 219–230

DAVIES, F.G., SHAW, T. and OCHIENG, P. (1975) Observations on the epidemiology of ephemeral fever in Kenya. *Journal of Hygiene, Cambridge*, **75**, 231–235

DAVIES, G. (1980) Animal disease surveillance. In: *Veterinary Epidemiology and Economics*. Proceedings of the Second International Symposium, Canberra, 7–11 May 1979. Eds Geering, W.A., Roe, R.T. and Chapman, L.A. Pp. 3–10. Australian Government Publishing Service, Canberra

DAVIES, G. (1983) The development of veterinary epidemiology. In: Society for Veterinary Epidemiology and Preventive Medicine, Proceedings. Southampton, 12–13 April 1983. Ed. Thrusfield, M.V. Pp. ix–xvi

DAVIES, O.L. and GOLDSMITH, P.L. (1972) *Statistical Methods in Research and Production*, 4th edn. Longman Group, New York and London

DE BOER, C.J. (1967) Studies to determine neutralizing

antibody in sera from animals recovered from African Swine Fever and laboratory animals inoculated with African virus adjuvants. *Archiv für die Gesamte Virusforschung,* **20**, 164–179

DE CANDOLLE, A.P.A. (1874) Constitution dans le regne vegetal de groupes physiologiques applicables a la geographie ancienne et moderne. *Archives des Sciences Physiques et Naturelles,* **50**, 5–42

DE KRUIF, A. (1978) Factors influencing the fertility of a cattle population. *Journal of Reproduction and Fertility,* **54**, 507–518

DE KRUIF, A. (1980) Efficiency of a fertility control programme in dairy herds. In: Proceedings of the Ninth International Congress on Animal Reproduction and Artificial Insemination, Madrid, 16–20 June 1980. Volume II. Pp. 381–388

DEGNER, R.L., RODAN, L.W., MATHIS, W.K. and GIBBS, E.P.J. (1983) The recreational and commercial importance of feral swine in Florida: relevance to the possible introduction of African Swine Fever into the U.S.A. *Preventive Veterinary Medicine,* **1**, 371–381

DIESCH, S.L. (1979) Disease recording at the farm level. In: Proceedings of an International Symposium on Animal Health and Disease Data Banks, 4–6 December 1978, Washington D.C. Pp. 97–100. United States Department of Agriculture, Miscellaneous Publications No. 1381

DIESCH, S.L. and ELLINGHAUSEN, H.C. (1975) Leptospiroses. In: *Diseases Transmitted from Animals to Man,* 6th edn. Eds Hubbert, W.T., McCulloch, W.F. and Schnurrenberger, P.R. Pp. 436–462. Charles C. Thomas, Springfield

DI SALVO, A.F. and JOHNSON, W.M. (1979) Histoplasmosis in South Carolina: support for the microfocus concept. *American Journal of Epidemiology,* **109**, 480–492

DIXON, W.J. (Ed.) (1983) *BMDP Statistical Software.* University of California Press, Berkeley

DOLL, R. (1959) Smoking and cancer. Report to the sub-committee for the study of the risks of cancer from air pollution and the consumption of tobacco. *Acta Uniaris Internationalis Contra Cancrum,* **15**, 1283–1296

DOLL, R. (1977) Strategy for detection of cancer hazards to man. *Nature,* **265**, 589–596

DOLL, R. and HILL, A.B. (1964a) Mortality in relation to smoking. Ten years' observations of British doctors. *British Medical Journal,* i, 1399–1410

DOLL, R. and HILL, A.B. (1964b) Mortality in relation to smoking. Ten years' observations of British doctors. *British Medical Journal,* i, 1460–1467

DONALDSON, A.I., GLOSTER, J., HARVEY, L.D.J. and DEANS, D.H. (1982) Use of prediction models to forecast and analyse airborne spread during the foot-and-mouth disease outbreaks in Brittany, Jersey and the Isle of Wight in 1981. *Veterinary Record,* **110**, 53–57

DONHAM, K.J., BERG, J.W. and SAWIN, R.S. (1980) Epidemiologic relationships of the bovine population and human leukemia in Iowa. *American Journal of Epidemiology,* **112**, 80–92

DORN, C.R. (1966) An animal tumour registry as a source of morbidity information. In: Proceedings of the United States Livestock Sanitation Association. Pp. 443–454

DORN, C.R. and PRIESTER, W.A. (1976) Epidemiologic analysis of oral and pharyngeal cancer in dogs, cats, horses and cattle. *Journal of the American Veterinary Medical Association,* **169**, 1202–1206

DORN, C.R., TAYLOR, D.O.N. and SCHNEIDER, R. (1971) Sunlight exposure and risk of developing cutaneous and oral squamous cell carcinomas in white cats. *Journal of the National Cancer Institute,* **46**, 1073–1081

DORN, C.R., TERBRUSCH, F.G. and HIBBARD, H.H. (1967) *Zoographic and Demographic Analysis of Dog and Cat Ownership in Alameda County, California, 1965.* State of California Department of Public Health, Berkeley

DOUGLAS, A. (1984) Disease prevention in pig herds. *In Practice,* **6**, 108–115

DRAPER, N. and SMITH, H. (1966) *Applied Regression Analysis,* 2nd edn. John Wiley and Sons, New York

DUBOS, R. (1965) *Man Adapting.* Yale University Press, New Haven

DUPPONG, B.L. and ETTINGER, S.J. (1983) The medical record. In: *Textbook of Veterinary Internal Medicine: Diseases of the Dog and Cat,* Vol. 2, 2nd edn. Ed. Ettinger, S.J. Pp. 3–29. W.B. Saunders Company, Philadelphia

EDWARDS, B. (1980) Foot lameness in cattle. *In Practice,* **2**, (4), 25–31

EGEBERG, R.O. (1954) Coccidioidomycosis: its clinical and climatological aspects with remarks on treatment. *American Journal of Medical Science,* **227**, 268–271

EGERTON, J.R. (1981) Foot-rot. In: Refresher Course on Sheep, 10–14 August. Post-graduate Committee in Veterinary Science, University of Sydney. Proceedings No. 58. Pp. 647–651

EJIGOU, A. and MCHUGH, R. (1977) On the factorization of the crude relative risk. *American Journal of Epidemiology,* **106**, 188–191

ELDER, J.K. (1976) A functional computer recording system for a veterinary diagnostic laboratory. *Australian Veterinary Journal,* **52**, 24–35

ELLIS, P.R. (1980) International aspects of animal disease surveillance. In: *Veterinary Epidemiology and Economics.* Proceedings of the Second International Symposium, Canberra, 7–11 May 1979. Eds Geering, W.A., Roe, R.T. and Chapman, L.A. Pp. 11–15. Australian Government Publishing Service, Canberra

ELLIS, P.R., JAMES, A.D. and SHAW, A.P. (1977) *Studies on the Epidemiology and Economics of Swine Fever Eradication in the E.E.C.* EUR 5738e. Commission of the European Communities, Luxembourg

ELTON, C.S. (1927) *Animal Ecology.* Macmillan, New York

ERICKSON, B.H. and NOSANCHUK, T.A. (1979) *Understanding Data.* Open University Press, Milton Keynes

ESSLEMONT, R.J., BAILIE, J.H. and COOPER, M.J. (1985) *Fertility Management in Dairy Cattle.* Collins Professional and Technical Books, London

EVANS, A.S. (1976) Causation and disease. The Henle-Koch postulates revisited. *Yale Journal of Biology and Medicine,* **49**, 175–195

EVANS-PRITCHARD, E.E. (1956) *Nuer Religion.* Oxford University Press, London

EWBANK, D. and WRAY, J.D. (1980) Population and public health. In *Maxcy-Rosenau: Public Health and Preventive Medicine.* 11th edn. Ed. Last, J.M. Pp. 1504–1548. Appleton-Century-Crofts, New York

FAHRMX (1984) FAHRMX dairy herd health management computer network. In: Proceedings of the Second Symposium on Computer Applications in Veterinary Medicine. College of Veterinary Medicine, Mississippi State University, 23–25 May 1984. Pp. 45–50

FAO (1983) *FAO Production Yearbook 1982,* Vol. 36. FAO Statistics Series No. 47. Food and Agriculture Organization of the United Nations, Rome

FAO/WHO (1967) *Report of a Joint Food and Agriculture Organization/World Health Organization Expert Committee on Zoonoses.* Technical Report Series No. 3. World Health Organization, Geneva

FAO-WHO-OIE (1984) *Animal Health Yearbook 1984.* Food and Agriculture Organization of the United Nations, World Health Organization, Office International des Epizooties. Food and Agriculture Organization of the United Nations, Rome

FEINSTEIN, A.R. (1973) The problems of the 'Problem-Oriented Medical Record'. *Annals of Internal Medicine*, **78**, 751–762

FELTON, M.R. and ELLIS, P.R. (1978) *Studies in the Control of Rinderpest in Nigeria.* Study No. 23. University of Reading

FENNER, F. and RATCLIFFE, F.N. (1965) Myxomatosis. Cambridge University Press, Cambridge

FERRIS, D.H. (1967) Epizootiology. *Advances in Veterinary Science*, **11**, 261–320

FERRIS, D.H. (1971) Epizootiologic features of transmissible swine gastroenteritis. *Journal of the American Veterinary Medical Association*, **159**, 184–194

FINNEGAN, D.J. (1976) *Bacterial Conjugation.* Meadowfield Press, Shildon

FINNEY, D.J. (1978) *Statistical Method in Biological Assay*, 3rd edn. Charles Griffin and Company, London and High Wycombe

FINNEY, D.J., HAZLEWOOD, T. and SMITH, M.J. (1955) Logarithms to base 2. *Journal of General Microbiology*, **12**, 222–225

FISK, D. (1959) *Dr. Jenner of Baltimore.* William Heinemann, London

FLEISS, J.L. (1981) *Statistical Methods for Rates and Proportions*, 2nd edn. John Wiley and Sons, New York

FOLEY, C.W., LASLEY, J.F. and OSWEILER, G.D. (1979) *Abnormalities of Companion Animals: Analysis of Heritability.* Iowa State University Press, Ames

FORSTER, F. (1966) Use of a demographic base map for the presentation of areal data in epidemiology. *British Journal of Preventive and Social Medicine*, **20**, 156–171

FOX, M.T. and SYKES, T.J. (1985) Establishment of the tropical dog tick, *Rhipicephalus sanguineus*, in a house in London. *Veterinary Record*, **116**, 661–662

FRANCIS, P.G., SUMNER, J. and JOYCE, D.A. (1979) *The Environment in Relation to Mastitis, A Field Study.* Agricultural Development Advisory Services, South-Western Region, UK

FRANTI, C.E., WIGGINS, A.D., LOPEZ-NIETO, E. and CRENSHAW, G. (1974) Factor analysis: a statistical tool useful in epizootiologic research, with an example from a study in dairy calves. *American Journal of Veterinary Research*, **35**, 649–655

FRASER, A.C. (1969) Advisory and preventive medicine in equine practice. *Veterinary Record*, **85**, 249–250

FRASER, A.F. (1976) *Topics in Theriogenology.* A supplementary handbook on special practical and clinical features of veterinary reproduction. Western College of Veterinary Medicine, Saskatoon

FRAUMENI, J.F. (1967) Stature and malignant tumours of bone in childhood and adolescence. *Cancer*, **20**, 967–973

FRITSCHEN, R.D. (1979) Housing and its effect on feet and leg problems. *The Pig Veterinary Society Proceedings*, **5**, 95–98

FROST, W.H. (1976) Some conceptions of epidemics in general. *American Journal of Epidemiology*, **103**, 141–151

GADDUM, J.H. (1933) *Reports of Biological Standards. III. Methods of Biological Assay Depending on a Quantal Response.* Special Report Series No. 183. Medical Research Council, London

GALEN, R.S. and GAMBINO, S.R. (1975) *Beyond Normality—The Predictive Value and Efficiency of Medical Diagnoses.* John Wiley and Sons, New York

GALUZO, I.G. (1975) Landscape epidemiology (epizootiology). *Advances in Veterinary Science and Comparative Medicine*, **19**, 73–96

GASKELL, C.J. (1983) Dilated pupil (Key-Gaskell) syndrome in cats. In: Society for Veterinary Epidemiology and Preventive Medicine, Proceedings, Southampton, 12–13 April 1983. Ed. Thrusfield, M.V. Pp. 99–100

GAUSE, G.F. (1934) *The Struggle for Existence.* Williams and Wilkins, Baltimore

GETTINBY, G. and McCLEAN, SALLY (1979) A matrix formulation of the life-cycle of liver fluke. *Proceedings of the Royal Irish Academy*, **79B**, 155–167

GETTINBY, G., BAIRDEN, K., ARMOUR, J. and BENITEZ-USHER, C. (1979) A prediction model for bovine ostertagiasis. *Veterinary Record*, **105**, 57–59

GIBSON, M. and WARREN, K.S. (1970) Capture of *Schistosoma mansoni* miracidia and cercariae by carnivorous aquatic vascular plants of the genus *Utricularia. Bulletin of the World Health Organization*, **42**, 833–835

GIBSON, T.E. (1978) The 'Mt' system for forecasting the prevalence of fascioliasis. In: *Weather and Parasitic Animal Disease.* Pp. 3–5. World Meteorological Organization Technical Note No. 159

GIBSON, T.E. and SMITH, L.P. (1978a) Forecasting the prevalence of nematodiriasis in England and Wales. In: *Weather and Parasitic Animal Disease.* Pp. 74–75. World Meteorological Organization Technical Note No. 159

GIBSON, T.E. and SMITH, L.P. (1978b) Forecasting outbreaks of parasitic gastroenteritis in ruminants in England and Wales. In: *Weather and Parasitic Animal Disease.* Pp. 76–77. World Meteorological Organization Technical Note No. 159

GITTINGER, J.P. (1972) *Economic Analysis of Agricultural Projects.* The Johns Hopkins University Press, Baltimore and London

GLICKMAN, L.T. (1980) Preventive medicine in kennel management. In: *Current Veterinary Therapy VII. Small Animal Practice.* Ed. Kirk, R.W. Pp. 67–76. W.B. Saunders Company, Philadelphia

GLICKMAN, L.T., DOMANSKI, L.M., MAGUIRE, T.G., DUBIELZIG, R.R. and CHURG, A. (1983) Mesothelioma in pet dogs associated with exposure of their owners to asbestos. *Environmental Research*, **32**, 305–313

GLICKMAN, L.T., DOMANSKI, L.M., PATRONEK, G.J. and VISINTAINER, F. (1985) Breed-related risk factors for canine parvovirus enteritis. *American Journal of Veterinary Research*, **187**, 589–594

GLOSTER, J., BLACKALL, R.M., SELLERS, R.F. and DONALDSON, A.I. (1981) Forecasting the airborne spread of foot-and-mouth disease. *Veterinary Record*, **108**, 370–374

GOGGIN, J.E., LI, A. and FRANTI, C.E. (1970) Canine intervertebral disc disease: characterization by age, sex, breed and anatomic site of involvement. *American Journal of Veterinary Research*, **31**, 1687–1692

GOODALL, E.A., McCAUGHEY, W.J., McMURRAY, C.H. and RICE, D. (1984) SIRO—a computer system for dairy herd recording. In: Society for Veterinary Epidemiology and Preventive Medicine, Proceedings, Edinburgh, 10–11 July 1984. Ed. Thrusfield, M.V. Pp. 174–183

GOODGER, W.J. and RUPPANNER, R. (1982) Why the dairy industry does not make greater use of veterinarians. *Journal of the American Veterinary Medical Association*, **181**, 706–710

GOODWIN, R.F.W. (1971a) The economics of enzootic pneumonia. *Veterinary Record*, **89**, 77–81

GOODWIN, R.F.W. (1971b) A procedure for investigating the influence of disease status on productivity efficiency in a pig herd. *Veterinary Record*, **88**, 387–392

GOPAL, T. (1977) Carcinogenesis. In: *Current Veterinary Therapy VI. Small Animal Practice*. Ed. Kirk, R.W. Pp. 164–166. W.B. Saunders Company, Philadelphia

GORDON, J.C. and ANGRICK, E.J. (1985) Stray dogs as sentinels for canine parvovirus. *Preventive Veterinary Medicine*, **3**, 311–316

GORDON SMITH, C.E. (1976) *Epidemiology and Infections*. Meadowfield Press, Shildon

GORDON SMITH, C.E. (1982) Major factors in the spread of infections. In: *Animal Disease in Relation to Animal Conservation*. Symposium of the Zoological Society of London No. 50. Eds Edwards, M.A. and McDonald, U. Pp. 207–235. Academic Press, London and New York

GORMAN, B.M., TAYLOR, J. and WALKER, P.J. (1979) Variation in arboviruses. In: *Arbovirus Research in Australia*. Proceedings of the Second Symposium, 17–19 July 1979. Eds St. George, T.D. and French, E.L. Pp. 71–76. The Commonwealth Scientific and Industrial Research Organization/Queensland Institute of Medical Research, Brisbane

GOULDEN, C.H. (1952) *Methods of Statistical Analysis*, 2nd edn. Chapman and Hall, London

GRACEY, J.F. (1960) *Survey of Livestock Diseases in Northern Ireland*. Her Majesty's Stationery Office, Belfast

GREENLAND, S. and KLEINBAUM, D.G. (1983) Correcting for misclassification in two-way tables and matched-pair studies. *International Journal of Epidemiology*, **12**, 93–97

GREENLAND, S., MORGENSTERN, H. and THOMAS, D.C. (1981) Considerations in determining matching criteria and stratum sizes for case-control studies. *International Journal of Epidemiology*, **10**, 389–392

GRINDLE, R.J. (1980) Appropriate methodology in economic analysis of disease control projects. In: *Veterinary Epidemiology and Economics*. Proceedings of the Second International Symposium, Canberra, 7–11 May 1979. Eds Geering, W.A., Roe, R.T. and Chapman, L.A. Pp. 506–510. Australian Government Publishing Service, Canberra

GRINDLE, R.J. (1986) The use and abuse of economic methods, as applied to veterinary problems. In: Proceedings of the Fourth International Symposium on Veterinary Epidemiology and Economics. Singapore, 18–22 November 1985. Singapore Veterinary Association. In press

GRINER, L.A. (1980) Storage and retrieval of necropsy records at San Diego zoo. In: *The Comparative Pathology of Zoo Animals*. Eds Montali, R.J. and Miguki, G. Pp. 663–667. Smithsonian Institution Press, Washington, D.C.

GROSS, L. (1955) Mouse leukaemia: an egg-borne virus disease (with a note on mouse salivary gland carcinoma). *Acta Haematologica*, **13**, 13–29

GRUNSELL, C.S., PENNY, R.H.C., WRAGG, S.R. and ALLCOCK, J. (1969) The practicability and economics of veterinary preventive medicine. *Veterinary Record*, **84**, 26–41

GUSTAVSSON, I. (1969) Cytogenetics, distribution and phenotypic effects of a translocation in Swedish cattle. *Hereditas*, **63**, 68–169

HABTEMARIAM, T., RUPPANNER, R., RIEMANN, H.P. and THEIS, J.H. (1983a) Evaluation of trypanosomiasis alternatives using an epidemiological simulation model. *Preventive Veterinary Medicine*, **1**, 147–156

HABTEMARIAM, T., RUPPANNER, R., RIEMANN, H.P. and THEIS, J.H. (1983b) An epidemiological systems analysis model for African trypanosomiasis. *Preventive Veterinary Medicine*, **1**, 125–136

HABTEMARIAM, T., RUPPANNER, R., RIEMANN, H.P. and THEIS, J.H. (1983c) Epidemic and endemic characterisation of trypanosomiasis in cattle: a simulation model. *Preventive Veterinary Medicine*, **1**, 137–145

HAELTERMAN, E.O. (1963) Epidemiological studies of transmissible gastroenteritis of swine. In: Proceedings of the 66th annual meeting of the United States Livestock Sanitary Association, 29 October–2 November 1962, Washington, D.C. Pp. 305–315

HAIG, D.A. (1977) Rabies in animals. In: *Rabies: The Facts*. Ed. Kaplan, C. Pp. 53–69. Oxford University Press, Oxford

HALL, S.A. (1978) Farm animal disease data banks. *Advances in Veterinary Science and Comparative Medicine*, **22**, 265–286

HALL, S.A., DAWSON, P.S. and DAVIES, G. (1980) VIDA II: a computerised diagnostic recording system for veterinary investigation centres in Great Britain. *Veterinary Record*, **106**, 260–264

HALLIWELL, R.E.W. (1978) Autoimmune disease in the dog. *Advances in Veterinary Science*, **22**, 221–263

HARRIS, R.E., REVFEIM, K.J.A. and HEATH, D.D. (1980) A decision-orientated simulation for comparing hydatid control strategies. In: *Veterinary Epidemiology and Economics*. Proceedings of the Second International Symposium, Canberra, 7–11 May 1979. Eds Geering, W.A., Roe, R.T. and Chapman, L.A. Pp. 613–616. Australian Government Publishing Service, Canberra

HATHAWAY, S.C. (1981) Leptospirosis in New Zealand: an ecological view. *New Zealand Veterinary Journal*, **29**, 109–112

HAYES, H.M. (1974a) Congenital umbilical and inguinal hernias in cattle, horses, swine, dogs and cats: risk by breed and sex among hospital patients. *American Journal of Veterinary Research*, **35**, 839–842

HAYES, H.M. (1974b) Ectopic ureter in dogs: epidemiologic features. *Teratology*, **10**, 129–132

HAYES, H.M. (1976) Canine bladder cancer: epidemiologic features. *American Journal of Epidemiology*, **104**, 673–677

HAYES, H.M. and FRAUMENI, J.F. (1975) Canine thyroid neoplasms: epidemiologic features. *Journal of the National Cancer Institute*, **55**, 931–934

HAYES, H.M. and FRAUMENI, J.F. (1977) Epidemiological features of canine renal neoplasms. *Cancer Research*, **37**, 2553–2556

HAYES, H.M. and PENDERGRASS, T.W. (1976) Canine testicular tumours: epidemiologic features. *International Journal of Cancer*, **18**, 482–487

HAYES, H.M., PRIESTER, W.A. and PENDERGRASS, T.W. (1975) Occurrence of nervous-tissue tumours in cattle, horses, cats and dogs. *International Journal of Cancer*, **15**, 39–47

HAYES, H.M., SELBY, L.A., WILSON, G.P. and HOHN, R.B. (1979) Epidemiologic observations on canine elbow disease (emphasis on dysplasia). *Journal of the American Animal Hospitals Association*, **15**, 449–453

HEIDELBERGER, C. (1978) Studies on the cellular mechanisms of chemical carcinogenesis. In: *Integration and Excision of DNA molecules*. 28. Colloquium der Gessellschaft für Biologische Chemie, 21–23 April 1977, Mosbach/Baden. Eds Hofschneider, P.H. and Starlinger, P. Pp. 106–111. Springer-Verlag, Berlin

HEIDT, G.A., FERGUSON, D.V. and LAMMERS, J. (1982) A profile of reported skunk rabies in Arkansas: 1977–79. *Journal of Wildlife Diseases*, **18**, 269–277

HELLE, O. (1971) The effect on sheep parasites of grazing in alternate years by sheep and cattle. A comparison with set-stocking, and the use of anthelmintics with these grazing arrangements. *Acta Veterinaria Scandinavica*, Suppl. 33, 1–59

HENDERSON, W.M. (1980) The priority for equine research. *Equine Veterinary Journal*, **12**, 50–53

HENDERSON, W.M. (1982) Priorities for research. In: *The Control of Infectious Diseases in Farm Animals*. British Veterinary Association Trust Project on the future of animal health control, London. Pp. 50–55

HERBERT, W.J. (1970) *Veterinary Immunology*. Blackwell Scientific Publications Limited, Oxford

HILL, A.B. (1971) *Principles of Medical Statistics*, 9th edn. The Lancet Limited, London

HIMSWORTH, H. (1970) *The Development and Organisation of Scientific Knowledge*. William Heinemann Medical Books, London

HINDSON, J. (1982) Sheep health schemes. *In Practice*, **4**, 53–58

HMSO (1954) *Mortality and Morbidity During the London Fog of December 1952*. Reports on Public Health and Medical Subjects, No. 95. Her Majesty's Stationery Office, London

HMSO (1968) *A Century of Agricultural Statistics, Great Britain, 1866–1966*. Ministry of Agriculture, Fisheries and Food; Department of Agriculture and Fisheries for Scotland. Her Majesty's Stationery Office, London

HMSO (1969) *Report of the Committee of Enquiry on Foot-and-Mouth Disease 1968. Part 1*. Her Majesty's Stationery Office, London

HMSO (1982) *Agricultural Statistics, United Kingdom 1980 and 1981*. Ministry of Agriculture, Fisheries and Food; Department of Agriculture and Fisheries for Scotland; Department of Agriculture for Northern Ireland; Welsh Agricultural Department. Her Majesty's Stationery Office, London

HOLLAND, W. (1984) A standard advisory system for lowland sheep flocks. In: Society for Veterinary Epidemiology and Preventive Medicine, Proceedings, Edinburgh, 10–11 July 1984. Ed. Thrusfield, M.V. Pp. 39–52

HOLT, P.E. (1976) *Toxocara canis*: An estimation of the incidence of infection in puppies in an industrial town. *Veterinary Record*, **98**, 383

HOOGSTRAAL, H. (1966) Ticks in relation to human diseases caused by viruses. *Annual Review of Entomology*, **11**, 261–308

HOPE-CAWDERY, M.J., GETTINBY, G. and GRAINGER, J.N. (1978) Mathematical models for predicting the prevalence of liver-fluke disease and its control from biological and meteorological data. In: *Weather and Parasitic Animal Disease*. Pp. 21–38. World Meteorological Organization Technical Note No. 159

HOURRIGAN, J.L. and KLINGSPORN, A.L. (1975) Epizootiology of bluetongue: the situation in the United States of America. *Australian Veterinary Journal*, **51**, 203–208

HOWE, K.S. (1976) *The Cost of Mortality in Sheep Production in the UK, 1971–74*. Report No. 198, Agricultural Economics Unit, University of Exeter

HOWE, K.S. (1985) An economist's view of animal disease. In: Society for Veterinary Epidemiology and Preventive Medicine, Proceedings, Reading, 27–29 March 1985. Ed. Thrusfield, M.V. Pp. 122–129

HUDSON, L. and HAY, E.C. (1981) *Practical Immunology*, 2nd edn. Blackwell Scientific, Oxford

HUGH-JONES, M.E. (1972) Epidemiological studies on the 1967/68 foot and mouth disease epidemic: Attack rates and cattle density. *Research in Veterinary Science*, **13**, 411–417

HUGH-JONES, M.E. (1975) Some pragmatic aspects of animal disease monitoring. In: *Animal Disease Monitoring*. Eds Ingram, D.G., Mitchell, W.F. and Martin, S.W. Pp. 220–236. Charles C. Thomas, Springfield

HUGH-JONES, M. (1983) Conclusions for the symposium and lessons for the future. In: Proceedings of the Third International Symposium on Veterinary Epidemiology and Economics. Arlington, Virginia, 6–10 September 1982. Pp. 650–654. Veterinary Medical Publishing Company, Edwardsville

HUGH-JONES, M.E., ELLIS, P.R. and FELTON, M.R. (1975a) An Assessment of the Eradication of Bovine Brucellosis in England and Wales. Study No. 19. University of Reading

HUGH-JONES, M.E., PARKIN, R.S. and WHITNEY, J.C. (1975b) The cost of premature death in young rabbits. *Veterinary Record*, **96**, 353–356

HUGH-JONES, M.E., ELLIS, P.R. and FELTON, M.R. (1976) The use of a computer model of brucellosis in the dairy herd. In: *New Techniques in Veterinary Epidemiology and Economics*. Proceedings of a symposium, University of Reading, 12–15 July 1976. Eds Ellis, P.R., Shaw, A.P.M. and Stephens, A.J. Pp. 96–112

HUGH-JONES, M.E. and WRIGHT, P.B. (1970) Studies on the 1967–68 foot-and-mouth disease epidemic. The relation of weather to spread of disease. *Journal of Hygiene, Cambridge*, **68**, 253–271

HURST, J.W. and WALKER, H.K. (Eds) (1972) *The Problem-Oriented System*. Medcom Inc., New York

IANOVICH, T.D., BLIZNICHENKO, A.G., ZABURINA, L.V., MSTIBOVSKII, S.A., BERKOVICH, A.I. and DUSHEVIN, I.P. (1957) Leptospirosis of the *canicola* type in one of the districts of Rostov-on-the-Don. *Journal of Microbiology, Epidemiology and Immunology*, **28**, 259–264

ISAACSON, R.E., MOON, H.W. and SCHNEIDER, R.A. (1978) Distribution and virulence of *Escherichia coli* in the small intestines of calves with and without diarrhoea. *American Journal of Veterinary Research*, **39**, 1750–1755

JACKSON, G.H. and BAKER, J.R. (1981) The occurrence of unthriftiness in piglets post-weaning. *The Pig Veterinary Society Proceedings*, **7**, 63–67

JAKAB, G.J. (1977) Pulmonary defense mechanisms and the interaction between viruses and bacteria in acute respiratory infections. *Bulletin Europeen de Physiopathologie Respiratoire*, **13**, 119–135

JARRETT, J.A. (Ed.) (1984) Symposium on bovine mastitis. *The Veterinary Clinics of North America*, **6**, 231–431

JARRETT, O. (1985) Update: feline leukaemia virus. *In Practice*, **7**, 125–126

JARRETT, W.F.H. (1980) Bracken fern and papilloma virus in bovine alimentary cancer. *British Medical Bulletin*, **36**, 79–81

JASPER, D.E., DELLINGER, J.D., ROLLINS, H. and HAKANSON,

H.D. (1979) Prevalence of mycoplasmal bovine mastitis in California. *American Journal of Veterinary Research*, **40**, 1043–1047

JERICHO, K.W.F. (1979) Update on pasteurellosis in young cattle. *Canadian Veterinary Journal*, **20**, 333–335

JOHNSON, R.E., CAMERON, T.P. and KINARD, R. (1968) Canine lymphoma as a potential model for experimental therapeutics. *Cancer Research*, **28**, 2562–2564

JOLLY, R.D. and TOWNSLEY, R.J. (1980) Genetic screening programmes: an analysis of benefits and costs using the bovine mannosidosis scheme as a model. *New Zealand Veterinary Journal*, **28**, 3–6

JOLLY, R.D., DODDS, W.J., RUTH, G.R. and TRAUNER, D.B. (1981) Screening for genetic diseases: principles and practice. *Advances in Veterinary Science and Comparative Medicine*, **25**, 245–275

JOLLY, R.D., TSE, C.A. and GREENWAY, R.M. (1973) Plasma α-mannosidase activity as a means of detecting mannosidosis heterozygotes. *New Zealand Veterinary Journal*, **21**, 64–69

JONES, D.R. and RUSHTON, L. (1982) Simultaneous inference in epidemiological studies. *International Journal of Epidemiology*, **11**, 276–282

JONES, G.E. and GILMOUR, J.S. (1983) Atypical pneumonia. In: *Diseases of Sheep*. Ed. Martin, W.B. Pp. 17–23. Blackwell, Oxford

JONES, W.H.S. (translator) (1923) *Hippocrates*, Vol. 1. The Loeb Classical Library. William Heinemann, London

JUBB, K.V.F. and KENNEDY, P.C. (1971) *Pathology of Domestic Animals*, 2nd edn. Academic Press, London and New York

JULIAN, A.F. (1981) Tuberculosis in the possum (*Trichosurus vulpecula*). In: Proceedings of the First Symposium on Marsupials in New Zealand. Ed. Bell, B.D. Pp. 163–174. Zoology Publications from Victoria University of Wellington No. 74. Victoria University, Wellington

KANEKO, J.J. (Ed.) (1980) *Clinical Biochemistry of Domestic Animals*, 3rd edn. Academic Press, London and New York

KAPLAN, M.M. (1982) Influenza in nature. In: *Animal Disease in Relation to Animal Conservation*. Symposium of the Zoological Society of London No. 50. Eds Edwards, M.A. and McDonald, U. Pp. 121–135. Academic Press, London and New York

KARBER, G. (1931) Beitrag zur kollektiven behandlung pharmakologischer reihenversuche. *Archiv für experimentelle Pathologie und Pharmakologie*, **162**, 480–487

KELLAR, J.A. (1983) Canada's bovine serum bank—a practical approach. In: Proceedings of the Third International Symposium on Veterinary Epidemiology and Economics. Arlington, Virginia, 6–10 September 1982. Pp. 138–143. Veterinary Medical Publishing Company, Edwardsville

KELLAR, J., MARRA, R. and MARTIN, W. (1976) Brucellosis in Ontario: a case-control study. *Canadian Journal of Comparative Medicine*, **40**, 119–128

KELLY, J.M. and WHITAKER, D.A. (1982) A dairy herd health and productivity service. In: Proceedings of the XIIth World Congress on Diseases of Cattle, Amsterdam, 7–10 September 1982. Pp. 659–664

KENDALL, M.G. and BUCKLAND, W.R. (1982) *A Dictionary of Statistical Terms*, 4th edn. Longman Group Limited, London and New York

KINGWILL, R.G., NEAVE, F.K., DODD, F.H., GRIFFIN, T.K. and WESTGARTH, D.R. (1970) The effect of a mastitis control system on levels of subclinical and clinical mastitis in two years. *Veterinary Record*, **87**, 94–100

KLEINBAUM, D.G., KUPPER, L.L. and MORGANSTERN, H. (1982) *Epidemiologic Research. Principles and Quantitative Measures*. Lifetime Learning Publications, Belmont

KNOX, G.A. (1964) The detection of space-time interactions. *Applied Statistics*, **13**, 25–29

KONIG, C.D.W. (1985) Bedrijfsdiergeneeskundige aspecten van de schapenhouderij (Planned animal health and production service on sheep farms. An inventory and evaluation). PhD thesis. University of Utrecht

KOVACS, A.B. and BEER, G.Y. (1979) The mechanical properties and qualities of floors for pigs in relation to limb disorders. *The Pig Veterinary Society Proceedings*, **5**, 99–104

KRABBE, H. (1864) Observations for Icelanders on hydatids and precautions against them. J. Schultz (Copenhagen). Translated by Maxwell, I.R. (1973). *Australian Veterinary Journal*, **49**, 395–401

KRAL, F. (1966) Canine pruritus (desire for scratching). *Animal Hospital*, **2**, 40–43

KUHN, T.S. (1970) *The Structure of Scientific Revolutions*. International Encyclopaedia of Unified Science, Vol. 2, No. 2, 2nd edn. University of Chicago Press, Chicago and London

KUPPER, L.L. and HOGAN, M.D. (1978) Interaction in epidemiologic studies. *American Journal of Epidemiology*, **103**, 447–453

LANGMUIR, A.D. (1965) Developing concepts in surveillance. *The Millbank Memorial Fund Quarterly*, **43**, (2), 369–372

LAST, J.M. (1983) *A Dictionary of Epidemiology*. Oxford University Press, New York

LEBEAU, A. (1953) L'age du chien et celui de l'homme. Essai de statistique sur la mortalite canine. *Bulletin de l'Academie Veterinaire de France*, **26**, 229–232

LEECH, A., HOWARTH, R.J., THORNTON, I. and LEWIS, G. (1982) Incidence of bovine copper deficiency in England and the Welsh borders. *Veterinary Record*, **111**, 203–204

LEECH, F.B. (1980) Relations between objectives and observations in epidemiological studies. In: *Veterinary Epidemiology and Economics*. Proceedings of the Second International Symposium, Canberra, 7–11 May 1979. Eds Geering, W.A., Roe, R.T. and Chapman, L.A. Pp. 254–257. Australian Government Publishing Services, Canberra

LEIMBACHER, F. (1978) Experience with the 'Mt' system of forecasting fascioliasis in France. In: *Weather and Parasitic Animal Disease*. Pp. 6–13. World Meteorological Organization Technical Note No. 159

LEPISSIER, H.E. and MacFARLANE, I.M. (1966) Organisation for African Unity. Scientific, Technical and Research Commission. Joint Campaign against rinderpest. Phase I Final Report, November 1965. *Bulletin of Epizootic Diseases of Africa*, **14**, 193–224

LESCH, T.E. (Ed.) (1981) Symposium on herd health management—dairy cow. *Veterinary Clinics of North America: Large Animal Practice*, **3**, 251–490

LEVINE, J.M. and HOHENBOKEN, W. (1982). Modelling of beef production systems. *World Animal Review*, **43**, 33–39

LIENHARDT, G. (1961) *Divinity and Experience, the Religion of the Dinka*. Oxford University Press, Oxford

LIESS, B. and PLOWRIGHT, W. (1964) Studies on the pathogenesis of rinderpest in experimental cattle. I. Correlations of clinical signs, viraemia and virus excretion by various routes. *Journal of Hygiene, Cambridge*, **62**, 81–100

LILIENFELD, A.M. and LILIENFELD, D.E. (1980) *Foundations of Epidemiology*, 2nd edn. Oxford University Press, New York

LILIENFELD, D.E. (1978) Definitions of epidemiology. *American Journal of Epidemiology*, **107**, 87–90

LINDEMANN, R.L. (1942) The trophic dynamic aspects of ecology. *Ecology*, **36**, 587–600

LINKLATER, K.A. and SPEEDY, A.W. (1980) Health and management programmes for lowland sheep flocks. Paper presented at the British Veterinary Association's annual congress, September 14, York. Unpublished

LISTER, D. and GREGORY, N.G. (Eds) (1978) *The Use of Blood Metabolites in Animal Production*. Proceedings of a symposium organized by the British Society of Animal Production, Harrogate, March 1976. BSAP occasional publication No. 1. British Society of Animal Production, Milton Keynes

LITTLE, I.M.D. and MIRRLEES, J.A. (1974) *Project Appraisal and Planning for Developing Countries*. Heinemann, London

LITTLE, T.W.A., SWAN, C., THOMPSON, H.V. and WILESMITH, J.W. (1982) Bovine tuberculosis in domestic and wild mammals in an area of Dorset. II. The badger population, its ecology and tuberculosis status. *Journal of Hygiene, Cambridge*, **89**, 211–224

LORD, R.D. (1983) Ecological strategies for the prevention and control of health problems. *Bulletin of the Pan American Health Organization*, **17**, 19–34

LORD, R.D., CALISHER, C.H., METZGER, W.R. and FISCHER, G.W. (1974) Urban St. Louis encephalitis surveillance through wild birds. *American Journal of Epidemiology*, **99**, 360–363

LORENZ, K. (1977) *Behind the Mirror: A Search for the Natural History of Human Knowledge*. Methuen, London

LORENZ, M.D. and SCHALL, W.D. (1977) Modified problem oriented record for 5 × 8 cards. *Journal of the American Animal Hospitals Association*, **13**, 323–327

LOTKA, A.J. (1925) *Elements of Physical Biology*. Williams and Wilkins, Baltimore

LUCEY, S., ROWLANDS, G.J. and RUSSELL, A.M. (1984) A statistical technique for quantifying short term effects of disease on milk yield. In: Society for Veterinary Epidemiology and Preventive Medicine Proceedings, Edinburgh, 10–11 July 1984. Ed. Thrusfield, M.V. Pp. 184–190

LUCKINS, A.G. and GRAY, A.R. (1983) Interference with anti-trypanosome immune responses in rabbits infected with cyclically-transmitted *Trypanosoma congolense*. *Parasite Immunology*, **5**, 547–556

LUTNAES, B. and SIMENSEN, E. (1983) An epidemiological study of abomasal bloat in young lambs. *Preventive Veterinary Medicine*, **1**, 335–345

MacDONALD, D.W. and BACON, P.J. (1980) To control rabies: vaccinate foxes. *New Scientist*, **87**, 640–645

MacKINTOSH, C.G., SCHOLLUM, L.M., HARRIS, R.E., BLACKMORE, D.K., WILLIS, A.F., COOK, N.R. *et al.* (1980) Epidemiology of leptospirosis in dairy farm workers in the Manawatu. Part I: A cross-sectional serological survey and associated occupational factors. *New Zealand Veterinary Journal*, **28**, 245–250

MacMAHON, B. (1972) Concepts of multiple factors. In: *Multiple Factors in the Causation of Environmentally Induced Disease*. Fogarty International Center Proceedings No. 12. Eds Lee, D.H.K. and Kotin, P. Pp. 1–12. Academic Press, New York and London

MacMAHON, B. and PUGH, T.F. (1970) *Epidemiology, Principles and Methods*. Little Brown and Company, Boston

MacVEAN, D.W., MONLUX, A.W., ANDERSON, P.S., SILBERG, S.L. and ROSZEL, J.F. (1978) Frequency of canine and feline tumours in a defined population. *Veterinary Pathology*, **15**, 700–715

MADDY, K.T. (1958) Disseminated coccidioidomycosis of the dog. *Journal of the American Veterinary Medical Association*, **132**, 483–489

MAF (1977) *Brucellosis: A Veterinarian's Guide to the Literature*. Ministry of Agriculture and Fisheries, Government Printer, Wellington, New Zealand

MAFF (1976) *Animal Disease Surveillance in Great Britain*. The Report of a Ministry of Agriculture, Fisheries and Food Working Party, May 1976

MAFF (1977) *Animal Disease Report*, **1**, (2), July 1977. Ministry of Agriculture, Fisheries and Food

MAFF/ADAS (1976a) Distribution of Cattle in England and Wales (map). Ministry of Agriculture, Fisheries and Food; Agricultural Development and Advisory Service

MAFF/ADAS (1976b) Distribution of Sheep in England and Wales (map). Ministry of Agriculture, Fisheries and Food; Agricultural Advisory and Development Service

MAFF/ADAS (1976c) Distribution of Pigs in England and Wales (map). Ministry of Agriculture, Fisheries and Food; Agricultural Development Advisory Service

MAFF/DAFS (1984) *Blood Characteristics and the Nutrition of Ruminants*. Ministry of Agriculture, Fisheries and Food; Department of Agriculture and Fisheries for Scotland. Reference book No. 260. Her Majesty's Stationery Office, London

MANTEL, H. and HAENZEL, W. (1959) Statistical aspects of the analysis of data from retrospective studies of disease. *Journal of the National Cancer Institute*, **22**, 719–748

MANTEL, N. (1967) The detection of disease clustering and a generalized regression approach. *Cancer Research*, **27**, 209–220

MARKUSFELD, O. (1985) Relationship between overfeeding, metritis and ketosis in high yielding dairy cows. *Veterinary Record*, **116**, 489–491

MARKUSH, R.E. (1977) Levin's attributable risk statistic for analytic studies and vital statistics. *American Journal of Epidemiology*, **105**, 401–406

MARMOR, M., WILLEBERG, P., GLICKMAN, L.T., PRIESTER, W.A., CYPESS, R.H. and HURVITZ, A.L. (1982) Epizootiologic patterns of diabetes mellitus in dogs. *American Journal of Veterinary Research*, **43**, 465–471

MARTIN, B., MAINLAND, D.D. and GREEN, M.A. (1982) VIRUS: A computer program for herd health and productivity. *Veterinary Record*, **110**, 446–448

MARTIN, C.M. (1964) Interactions of hydrocarbon carcinogens with viruses and nucleic acids in vivo and in vitro. *Progress in Experimental Tumor Research*, **5**, 134–156

MARTIN, P.M., COTARD, M., MIALOT, J.-P., ANDRE, F. and RAYNAUD, J.-P. (1984) Animal models for hormone-dependent human breast cancer. Relationship between steroid receptor profiles in canine and feline mammary tumors and survival rate. *Cancer Chemotherapy and Pharmacology*, **12**, 13–17

MARTIN, S.W. (1977) The evaluation of tests. *Canadian Journal of Comparative Medicine*, **41**, 19–25

MARTIN, S.W. and WIGGINS, A.D. (1973) A model of the economic costs of dairy calf mortality. *American Journal of Veterinary Research*, **34**, 1027–1031

MARTIN, S.W., MEEK, A.H., DAVIS, D.G., JOHNSON, J.A. and CURTIS, R.A. (1982) Factors associated with mortality and treatment costs in feedlot calves: The Bruce County beef project, years 1978, 1979, 1980. *Canadian Journal of Comparative Medicine*, **46**, 341–349

MASLAKOV, V.I. (1968) On the problem of the elimination of communicable diseases. *Zeichift für Mikrobiologie, Epidemiologie und Immunologie*, **45**, 118–122

McALLUM, H.J.F. (1985) Stress and postcapture myopathy in red deer. In: *Biology of Deer Production*. Proceedings of an international conference, Dunedin, New Zealand, 13–18 February 1983. Eds Fennessy, P.F. and Drew, K.R. Pp. 65–72. Bulletin 22. The Royal Society of New Zealand, Wellington

McCAULEY, E.H. (1985) Hog cholera in Honduras. Evaluation of the economic and technical aspects of the impact on production and consequences of vaccination programs; and report of 1985 owner survey results, February–April 1985. College of Veterinary Medicine, Department of Large Animal Clincal Sciences, University of Minnesota

McCAULEY, E.H., AULAQI, N.A., SUNDQUIST, W.B., NEW, J.C. and MILLER, W.M. (1977). A study of the potential economic impact of foot-and-mouth disease in the United States. *Proceedings of the Annual Meeting of the United States Animal Health Association*, **81**, 284–296

McCAULEY, E.H., MAJID, A.A., TAYEB, A. and BUSHARA, H.O. (1983a) Clinical diagnosis of schistosomiasis in Sudanese cattle. *Tropical Animal Health and Production*, **15**, 129–136

McCAULEY, E.H., TAYEB, A. and MAJID, A.A. (1983b) Owner survey of schistosomiasis mortality in Sudanese cattle. *Tropical Animal Health and Production*, **15**, 227–233

McCREA, C.T. and HEAD, K.W. (1978) Sheep tumours in north-east Yorkshire. I. Prevalence on seven moorland farms. *British Veterinary Journal*, **134**, 454–461

McCREA, C.T. and HEAD, K.W. (1981) Sheep tumours in north-east Yorkshire. II. Experimental production of tumours. *British Veterinary Journal*, **137**, 21–30

McKINNELL, R.G. and ELLIS, V.L. (1972) Epidemiology of the frog renal tumour and the significance of tumour nuclear transplantation studies to a viral aetiology of the tumour—a review. In: *Oncogenesis and Herpesviruses*. Proceedings of a symposium held at Christ's College, Cambridge, 20–25 June 1971. Eds Biggs, P.M., de-The, G. and Payne, L.N. IARC Scientific Publications No. 2. International Agency for Research on Cancer, Lyon

McLAUCHLAN, J.D. and HENDERSON, W.M. (1947) The occurrence of foot-and-mouth disease in the hedgehog under natural conditions. *Journal of Hygiene, Cambridge*, **45**, 474–479

McMILLAN, B.C. and HANSON, R.P. (1983) Oligonucleotide fingerprinting—a tool for Newcastle Disease virus epidemiology. In: Proceedings of the Third International Symposium on Veterinary Epidemiology and Economics. Arlington, Virginia, 6–10 September 1982. Pp. 577–580. Veterinary Medical Publishing Company, Edwardsville

McNEIL, P.H., RHODES, A.P. and WILLIS, B.H. (1984) *A Flock Health and Productivity Service for New Zealand*. Report of a trial involving ten farms in the Dannevirke area, November 1979–June 1983. Veterinary Services Council, New Zealand

McTAGGART, H.S., LAING, A.H., IMLAH, P., HEAD, K.W. and BROWNLIE, S.E. (1979) The genetics of hereditary lymphosarcoma of pigs. *Veterinary Record*, **105**, 36

MEISCHKE, H.R.C., RAMSEY, W.R. and SHAW, F.D. (1974) The effect of horns on bruising in cattle. *Australian Veterinary Journal*, **50**, 432–434

MELLAART, J.C. (1967) *Catal Huyuk*. McGraw-Hill, New York

MELLOR, P.S., JENNINGS, D.M., WILKINSON, P.J. and BOORMAN, J.P.T. (1985) *Culicoides imicola*: a bluetongue virus vector in Spain and Portugal. *Veterinary Record*, **116**, 589–590

MERRIAM, C.H. (1893) *The Geographic Distribution of Life in North America*. Smithsonian Institute Annual Report. Pp. 365–415

MERRY, D.L. and KOLAR, J.R. (1984) A comparative study of four rabies vaccines. *Veterinary Medicine and Small Animal Clinician*, **79**, 661–664

MIETTINEN, O.S. (1970) Matching and design efficiency in retrospective studies. *American Journal of Epidemiology*, **91**, 111–118

MIETTINEN, O.S. (1972) Components of the crude risk ratio. *American Journal of Epidemiology*, **96**, 168–172

MIETTINEN, O.S. (1974) Proportion of disease caused or prevented by a given exposure, trait or intervention. *American Journal of Epidemiology*, **99**, 325–332

MIETTINEN, O.S. (1976) Estimability and estimation in case-referent studies. *American Journal of Epidemiology*, **103**, 226–235

MILLAR, R. and FRANCIS, J. (1974) The relation of clinical and bacteriological findings to fertility in thoroughbred mares. *Australian Veterinary Journal*, **50**, 351–355

MILNE, A. (1950) The ecology of the sheep tick, *Ixodes ricinus* (L.). Spatial distribution. *Parasitology*, **41**, 189–207

MIMS, C.A. (1982) *The Pathogenesis of Infectious Disease*, 2nd edn. Academic Press, London and New York

MISHAN, E.J. (1976) *Elements of Cost-Benefit Analysis*. George Allen and Unwin, London

MONAGHAN, M.L.M. and HANNAN, J. (1983) Abattoir survey of bovine kidney disease. *Veterinary Record*, **113**, 55–57

MONATH, T.P., NEWHOUSE, V.F., KEMP, G.E., SETZER, H.W. and CACCIAPUOTI, A. (1974) Lassa virus isolation from *Mastomys natalensis* rodents during an epidemic in Sierra Leone. *Science*, **185**, 263–265

MONTGOMERY, R.D., STEIN, G., STOTTS, V.D. and SETTLE, F.H. (1979) The 1978 epornitic of avian cholera on the Chesapeake Bay. *Avian Diseases*, **23**, 966–978

MOORHOUSE, P.D. and HUGH-JONES, M.E. (1981) Serum banks. *The Veterinary Bulletin*, **51**, 277–290

MORANT, S.V. (1984) Factors affecting reproductive performance including the importance and effect of problem cows. In: *Dairy Cow Fertility*. Proceedings of a joint British Veterinary Association and British Society of Animal Production conference, Bristol University, 28–29 June 1984. Eds Eddy, R.G. and Ducker, M.J. Pp. 15–23. British Veterinary Association, London

MORGENSTERN, H., KLEINBAUM, D.G. and KUPPER, L. (1980) Measures of disease incidence used in epidemiologic research. *International Journal of Epidemiology*, **9**, 97–104

MORLEY, F.H.W., WATT, B.R., GRANT, I.McL. and GALLOWAY, D.B. (1983) A flock health and production program for sheep. In: Proceedings of the Third International Symposium on Veterinary Epidemiology and Economics. Arlington, Virginia, 6–10 September 1982. Pp.

186–194. Veterinary Medical Publishing Company, Edwardsville

MORRIS, R.S. (1982) New techniques in veterinary epidemiology—providing workable answers to complex problems. In: *Epidemiology in Animal Health*. Proceedings of a symposium held at the British Veterinary Association's Centenary Congress, Reading, 22–25 September 1982. Pp. 1–16. Society for Veterinary Epidemiology and Preventive Medicine

MORRIS, R.S. and MEEK, A.H. (1980) Measurement and evaluation of the economic effects of parasitic disease. *Veterinary Parasitology*, **6**, 165–184

MORRIS, R.S., WILLIAMSON, N.B., BLOOD, D.C., CANNON, R.M. and CANNON, C.M. (1978a) A health program for commercial dairy herds. 3. Changes in reproductive performance. *Australian Veterinary Journal*, **54**, 231–246

MORRIS, R.S., BLOOD, D.C., WILLIAMSON, N.B., CANNON, C.M. and CANNON, R.M. (1978b) A health program for commercial dairy herds. 4. Changes in mastitis prevalence. *Australian Veterinary Journal*, **54**, 247–251

MORRISON, R.B. and MORRIS, R.S. (1985) RESPITE: A computer-aided guide to the prevalence of pneumonia in pig herds. *Veterinary Record*, **117**, 268–271

MORROW, D.A. (1980) Examination schedule for a dairy reproductive health programme. In: *Current Therapy in Theriogenology*, Ed. Morrow, D.A. Pp. 549–562. W.B. Saunders Company, Philadelphia, London, Toronto

MOULDER, J.W. (1974) Intracellular parasitism: life in an extreme environment. *Journal of Infectious Diseases*, **130**, 300–306

MUIRHEAD, M.R. (1976) Veterinary problems of intensive pig husbandry. *Veterinary Record*, **99**, 288–292

MUIRHEAD, M.R. (1978a) Veterinary services in intensive pig production in England. *The Pig Veterinary Society Proceedings*, **3**, 1–19

MUIRHEAD, M.R. (1978b) Intensive pig production: studies in preventive medicine. Fellowship thesis. Royal College of Veterinary Surgeons

MUIRHEAD, M.R. (1980) The pig advisory visit in preventive medicine. *Veterinary Record*, **106**, 170–173

MURRAY, J. (1968) Some aspects of ovicaprid and pig breeding in neolithic Europe. In: *Studies in Ancient Europe. Essays presented to Stuart Piggott*. Eds Coles, J.M. and Simpson, D.A.A. Pp. 71–81. Leicester University Press, Leicester

MURRAY, M., MORRISON, W.I., MURRAY, P.K., CLIFFORD, D.J. and TRAIL, J.C.M. (1979) Trypanotolerance—a review. *World Animal Review*, **31**, 2–12

MUSSMAN, H.C., McCALLON, W.R. and OTTO, E. (1980) Planning and implementation of animal disease control programs in developing countries. In: *Veterinary Epidemiology and Economics*. Proceedings of the Second International symposium, Canberra, 7–11 May 1979. Eds Geering, W.A., Roe, R.T. and Chapman, L.A. Pp. 551–557. Australian Government Publishing Service, Canberra

NEITZ, W.O. (1948) Immunological studies on bluetongue in sheep. *Onderstepoort Journal of Veterinary Science*, **23**, 93–135

NEWELL, K.W., ROSS, A.D. and RENNER, R.M. (1984) Phenoxy and picolinic acid herbicides and small intestinal adenocarcinoma in sheep. *Lancet*, ii, 1301–1305

NICHOLLS, T.J., BARTON, M.G. and ANDERSON, B.P. (1981) An outbreak of mastitis in dairy cows due to *Pseudomonas aeruginosa* contamination of dry-cow therapy at manufacture. *Veterinary Record*, **108**, 93–96

NIE, N.H., HULL, C.H., JENKINS, J.G., STEINBRENNER, K. and BRENT, D.A. (1977) *Statistical Packages for the Social Sciences*. McGraw Hill, New York

NILSSON, S.A. (1978) Bovine laminitis and sequelae of it. In: Report on the Second Symposium on Bovine Digital Disease, 25–28 September 1978, Skara, Sweden. Unpaginated

NOORDHUIZEN, J.P.T.M. (1984) Veterinary herd health and production control on dairy farms. Offsetdrukkerij Kanters B.V. (Alblasserdam, The Netherlands). PhD thesis. University of Utrecht

NOORDHUIZEN, J.P.T.M. and BUURMAN, J. (1984) Veterinary automated management and production control programme for dairy herds (VAMPP). The application of MUMPS for data processing. *The Veterinary Quarterly*, **6**, 62–77

NORDENSTAM, T. and TORNEBOHM, H. (1979) Research, ethics and development. *Zeitschrift für Allgemeine Wissensschaftstheorie*, **10**, 54–66

NORTON-GRIFFITHS, M. (1978) *Counting Animals*. 2nd edn. African Wildlife Leadership Foundation, Nairobi

ODEND'HAL, S. (1983) *The Geographical Distribution of Animal Viral Diseases*. Academic Press, New York and London

OLDHAM, P.D. (1968) *Measurement in Medicine. The Interpretation of Numerical Data*. The English Universities Press Limited, London

OLLERENSHAW, C.B. (1966) The approach to forecasting the incidence of fascioliasis over England and Wales, 1958–1962. *Agricultural Meteorology*, (**1/2**), 35–54

OLLERENSHAW, C.B. and ROWLANDS, W.T. (1959) A method of forecasting the incidence of fascioliasis in Anglesey. *Veterinary Record*, **71**, 591–598

OSBORNE, C.A. (1975) The transition of quality patient care from an art to a science: The problem oriented concept. *Journal of the American Animal Hospitals Association*, **11**, 250–260

OWEN, J.M. (1985) Preventive medicine in stud and stable. In: Society for Veterinary Epidemiology and Preventive Medicine, Proceedings, Reading, 27–29 March 1985. Ed. Thrusfield, M.V. Pp. 56–60

*OXFORD ENGLISH DICTIONARY* (1972) *A Supplement to the Oxford English Dictionary*. Ed. Burchfield, R.W. Oxford University Press, London

PAGE, E.S. (1961) Cumulative sum charts. *Technometrics*, **3**, 1–9

PARSONS, J.H. (1982) Funding of control measures. In: *The Control of Infectious Diseases in Farm Animals*. British Veterinary Association Trust Project on the future of animal health control, London. Pp. 58–62

PATON, G. and GETTINBY, G. (1983) The control of a parasitic nematode population in sheep represented by a discrete time network with stochastic inputs. *Proceedings of the Royal Irish Academy*, **83B**, 267–280

PATON, G. and GETTINBY, G. (1985) Comparing control strategies for parasitic gastro-enteritis in lambs grazed on previously contaminated pasture: a network modelling approach. *Preventive Veterinary Medicine*, **3**, 301–310

PATTERSON, D.F. (1968) Epidemiologic and genetic studies of congenital heart disease in the dog. *Circulation Research*, **23**, 171–202

PATTERSON, D.F. (1980) A catalog of genetic disorders of

the dog. In: *Current Veterinary Therapy VII. Small Animal Practice*. Ed. Kirk, R.W. Pp. 82–103. W.B. Saunders Company, Philadelphia

PATTERSON, D.F. and MEDWAY, W. (1966) Hereditary diseases of the dog. *Journal of the American Veterinary Medical Association*, **149**, 1741–1754

PAUL, J.R. and WHITE, C. (Eds) (1973) *Serological Epidemiology*. Academic Press, New York and London

PAVLOVSKY, E.N. (1964) *Prirodnaya Ochagovost' Transmissivnykh Bolezney v Svyazi s Landshaftnoy Epidemiologiey Zooantroponozo*. Translated as *Natural Nidality of Transmissible Disease with Special Reference to the Landscape Epidemiology of Zooanthroponoses*. F.K. Plous (translator), N.D. Levine (editor) 1966. University of Illinois Press, Urbana

PAYNE, A.M. (1963) Basic concepts of eradication. *American Review of Respiratory Diseases*, **88**, 449–455

PAYNE, J.M., DEW, SALLY M., MANSTON, R. and FAULKS, MARGARET (1970) The use of a metabolic profile test in dairy herds. *Veterinary Record*, **87**, 150–158

PAYNE, L.N. (1982) Breeding resistant stock. In: *The Control of Infectious Diseases in Farm Animals*. British Veterinary Association Trust Project on the future of animal health control, London. Pp. 37–42

PEARCE, D.W. (1971) *Cost-Benefit Analysis*. The Macmillan Press Limited, London

PEARCE, D.W. and STURMEY, S.G. (1966) Private and social costs and benefits: a note on terminology. *Economic Journal*, March, pp. 152–158

PEARSON, R.A. (1983) Prevention of foot lesions in broiler breeder hens kept in individual cages. *British Poultry Science*, **24**, 183–190

PENNY, R.H.C., CAMERON, R.D.A., JOHNSON, S., KENYON, P.J., SMITH, H.A., BELL, A.W.P. *et al.* (1980) Foot rot of pigs: the influence of biotin supplementation on foot lesions in sows. *Veterinary Record*, **107**, 350–351

PERAINO, C., FRY, R.J.M. and STAFFELDT, E. (1977) Effects of varying the onset and duration of exposure to phenobarbital on its enhancement of 2-acetylaminofluorene-induced hepatic tumorigenesis. *Cancer Research*, **37**, 3623–3627

PERALTA, E.A., CARPENTER, T.E. and FARVER, T.B. (1982) The application of time series analysis to determine the pattern of foot-and-mouth disease in cattle in Paraguay. *Preventive Veterinary Medicine*, **1**, 27–36

PERRY, B.D. and McCAULEY, E.H. (1984) Owner interview surveys as a basis for estimating animal productivity and disease impact in developing countries. In: Society for Veterinary Epidemiology and Preventive Medicine, Proceedings, Edinburgh, 10–11 July 1984. Ed. Thrusfield, M.V. Pp. 54–62

PERRY, B.D., MATTHEWMAN, R.W., EICHER, E. and SNACKEN, M. (1983) An evaluation of the efficacy of a questionnaire survey by comparison with data from sentinel herds. In: Proceedings of the Third International Symposium on Veterinary Epidemiology and Economics. Arlington, Virginia, 6–10 September, 1982. P. 667. Veterinary Medical Publishing Company, Edwardsville

PERRY, B.D., MWANAUMA, B., SCHELS, H.F., EICHER, E. and ZAMAN, M.R. (1984a) A study of health and productivity in traditionally managed cattle in Zambia. *Preventive Veterinary Medicine*, **2**, 633–653

PERRY, B.D., PALMER, J.E., BIRCH, J.B., MAGNUSSON, R.A., MORRIS, D. and TROUTT, H.F. (1984b) Epidemiological characterization of an acute equine diarrhoea syndrome: the case-control approach. In: Society for Veterinary Epidemiology and Preventive Medicine, Proceedings, Edinburgh, 10–11 July 1984. Ed. Thrusfield, M.V. Pp. 148–153

PERRY, B.D., PALMER, J.E., TROUTT, H.F., BIRCH, J.B., MORRIS, D., EHRICH, M. and RIKIHISA, Y. (1986) A case-control study of Potomac horse fever. *Preventive Veterinary Medicine*. In press

PETERS, A.R. (1985) An estimation of the economic impact of an outbreak of *Salmonella dublin* in a calf rearing unit. *Veterinary Record*, **117**, 667–668

PETERS, J.A. (1969) Canine mastocytoma: excess risk as related to ancestry. *Journal of the National Cancer Institute*, **42**, 435–443

PETERSE, D.J. and ANTONISSE, W. (1981) Genetic aspects of feet soundness in cattle. *Livestock Production Science*, **8**, 253–261

PETERSEN, G.V. (1983) The effect of swimming lambs and subsequent resting periods on the ultimate pH of meat. *Meat Science*, **9**, 237–246

PETO, R. (1977) Epidemiology, multistage models and short-term mutagenicity tests. In: *Origins of Human Cancer*. Eds Hiatt, H.H., Watson, J.D. and Winsten, J.A. Pp. 1403–1429. Cold Spring Harbor Laboratory, New York

PHARO, H.J. (1983) DAISY—Health and fertility monitoring for dairy herds. In: Society for Veterinary Epidemiology and Preventive Medicine, Proceedings, Southampton, 12–13 April 1983. Ed. Thrusfield, M.V. Pp. 37–44

PHARO, H.J., ESSLEMONT, R.J. and PUTT, S.N.H. (1984) Assessing the benefits and costs of a computerised information system in dairy herd management. In: Society for Veterinary Epidemiology and Preventive Medicine, Proceedings, Edinburgh, 10–11 July 1984. Ed. Thrusfield, M.V. Pp. 80–89

PIERREPOINT, C.G. (1985) Possible benefits to veterinary medicine of considering the dog as a model for human cancer. *Journal of Small Animal Practice*, **26**, 43–47

PIERREPOINT, C.G., THOMAS, S. and EATON, C.L. (1984) Hormones and cancer. In: *Progress in Cancer Research and Therapy*, Vol. 31. Eds Bresciani, F., King, R.J.B., Lippman, M.E., Namer, M. and Raynaud, J.-P. Pp. 357–365. Raven Press, New York

PIKE, M.C. and CASAGRANDE, J.T. (1979) Re: cost considerations and sample size requirements in cohort and case-control studies (letter). *American Journal of Epidemiology*, **110**, 100–102

PIKE, M.C. and SMITH, P.G. (1968) Disease clustering: a generalization of Knox's approach to the detection of space-time interactions. *Biometrics*, **24**, 541–556

PILCHARD, E.I. (1979) The world situation for animal health and disease information. *Journal of the American Veterinary Medical Association*, **175**, 1297–1300

PINNEY, M.E. (1981) How I learned to live with the computer. *Veterinary Record*, **109**, 431–432

PISANO, R.G. and STORER, T.I. (1948) Burrows and feeding of the Norway rat. *Journal of Mammalogy*, **29**, 374–383

PIVNICK, H. and NURMI, E. (1982) The Nurmi concept and its role in the control of *Salmonellae* in poultry. In: *Developments in Food Microbiology—1*. Ed. Davies, R. Pp. 41–70. Applied Science Publishers Ltd, Barking

PLACKETT, P. and ALTON, G.G. (1975) A mechanism for prozone formation in the complement fixation test for bovine brucellosis. *Australian Veterinary Journal*, **52**, 136–140

PLACKETT, R.L. (1981) *The Analysis of Categorical Data*, 2nd edn. Charles Griffin and Company, London

PLOWRIGHT, R.C. and PALOHEIMO, J.E. (1977) A theoretical study of population dynamics in the sheep tick. *Theoretical Population Biology*, **12**, 286–297

PLOWRIGHT, W., FERRIS, R.D. and SCOTT, G.R. (1960) Blue wildebeest and the aetiological agent of bovine malignant catarrhal fever. *Nature, London*, **188**, 1167–1169

PLOWRIGHT, W., PERRY, C.T. and GREIG, A. (1974) Sexual transmission of African swine fever virus in the tick, *Ornithodoros moubata porcinus*, Walton. *Research in Veterinary Science*, **17**, 106–113

POLLARD, J.H. (1966) On the use of the direct matrix product in analysing certain stochastic population models. *Biometrika*, **53**, 397–415

POLLITZER, R. and MEYER, K.F. (1961) The ecology of plague. In: *Studies in Disease Ecology*. Ed. May, J.M. Pp. 433–510. Hafner Publishing Company, New York

PORTER, P. (1979) Hazards of recycling enteropathogens (letter). *Veterinary Record*, **105**, 515–516

POWELL, D.G. (1985) International movement of horses and its influence on the spread of infection. In: Society for Veterinary Epidemiology and Preventive Medicine, Proceedings, Reading 27–29 March 1985. Ed. Thrusfield, M.V. Pp. 90–94

PRABHAKARAN, P., SOMAN, M., IYER, R.P. and ABRAHAM, J. (1980) Common disease conditions among cattle slaughtered in Trichur municiple slaughterhouse, a preliminary study. *Kerala Journal of Veterinary Science*, **11**, 159–163

PRATT, D.J., GREENWAY, P.J. and GWYNNE, M.D. (1966) A classification of East African rangeland, with an appendix on terminology. *Journal of Applied Ecology*, **3**, 369–382

PRIESTER, W.A. (1964) *Standard Nomenclature of Veterinary Diseases and Operations*. USHEW/PHS National Cancer Institute, Bethesda, Md. 1st edition revised 1966. 2nd (abridged) edition 1975

PRIESTER, W.A. (1971) *Coding Supplement to Standard Nomenclature of Veterinary Diseases and Operations*. USHEW/PHS National Cancer Institute, Bethesda, Md. Revised 1977

PRIESTER, W.A. (1974a) Canine progressive retinal atrophy: occurrence by age, breed and sex. *American Journal of Veterinary Research*, **35**, 571–574

PRIESTER, W.A. (1974b). Data from eleven United States and Canadian colleges of Veterinary Medicine on pancreatic carcinoma in domestic animals. *Cancer Research*, **34**, 1372–1375

PRIESTER, W.A. (1975) Collecting and using veterinary clinical data. In: *Animal Disease Monitoring*. Eds Ingram, D.G., Mitchell, W.F. and Martin, S.W. Pp. 119–128. Charles C. Thomas, Springfield

PRIESTER, W.A. and MANTEL, N. (1971) Occurrence of tumours in domestic animals. Data from twelve United States and Canadian colleges of Veterinary Medicine. *Journal of the National Cancer Institute*, **47**, 1333–1344

PRIESTER, W.A. and McKAY, F.W. (1980) *The Occurrence of Tumours in Domestic Animals*. National Cancer Institute Monograph Number 54. United States Department of Health and Human Services. National Cancer Institute, Bethesda

PRIMROSE, S.B. (1976) *Bacterial Transduction*. Meadowfield Press, Shildon

PRITCHARD, D.G., CARPENTER, G.A., MORZARIA, S.P., HARKNESS, J.W., RICHARDS, M.S. and BREWER, J.I. (1981) Effect of air filtration on respiratory disease in intensively housed veal calves. *Veterinary Record*, **109**, 5–9

PRITCHARD, D.G., EDWARDS, S., MORZARIA, S.P., ANDREWS, A.H., PETERS, A.R. and GILMOUR, N.J.L. (1983) Case-control studies in the evaluation of serological data from respiratory disease outbreaks in cattle. In: Society for Veterinary Epidemiology and Preventive Medicine, Proceedings, Southampton, 12–13 April 1983. Ed. Thrusfield, M.V. Pp. 131–138

PRITCHARD, D.G., LITTLE, T.W.A., WRATHALL, A.E. and JONES, P. (1985) Epidemiology of leptospirosis in relation to reproductive disease in pigs. *The Pig Veterinary Society Proceedings*, **12**, 65–82

PROTHRO, R.M. (1977) Disease and mobility: a neglected factor in epidemiology. *International Journal of Epidemiology*, **6**, 259–267

PUGSLEY, S.L. (1981) The veterinary computer system at London zoo. In: *A Computerised Veterinary Clinical Data Base*. Ed. Thrusfield, M.V. Proceedings of a symposium, Edinburgh, 30 September 1981. P. 55. Department of Animal Health, Royal (Dick) School of Veterinary Studies, Edinburgh

PURVIS, G.M., OSTLER, D.C., STARR, J., BAXTER, J., BISHOP, J., JAMES, A.D. *et al.* (1979) Lamb mortality in a commercial lowland sheep flock with reference to the influence of climate and economics. *Veterinary Record*, **104**, 241–242

RADOSTITS, O.M. (Ed.) (1983) Symposium on herd health management—cow-calf and feedlot. *Veterinary Clinics of North America: Large Animal Practice*, **5**, 1–209

RADOSTITS, O.M. and BLOOD, D.C. (1985) *Herd Health. A Textbook of Health and Production Management of Agricultural Animals*. W.B. Saunders Company, Philadelphia

REECE, R.L. and BEDDOME, V.D. (1983) Causes of culling and mortality in three flocks of broiler chickens in Victoria during 1979. *Veterinary Record*, **112**, 450–452

REID, J.F.S. and ARMOUR, J. (1978) An economic appraisal of helminth parasites in sheep. *Veterinary Record*, **102**, 4–7

REIF, J.S. (1976) Seasonality, natality and herd immunity in feline panleukopenia. *American Journal of Epidemiology*, **103**, 81–87

REIF, J.S. (1983) Ecologic factors and disease. In: *Textbook of Veterinary Internal Medicine. Volume 1. Diseases of the Dog and Cat*, 2nd edn. Ed. Ettinger, S.J. Pp. 147–173. W.B. Saunders Company, Philadelphia

REIF, J.S. and COHEN, D. (1970) II Retrospective radiographic analysis of pulmonary disease in rural and urban dogs. *Archives of Environmental Health*, **20**, 684–689

REIF, J.S. and COHEN, D. (1971) The environmental distribution of canine respiratory tract neoplasms. *Archives of Environmental Health*, **22**, 136–140

REIF, J.S. and COHEN, D. (1979) Canine pulmonary disease: a spontaneous model for environmental epidemiology. In: *Animals as Monitors of Environmental Pollutants*. Pp. 241–250 National Academy of Sciences, Washington, D.C.

REIF, J.S., MAGUIRE, T.G., KENNEY, R.M. and BRODEY, R.S. (1979) A cohort study of canine testicular neoplasia. *Journal of the American Veterinary Medical Association*, **175**, 719–723

REUTLINGER, S. (1970) *Techniques for Project Appraisal Under Uncertainty*. World Bank Staff Occasional Paper No. 10, Washington, D.C.

RICE, L. (1980a) Reproductive health management in beef cows. In: *Current Therapy in Theriogenology: Diagnosis, Treatment and Prevention of Reproductive Diseases in Animals.* Ed. Morrow, D. Pp. 534–545. W.B. Saunders Company, Philadelphia, London and Toronto

RICE, L. (1980b) Reproductive health program for beef cattle. In: *Current Therapy in Theriogenology: Diagnosis, Treatment and Prevention of Reproductive Diseases in Animals.* Ed. Morrow, D. Pp. 545–548. W.B. Saunders Company, Philadelphia, London and Toronto

RISER, W.H. (1974) Canine hip dysplasia: cause and control. *Journal of the American Veterinary Medical Association,* **164,** 360–362

ROBERTS, D.S. (1969) Synergic mechanisms in certain mixed infections. *Journal of Infectious Diseases,* **120,** 720–724

ROBERTS, L., LAWSON, G.H.K., ROWLAND, A.C. and LAING, A.H. (1979) Porcine intestinal adenomatosis and its detection in a closed pig herd. *Veterinary Record,* **104,** 366–368

ROBERTSON, F.J. (1971) Brucellosis: a possible symptomless carrier. *Veterinary Record,* **88,** 313–314

ROE, R.T. (1980) Features of the Australian National Animal Disease Information System. In: *Veterinary Epidemiology and Economics.* Proceedings of the Second International Symposium, Canberra, 7–11 May 1979. Eds Geering, W.A., Roe, R.T. and Chapman, L.A. Pp. 26–34. Australian Government Publishing Service, Canberra

ROGAN, W.J. and GLADEN, B. (1978) Estimating prevalence from the results of a screening test. *American Journal of Epidemiology,* **107,** 71–76

ROITT, I.M. (1984) *Essential Immunology,* 4th edn. Blackwell Scientific Publications, Oxford

ROSE, N.R. and FRIEDMAN, H. (1980) *Manual of Clinical Immunology,* 2nd edn. American Society for Microbiology, Washington

ROSENBERG, F.J., ASTUDILLO, V.M. and GOIC, R. (1980) Regional strategies for the control of foot-and-mouth disease—an ecological outlook. In: *Veterinary Epidemiology and Economics.* Proceedings of the Second International Symposium, Canberra, 7–11 May 1979. Eds Geering, W.A., Roe, R.T. and Chapman, L.A. Pp. 587–596. Australian Government Publishing Service, Canberra

ROSS, J.G. (1978) Stormont 'wet-day' fluke forecasting. In *Weather and Parasitic Animal Disease.* Pp. 14–20. World Meteorological Organization Technical Note No. 159

ROSSITER, P.B., JESSETT, D.M., WAFULA, J.S., KARSTAD, L., CHEMA, S., TAYLOR, A. *et al.* (1983) Re-emergence of rinderpest as a threat in East Africa since 1979. *Veterinary Record,* **113,** 459–461

ROTH, H.H., KEYMER, I.F. and APPLEBY, E.C. (1973) Computerised data recording from captive and free-living wild animals. *International Zoo Yearbook,* **13,** 252–257

ROTHMAN, K.J. (1975) A pictorial representation of confounding in epidemiologic studies. *Journal of Chronic Diseases,* **28,** 101–108

ROTHMAN, K.J. (1976) Causes. *American Journal of Epidemiology,* **104,** 587–592

ROTHMAN, K.J. (1978) A show of confidence (editorial). *New England Journal of Medicine,* **299,** 1362–1363

ROTHMAN, K.J. and BOICE, J.D. (1982) *Epidemiologic Analysis with a Programmable Calculator.* Epidemiology Resources Inc., Boston

ROUECHÉ, B. (1967) *Annals of Epidemiology.* Little, Brown and Company, Boston

ROWLANDS, G.J. and RUSSELL, A.M. (1985) Remote use of COSREEL over the British Telecom PSS network. In: Society for Veterinary Epidemiology and Preventive Medicine, Proceedings, Reading, 27–29 March 1985. Ed. Thrusfield, M.V. Pp. 115–119

ROY, J.H.B. (1980) *The Calf. Studies in the Agricultural and Food Sciences,* 4th edn. Butterworths, London and Boston

RUPPANNER, R. (1972) Measurement of disease in animal populations based on interviews. *Journal of the American Veterinary Medical Association,* **161,** 1033–1038

RUSSEL, A. (1985) Nutrition of the pregnant ewe. *In Practice,* **7,** 23–28

RUSSELL, A.M. and ROWLANDS, G.J. (1983). COSREEL: Computerised recording system for herd health information management. *Veterinary Record,* **112,** 189–193

RUSSELL, A.M., ROWLANDS, G.J., SHAW, S.R. and WEAVER, A.D. (1982a) Survey of lameness in British dairy cattle. *Veterinary Record,* **111,** 155–160

RUSSELL, A.M., ROWLANDS, G.J. and LUCEY, S. (1982b) *COSREEL Veterinary Coding Manual.* A.R.C. Institute for Research on Animal Diseases, Compton, Berkshire

RUTTER, J.M. (1975) *Escherichia coli* infections in piglets: Pathogenesis, virulence and vaccination. *Veterinary Record,* **96,** 171–175

RUTTER, J.M. (1982) Diseases caused by mixed agents and factors. In: *The Control of Infectious Diseases in Farm Animals.* British Veterinary Association Trust Project on the future of animal health control, London. Pp. 5–10

RYAN, B.F., JOINER, B.L. and RYAN, T.A. (1985) *'Minitab' Handbook,* 2nd edn. Prindle, Weber and Schmidt, Boston

SACKETT, D.I. (1979) Bias in analytic research. *Journal of Chronic Diseases,* **32,** 51–68

SAIDLA, J.F. (1983) Problem-oriented veterinary medical record. In: *Textbook of Veterinary Internal Medicine: Diseases of the Dog and Cat,* Vol. 1, 2nd edn. Ed. Ettinger, S.J. Pp. 29–37. W.B. Saunders Company, Philadelphia

SARD, D.M. (1979) *Dealing with Data. The Practical Use of Numerical Information.* British Veterinary Association Publications, London

SARTWELL, P.E. (1950) The distribution of incubation periods of infectious disease. *American Journal of Hygiene,* **51,** 310–318

SARTWELL, P.E. (1966) The incubation period and the dynamics of infectious disease. *American Journal of Epidemiology,* **83,** 204–216

SARTWELL, P.E. (1973) *Preventive Medicine and Public Health.* Appleton-Century-Crofts, New York

SCHACHTER, J., SUGG, N. and SUNG, M. (1978). Psittacosis: the reservoir persists. *Journal of Infectious Diseases,* **137,** 44–49

SCHEAFFER, R.L., MENDENHALL, W. and OTT, L. (1979) *Elementary Survey Sampling,* 2nd edn. Duxbury Press, Belmont

SCHERER, W.F., MOYER, J.T., IZUMI, T., GRESSER, I. and McCOWN, J. (1959) Ecologic studies of Japanese Encephalitis virus in Japan. VI. Swine infection. *American Journal of Tropical Medicine and Hygiene,* **8,** 698–706

SCHLESSELMAN, J.J. (1982) *Case-control Studies: Design, Conduct, Analysis.* Oxford University Press, New York

SCHMELZER, L.L. and TABERSHAW, I.R. (1968) Exposure factors in occupational coccidioidomycosis. *American Journal of Public Health*, **58**, 107–113

SCHNEIDER, R. (1970) Comparison of age, sex, and incidence rates in human and canine breast cancer. *Cancer*, **26**, 419–426

SCHNEIDER, R. and VAIDA, M.L. (1975) Survey of canine and feline populations: Alameda and Contra Costa Counties, California, 1970. *Journal of the American Veterinary Medical Association*, **167**, 481–486

SCHNEIDER, R., DORN, C.R. and TAYLOR, D.O.N. (1969) Factors influencing canine mammary cancer development and postsurgical survival. *Journal of the National Cancer Institute*, **43**, 1249–1261

SCHNURRENBERGER, P.R., KANGILASKI, E., BERG, L.E. and BASHE, W.J. (1961) Characteristics of a rural Ohio dog population. *Veterinary Medicine*, **56**, 519–523

SCHWABE, C.W. (1980a) Animal disease control. Part I. Developments prior to 1960. *Sudan Journal of Veterinary Science and Animal Husbandry*, **21**, 43–54

SCHWABE, C.W. (1980b) Animal disease control. Part II. Newer methods, with possibility for their application in the Sudan. *Sudan Journal of Veterinary Science and Animal Husbandry*, **21**, 55–65

SCHWABE, C. (1982) The current epidemiological revolution in veterinary medicine. Part 1. *Preventive Veterinary Medicine*, **1**, 5–15

SCHWABE, C.W. (1984) *Veterinary Medicine and Human Health*, 3rd edn. Williams and Wilkins, Baltimore and London

SCHWABE, C.W., RIEMANN, H.P. and FRANTI, C.E. (1977) *Epidemiology in Veterinary Practice*. Lea and Febiger, Philadelphia

SCOTT, R.J. (1981) Zoonoses in the abattoir. In: *Advances in Veterinary Public Health*, Vol. 2. Ed. Senevirata, P. Pp. 68–72. Australian College of Veterinary Scientists, Brisbane

SELBY, L.A., CORWIN, R.M. and HAYES, H.M. (1980) Risk factors associated with canine heartworm infection. *Journal of the American Veterinary Medical Association*, **176**, 33–35

SELBY, L.A., EDMONDS, L.D., PARKE, D.W., STEWART, R.W., MARIENFELD, C.J. and HEIDLAGE, W.F. (1973) Use of mailed questionnaire data in a study of swine congenital malformations. *Canadian Journal of Comparative Medicine*, **37**, 413–417

SELBY, L.A., EDMONDS, L.D. and HYDE, L.D. (1976) Epidemiological field studies of animal populations. *Canadian Journal of Comparative Medicine*, **40**, 135–141

SELLERS, R.F. (1982) Eradication—local and national. In: *The Control of Infectious Diseases in Farm Animals*. British Veterinary Association Trust Project on the future of animal health control, London. Pp. 18–21

SELLERS, R.F. and GLOSTER, J. (1980) The Northumberland epidemic of foot-and-mouth disease, 1966. *Journal of Hygiene, Cambridge*, **85**, 129–140

SELLERS, R.F., PEDGLEY, D.E. and TUCKER, M.R. (1978) Possible windborne spread of bluetongue to Portugal, June–July, 1956. *Journal of Hygiene, Cambridge*, **81**, 189–196

SELYE, H. (1936) A syndrome produced by diverse nocuous agents. *Nature*, **138**, 32

SELYE, H. (1946) The general adaptation syndrome and the diseases of adaptation. *Journal of Clinical Endocrinology*, **6**, 117–230

SHEPS, M.C. (1966) On the person years concept in epidemiology and demography. *Millbank Memorial Fund Quarterly*, **44**, 69–91

SHEWHART, W.A. (1931) *The Economic Control of the Quality of the Manufactured Product*. Macmillan and Company Limited, New York

SIEGEL, S. (1956) *Nonparametric Statistics for the Behavioral Sciences*. McGraw-Hill, New York

SIMMONS, A. and CUTHBERTSON, J.C. (1985) Time series analysis of ovine pneumonia using Scottish slaughterhouse data. In: Society for Veterinary Epidemiology and Preventive Medicine, Proceedings, Reading, 27–29 March 1985. Ed. Thrusfield, M.V. Pp. 130–141

SIMPSON, B.H. (1972) The geographic distribution of carcinomas of the small intestine in New Zealand sheep. *New Zealand Veterinary Journal*, **20**, 24–28

SIMPSON, B.H. and WRIGHT, D.F. (1980) The use of questionnaires to assess the importance of clinical disease in sheep. In: *Veterinary Epidemiology and Economics*. Proceedings of the Second International Symposium, Canberra, 7–11 May 1979. Eds Geering, W.A., Roe, R.T. and Chapman, L.A. Pp. 97–105. Australian Government Publishing Service, Canberra

SINGH, K.P.R., KHORSHED, M.P. and ANDERSON, C.R. (1964) Transmission of Kyasanur Forest Disease virus by *Haemaphysalis turturis*, *Haemaphysalis papuana kinreari* and *Haemaphysalis minuta*. *Indian Journal of Medical Research*, **52**, 566–573

SINNECKER, H. (1976) *General Epidemiology* (translated by Walker, N.). John Wiley and Sons, London

SLOCOMBE, J.O.D. (1975) Surveillance for parasitism in domestic animals. In: *Animal Disease Monitoring*. Eds Ingram, D.G., Mitchell, W.F. and Martin, S.W. Pp. 129–135. Charles C. Thomas, Springfield

SMITH, E.J., KELLY, J.M. and WHITAKER, D.A. (1983) Health and fertility data recorded by members of the Dairy Herd Health and Productivity Service. In: Society for Veterinary Epidemiology and Preventive Medicine, Proceedings, Southampton, 12–13 April 1983. Ed. Thrusfield, M.V. Pp. 8–12

SMITH, J.E. (1977) Analysis of autopsy data on pig respiratory disease by multivariate methods. *British Veterinary Journal*, **133**, 281–291

SMITH, K.G.V. (Ed.) (1973) *Insects and Other Arthropods of Medical Importance*. The Trustees of the British Museum (Natural History), London

SMITH, L.P. and HUGH-JONES, M.E. (1969) The weather factor in foot-and-mouth disease epidemics. *Nature*, **223**, 712–715

SMITH, W.J. (1981) Rectal prolapse in swine. *The Pig Veterinary Society Proceedings*, **7**, 68–72

SMITHCORS, J.F. (1957) *Evolution of the Veterinary Art*. Veterinary Medicine Publishing Company, Kansas

SNEDECOR, G.W. and COCHRAN, W.G. (1980) *Statistical Methods*, 7th edn. Iowa State University Press, Ames, Iowa

SNODGRASS, D.R. (1974) Studies on bovine petechial fever and tick-borne fever. PhD thesis. University of Edinburgh

SNOW, J. (1855) *On the Mode of Communication of Cholera*, 2nd edn. Churchill, London. Reproduced in *Snow on Cholera*. Commonwealth Fund, New York, 1936. Reprinted by Hafner, New York, 1965

SOULSBY, E.J.L. (1982) *Helminths, Arthropods and Protozoa of Domestic Animals*, 7th edn. Baillière Tindall, London

SOUTHWOOD, T.R.E. (1978) *Ecological Methods with Particular Reference to the Study of Insect Populations*, 2nd edn. Chapman and Hall, London

SPEARMAN, C. (1908) The method of 'right and wrong' cases ('constant stimuli') without Gauss's formulae. *British Journal of Psychology*, **2**, 227–242

SPONENBERG, D.P. (1979) The inheritance of pathological conditions in dairy bulls. PhD thesis. Cornell University

STALLBAUMER, M.F. (1983) The prevalence of *Cysticercus tenuicollis* in slaughtered sheep in Britain. In: Society for Veterinary Epidemiology and Preventive Medicine, Proceedings, Southampton, 12–13 April 1983. Ed. Thrusfield, M.V. Pp. 124–130

STEELE, J.H., HENDRICKS, S.L., BARR, R. and PARKER, R.L. (1972) Brucellosis in the United States, 1970. *Archives of Environmental Health*, **25**, 66–72

STEIN, T., MOLITOR, T., JOO, H.S. and LEMAN, A.D. (1982) Porcine parvovirus infection and its control. *The Pig Veterinary Society Proceedings*, **9**, 158–167

STEPHEN, L.E. (1980) An index for coding and recording veterinary diseases and pathological states, according to body system(s) involved and aetiology or indicated cause. In: *Veterinary Epidemiology and Economics*. Proceedings of the Second International Symposium, Canberra, 7–11 May 1979. Eds Geering, W.A., Roe, R.T. and Chapman, L.A. Pp. 247–249. Australian Government Publishing Service, Canberra

STITES, D.P., STOBO, J.D., FUNDENBERG, H.H. and WELLS, J.V. (1982) *Basic and Clinical Immunology*, 4th edn. Lange Medical Publications, Los Altos

STUART-HARRIS, C.H. and SCHILD, G.C. (1976) *Influenza, the Viruses and the Disease*. Edward Arnold Limited, London

SUGDEN, R. and WILLIAMS, A. (1978) *The Principles of Practical Cost-Benefit Analysis*. Oxford University Press, London

SUMMERS, M. (1961) *The Vampire in Europe*. University Books, New York

SUNGUYA, F.P.A. (1981) Disease surveillance, economic losses and trace back of pigs in the abattoir. MSc thesis. University of Edinburgh

TAKIZAWA, T. and ITO, T. (1977) Secular trends of annual morbidities of animal infectious diseases. *National Institute of Animal Health Quarterly*, **17**, 179–183

TAKIZAWA, T., ITO, T. and KOSUGE, M. (1977) Prototype of simulation models for epizootics in domestic animals. *National Institute of Animal Health Quarterly*, **17**, 171–178

TAKIZAWA, T., ITO, T., KOSUGE, M. and MIZUMURA, Y. (1978a) Computer simulation of Gumboro Disease outbreak: I. Construction of models G-1 and G-2. *National Institute of Animal Health Quarterly*, **18**, 164–169

TAKIZAWA, T., ITO, T., KOSUGE, M., TANAKA, T. and MIZUMURA, Y. (1978b) Computer simulation of Gumboro Disease outbreak: II. Results obtained with models G-1 and G-2. *National Institute of Animal Health Quarterly*, **18**, 170–175

TAKIZAWA, T., ITO, T., TANAKA, T. and MIZUMURA, Y. (1980a) Computer simulation of Gumboro Disease outbreak: III. Construction of model G-4. *National Institute of Animal Health Quarterly*, **20**, 60–67

TAKIZAWA, T., ITO, T., TANAKA, T. and MIZUMURA, Y. (1980b) Computer simulation of Gumboro Disease outbreak: IV. Epizootics obtained by Model G-4 with flock size, age and immunity charged. *National Institute of Animal Health Quarterly*, **20**, 68–74

TANSLEY, A.G. (1935) The use and abuse of vegetational concepts and terms. *Ecology*, **16**, 284–307

TAYLOR, H.M. (1968) Some models in epidemic control. *Mathematical Biosciences*, **3**, 383–398

TAYLOR, R. (1967) Causation. In: *The Encyclopaedia of Philosophy*, Vol. 2. Ed. Edwards, P. The Macmillan Company and The Free Press, New York

TAYLOR, W.P. and MARSHALL, I.E. (1975) Adaptation studies with Ross River virus: retention of field level virulence. *Journal of General Virology*, **28**, 73–83

TEDOR, J. and REIF, J.S. (1978) Natal patterns among registered dogs in the United States. *Journal of the American Veterinary Medical Association*, **172**, 1179–1185

TERRIS, M. (1962) Scope and methods of epidemiology. *American Journal of Public Health*, **52**, 1371–1376

THE TIMES (1983) Running dogs banned. *The Times*, 13 October 1983, p. 6

THODAY, K.L. (1980) Canine pruritus: an approach to diagnosis. Stage I. Preliminary investigation. *Journal of Small Animal Practice*, **21**, 399–408

THOMAS, R.J. (1978) Forecasting the onset of nematodiriasis in sheep. In: *Weather and Parasitic Animal Disease*. Pp. 68–73. World Meteorological Organization Technical Note No. 159

THOMAS, S.E. and PIERREPOINT, C.G. (1983) Cytoplasmic steroid effects of nuclear RNA polymerase activity in canine mammary carcinomas. *European Journal of Cancer and Clinical Oncology*, **19**, 377–382

THORBURN, M.A., CARPENTER, T.E., JASPER, D.E. and THOMAS, C.B. (1983) The use of the log-linear model to evaluate the effects of three herd factors on *Streptococcus agalactiae* mastitis occurrence in California, 1977. *Preventive Veterinary Medicine*, **1**, 243–256

THORNS, C.J. and MORRIS, J.A. (1983) The immune spectrum of *Mycobacterium bovis* infection in some mammalian species: a review. *Veterinary Bulletin*, **53**, 543–550

THRUSFIELD, M.V. (Ed.) (1981) *A Computerised Veterinary Clinical Data Base*. Proceedings of a symposium, Edinburgh, 30 September 1981. Department of Animal Health, Royal (Dick) School of Veterinary Studies, Edinburgh

THRUSFIELD, M.V. (1983a) Recording and manipulating clinical data. *Journal of Small Animal Practice*, **24**, 703–717

THRUSFIELD, M.V. (1983b) Application of computer technology to the collection, analysis and use of veterinary data. *Veterinary Record*, **112**, 538–543

THRUSFIELD, M.V. (1985a) How to use a knowledge of epidemiology in practice. *The Pig Veterinary Society Proceedings*, **12**, 25–37

THRUSFIELD, M.V. (1985b) Data recording in general practice. *In Practice*, **7**, 128–138

THRUSFIELD, M.V. (1985c) Association between urinary incontinence and spaying in bitches. *Veterinary Record*, **116**, 695

THRUSFIELD, M.V. and HINXMAN, A.I. (1981) A computerized system for storing and querying clinical case record summaries. *Journal of Small Animal Practice*, **22**, 669–679

THRUSFIELD, M.V. and GETTINBY, G. (1984) An introduction to techniques of veterinary modelling. In: Society for Veterinary Epidemiology and Preventive Medicine. Proceedings, Edinburgh, 10–11 July 1984. Ed. Thrusfield, M.V. Pp. 114–138. (Also published separately, ISBN: 0 948073 01 2)

THRUSFIELD, M.V., AITKEN, C.G.G. and DARKE, P.G.G. (1985) Observations on breed and sex in relation to canine heart valve incompetence. *Journal of Small Animal Practice*, **26**, 709–717

THURMOND, M.C., PORTIER, K.M., PUHR, D.M. and BURRIDGE, M.J. (1983) A prospective investigation of bovine leukemia virus infection in young dairy cattle, using survival methods. *American Journal of Epidemiology*, **117**, 621–631

TIMBS, D.V. (1980) The New Zealand national bovine serum bank. In: *Veterinary Epidemiology and Economics*. Proceedings of the Second International Symposium, Canberra, 7–11 May 1979. Eds Geering, W.A., Roe, R.T. and Chapman, L.A. Pp. 76–80. Australian Government Publishing Service, Canberra

TINLINE, R. (1970) Lee wave hypothesis for the initial pattern of spread during the 1967–68 foot-and-mouth disease epizootic. *Nature*, **227**, 860–862

TINLINE, R. (1972) A simulation study of the 1967–68 foot-and-mouth epizootic in Great Britain. PhD thesis. University of Bristol

TIZARD, I.R. (1982) *An Introduction to Veterinary Immunology*, 2nd edn. W.B. Saunders, Philadelphia

TJALMA, R.A. (1966) Canine bone sarcoma: estimation of relative risk as a function of body size. *Journal of the National Cancer Institute*, **36**, 1137–1150

TREWHELLA, W.R. and ANDERSON, R.M. (1983) Modelling bovine tuberculosis in badgers. In: Society for Veterinary Epidemiology and Preventive Medicine, Proceedings, Southampton, 12–13 April 1983. Ed. Thrusfield, M.V. Pp. 78–84

TROTTER, W. (1930) Observation and experiment and their use in the medical sciences. *British Medical Journal*, ii, 129–134

TROTTER, W. (1932) *Art and Science in Medicine* (quoted by Himsworth, 1970)

TUKEY, J.W. (1977) *Exploratory Data Analysis*. Addison-Wesley Publishing Co., Philippines

TURNER, T. and PEGG, E. (1977) A survey of patent nematode infestations in dogs. *Veterinary Record*, **100**, 284–285

URQUHART, G.M. (1980) Application of immunity in the control of parasitic disease. *Veterinary Parasitology*, **6**, 217–239

USDA (1982) *International Directory of Animal Health and Disease Data Banks*. National Agricultural Library, United States Department of Agriculture. Miscellaneous Publication No. 1423

VANDEGRAAFF, R. (1980) The use of discriminant analysis in a case-control study of salmonellosis in East Gippsland dairy herds. In: *Veterinary Epidemiology and Economics*. Proceedings of the Second International Symposium, Canberra, 7–11 May 1979. Eds Geering, W.A., Roe, R.T. and Chapman, L.A. Pp. 258–263. Australian Government Publishing Service, Canberra

VARLEY, E.M. (1984) The use and potential of VIEWDATA for the veterinary profession. In: Society for Veterinary Epidemiology and Preventive Medicine, Proceedings, Edinburgh, 10–11 July 1984. Ed. Thrusfield, M.V. Pp. 63–70

VECCHIO, T.J. (1966) Predictive value of a single diagnostic test in unselected populations. *New England Journal of Medicine*, **274**, 1171–1173

VERBERNE, L.R.M. and MIRCK, M.H. (1976). A practical health programme for prevention of parasitic and infectious diseases in horses and ponies. *Equine Veterinary Journal*, **8**, 123–125

WALTER, S.D. (1977) Determination of significant relative risks and optimal sampling procedures in prospective and retrospective comparative studies of various sizes. *American Journal of Epidemiology*, **105**, 387–397

WALTERS, J.R. (1978) Problems associated with the movement and marketing of weaners. *The Pig Veterinary Society Proceedings*, **3**, 37–44

WALTNER-TOEWS, D. (1983) Questionnaire design and administration. In: Proceedings of the Third International Symposium on Veterinary Epidemiology and Economics. Arlington, Virginia, 6–10 September 1982. Pp. 31–37. Veterinary Medical Publishing Company, Edwardsville

WALTNER-TOEWS, D., MARTIN, S.W. and MEEK, A.H. (1986) Estimating disease prevalence using a test with no false positives. In: Proceedings of the 4th International Symposium on Veterinary Epidemiology and Economics. Singapore, 18–22 November 1985. Singapore Veterinary Association. In press

WANG, C.Y., CHIU, C.W., PAMUKCU, A.M. and BRYAN, G.T. (1976) Identification of carcinogenic tannin isolated from bracken fern (*Pteridium aquilinum*). *Journal of the National Cancer Institute*, **56**, 33–36

WATHES, C.M., JONES, C.D.R. and WEBSTER, A.J.F. (1983) Ventilation, air hygiene and animal health. *Veterinary Record*, **113**, 554–559

WATSON, J.C. (1982) Food hygiene. Methods of linking meat inspection findings with disease on the farm and in human populations. In: *Epidemiology in Animal Health*. Proceedings of a symposium held at the British Veterinary Association's Centenary Congress, Reading, 22–25 September 1982. Pp. 131–140. Society for Veterinary Epidemiology and Preventive Medicine

WATT, G.E.L. (1980) An approach to determining the prevalence of liver fluke in a large region. In: *Veterinary Epidemiology and Economics*. Proceedings of the Second International Symposium, Canberra, 7–11 May 1979. Eds Geering, W.A., Roe, R.T. and Chapman, L.A. Pp. 152–155. Australian Government Publishing Service, Canberra

WEBB, J.S., THORNTON, I., THOMPSON, M., HOWARTH, R.J. and LOWENSTEIN, P.L. (1978) *The Wolfston Geochemical Atlas of England and Wales*. Oxford University Press, London

WEBSTER, A.J.F. (1981) Weather and infectious disease in cattle. *Veterinary Record*, **108**, 183–187

WEBSTER, A.J.F. (1982) Improvements of environment, husbandry and feeding. In: *The Control of Infectious Diseases in Farm Animals*. British Veterinary Association Trust Project on the future of animal health control, London. Pp. 28–35

WEED, L.L. (1970) *Medical Records, Medical Education and Patient Care. The Problem-oriented Record as a Basic Tool*. Year Book Medical Publishers Inc., Chicago

WEINBERG, R.A. (1983) A molecular basis of cancer. *Scientific American*, **249**, (5), 102–116

WEST, G.P. (1972) *Rabies in Animals and Man*. David and Charles, Newton Abbot

WETHERILL, G.B. (1969) *Sampling Inspection and Quality Control*. Methuen, London

WHEELWRIGHT, S.C. and MAKRIDAKIS, S. (1973) *Forecasting Methods for Management*. Wiley-Interscience, New York

WHITAKER, D.A. (1978) Herd health programmes in dairy cattle. MVSc thesis. University of Sydney

WHITAKER, D.A., KELLY, J.M. and SMITH, E.J. (1983a) Incidence of lameness in dairy cows. *Veterinary Record*, **113**, 60–62

WHITAKER, D.A., KELLY, J.M. and SMITH, E.J. (1983b) Subclinical ketosis and serum beta hydroxybutyrate levels in dairy cattle. *British Veterinary Journal*, **139**, 462–463

WHITE, M.E. and VELLAKE, E. (1980) A coding system for veterinary clinical signs. *Cornell Veterinarian*, **70**, 160–182

WHO (1959) *Immunological and Haematological Surveys*. Report of a study group. World Health Organization Technical Report Series No. 181

WHO (1970) *Multipurpose Serological Surveys and WHO Serum Reference Banks*. Report of a World Health Organization scientific group. World Health Organization Technical Report Series No. 454

WHO (1973) *Adequacy of Sample Size*. Health Statistical Methodology Unit. World Health Organization Publication HSM/73.1. World Health Organization, Geneva

WHO (1978) Proposals for the nomenclature of salivarian trypanosomes and for the nomenclature of reference collections. *Bulletin of the World Health Organization*, **56**, 467–480

WHO (1980) A revision of the system of nomenclature for influenza A viruses: a WHO memorandum. *Bulletin of the World Health Organization*, **58**, 585–591

WIERUP, M. (1983) The Swedish canine parvovirus epidemic—an epidemiological study in a dog population of defined size. *Preventive Veterinary Medicine*, **1**, 273–288

WILESMITH, J.W., LITTLE, T.W.A., THOMPSON, H.V. and SWAN, C. (1982) Bovine tuberculosis in domestic and wild mammals in an area of Dorset. I. Tuberculosis in cattle. *Journal of Hygiene, Cambridge*, **89**, 195–210

WILLEBERG, P. (1975a) A case-control study of some fundamental determinants in the epidemiology of the feline urological syndrome. *Nordisk Veterinaermedicin*, **27**, 1–14

WILLEBERG, P. (1975b) Diets and the feline urological syndrome, a retrospective case-control study. *Nordisk Veterinaermedicin*, **27**, 15–19

WILLEBERG, P. (1975c) Outdoor activity level as a factor in the feline urological syndrome. *Nordisk Veterinaermedicin*, **27**, 523–524

WILLEBERG, P. (1976) Interaction effects of epidemiologic factors in the feline urological syndrome. *Nordisk Veterinaermedicin*, **28**, 193–200

WILLEBERG, P. (1977) Animal disease information processing: epidemiologic analyses of the feline urological syndrome. *Acta Veterinaria Scandinavica*, **18**, Suppl. 64, 1–48

WILLEBERG, P. (1979) The Danish swine slaughter inspection data bank and some epidemiological applications. In: Proceedings of an international symposium on animal health and disease data banks, 4–6 December 1978, Washington D.C. Pp. 133–145. United States Department of Agriculture. Miscellaneous Publication Number 1381

WILLEBERG, P. (1980a) Abattoir surveillance in Denmark. *The Pig Veterinary Society Proceedings*, **6**, 43–54

WILLEBERG, P. (1980b) The analysis and interpretation of epidemiological data. In: *Veterinary Epidemiology and Economics*. Proceedings of the Second International Symposium on Veterinary Epidemiology and Economics, Canberra, 7–11 May 1979. Eds Geering, W.A., Roe, R.T. and Chapman, L.A. Pp. 185–198. Australian Government Publishing Service, Canberra

WILLEBERG, P. (1981) Epidemiology of the feline urological syndrome. *Advances in Veterinary Science*, **25**, 311–344

WILLEBERG, P. and PRIESTER, W.A. (1976) Feline urological syndrome: association with some time, space, and individual patient factors. *American Journal of Veterinary Research*, **37**, 975–978

WILLEBERG, P., GERBOLA, M-A., MADSEN, A., MANDRUP, M., NIELSEN, E.K., RIEMANN, H.P. *et al*. (1978) A retrospective study of respiratory disease in a cohort of bacon pigs: I. Clinico-epidemiological analyses. *Nordisk Veterinaermedicin*, **30**, 513–525

WILLEBERG, P., GERBOLA, M-A., KIRKEGAARD PETERSEN, B. and ANDERSEN, J.B. (1984) The Danish pig health scheme; nationwide computer-based abattoir surveillance and follow-up at the herd level. *Preventive Veterinary Medicine*, **3**, 79–91

WILLIAMS, G.W. (1984) Time-space clustering of disease. In: *Statistical Methods for Cancer Studies*. Ed. Cornell, R.G. Pp. 167–227. Marcel Dekker Inc., New York and Basel

WILLIAMSON, M.H. and WILSON, R.A. (1978) The use of mathematical models for predicting the incidence of fascioliasis. In: *Weather and Parasitic Animal Disease*. Pp. 39–48. World Meteorological Organization Technical Note No. 159

WILLIAMSON, N.B. (1980) The economic efficiency of a veterinary preventive medicine and management program in Victorian dairy herds. *Australian Veterinary Journal*, **56**, 1–9

WILLIAMSON, N.B., CANNON, R.M., BLOOD, D.C. and MORRIS, R.S. (1978) A health program for commercial dairy herds. 5. The occurrence of specific disease entities. *Australian Veterinary Journal*, **54**, 252–256

WILSON, C.D., RICHARDS, M.S., STEVENSON, F.J. and DAVIES, G. (1983) *The National Mastitis Survey*. A survey of udder infection and related factors in the British dairy herd 1977. Ministry of Agriculture, Fisheries and Food, Agricultural Development Advisory Services Booklet No. 2433

WILSON, T.M. and HOWES, B. (1980) An epizootic of bovine tuberculosis in Barbados, West Indies. Proceedings of the Second International Symposium of Veterinary Laboratory Diagnosticians, 24–26 June 1980, Lucerne, Switzerland, **1**, 136–144

WINKLER, W.G. (1975) Fox rabies. In: *The Natural History of Rabies*, Vol. 2. Ed. Baer, G.M. Pp. 3–22. Academic Press, New York

WITTS, L.J. (Ed.) (1964) *Medical Surveys and Clinical Trials*, 2nd edn. Oxford University Press, London

WONG, W.T. and LEE, M.K.C. (1985) Some observations on the population and natal patterns among purebred dogs in Malaysia. *Journal of Small Animal Practice*, **26**, 111–119

WOOD, E.N. (1978) The incidence of stillborn piglets associated with high atmospheric carbon monoxide levels. *The Pig Veterinary Society Proceedings*, **3**, 117–118

WOODRUFF, A.W. (1976) Toxocariasis as a public health problem. *Environmental Health*, **84**, 29–31

WOODS, J.M. and HOWARD, T.H. (1980) Reproductive

management in large dairy herds. In: *Current Therapy in Theriogenology: Diagnosis, Treatment and Prevention of Reproductive Diseases in Animals*. Ed. Morrow, D.A. Pp. 524–528. W.B. Saunders Company, Philadelphia, London and Toronto

WOODWARD, R.H. and GOLDSMITH, P.L. (1964) *Cumulative Sum Techniques*. Imperial Chemical Industries Mathematical and Statistical Techniques for Industry Monograph No. 3. Oliver and Boyd, Edinburgh

WORTHINGTON, R.W. (1982) Serology as an aid to diagnosis: uses and abuses. *New Zealand Veterinary Journal*, **30**, 93–97

WRATHALL, A.E. (1975) *Reproductive Disorders in Pigs*. Review Series No. 11 of the Commonwealth Bureau of Animal Health. Commonwealth Agricultural Bureaux, Farnham Royal

WRATHALL, A.E. and HEBERT, C.N. (1983) Monitoring reproductive performance in the pig herd. *The Pig Veterinary Society Proceedings*, **9**, 136–148

WRIGHT, S. (1959) Genetics and hierarchy of biological sciences. *Science, New York*, **130**, 959–965

WYNNE-EDWARDS, V.C. (1962) *Animal Dispersion in Relation to Social Behaviour*. Oliver and Boyd, Edinburgh

YATES, F. (1981) *Sampling Methods for Censuses and Surveys*, 4th edn. Charles Griffin and Company Limited, London and High Wycombe

YEKUTIEL, P. (1980) *Eradication of Infectious Disease—A Critical Study*. Contributions to Epidemiology and Biostatistics Vol. 2. S. Karger, Basel

YOUNG, G.B., LEE, G.J., WADDINGTON, D., SALES, D.I., BRADLEY, J.S. and SPOONER, R.L. (1983) Culling and wastage in dairy cows in East Anglia. *Veterinary Record*, **113**, 107–111

ZUCKERMAN, LORD (1980) *Badgers, Cattle and Tuberculosis*. Report to the Right Honourable Peter Walker. Her Majesty's Stationery Office, London

# Index

Abattoirs, as sources of data, 117
Abomasal mucosal hyperplasia, 24
Abortive reaction, 54
Actinobacillosis, 12, 20
*Actinobacillus lignieresi*, 12, 25
Adjusted (standardized) measures of
  disease, 38
*Aedes africanus*, 87
*Aedes simpsoni*, 87
African horse sickness, 53, 217
African swine fever, 21, 68, 70, 153,
  181
Age, disease and, 48
Age-specific rates, 49
Agricultural organizations, as sources
  of data, 119
Anaemia, in dogs, 72
Analytical epidemiology, 14
Anaplasmosis, 72
Animals,
  *See also* Populations, separate
    species, etc.
  feeding habits, 84
  group behaviour, 80
  movement of, 83
    in control of disease, 217
  predator/prey relationships, 86
  relationships between types, 83
  size of, food webs and, 83
  territorality, 80
Animal plagues,
  current problems, 6
  dates of occurrence, 4
Animal-years at risk, 33
Anthrax, 3, 68
  in cattle, 41
  plague, 4
Anthropurgic ecosystems, 87
Antibodies, 229
  assaying, 175
  blocking, 181
  comparison of levels, 178

Antibodies (*cont.*)
  detecting presence of, 178
  half-life, 184
  mean titres, 176
  measurement, 175
  methods of expressing amounts of,
    175
  multiple serial dilution assay, 177
  prevalence, 184
  quantal assay, 176
  single serial dilution assay, 177
  Spearman-Kärber titration, 177
  titres, 175, 176
Antigens, 179, 181, 229
Area incidence ratio, 36
Arthropods, transmission of infection
  in, 72
Association, 229
  demonstrating, 141–152
    aetiological fraction, 147
    attributable risk, 146
    basic techniques, 141
    $x^2$-test, 144, 236
    correlation, 149
    degrees of freedom, 143
    errors of inference, 142
    estimation of risk, 145
    interval estimation, 142
    measures of occurrence, 147
    multivariate analysis, 151
    non-parametric tests, 150
    null hypothesis, 142
    odds ratio, 145
    one- and two-tailed tests, 142
    relative risk, 145
    significance tests, 141
    Student's $t$-test, 142, 235
    variables, 141
  measures of, 147
    interpreting results, 168
    used in observational studies, 167
  non-statistical, 23

Association (*cont.*)
  statistical, 24
  types of, 23
Atrophic rhinitis, 58
Attack rate, 35, 37
Australia,
  control of screw-worm fly in, 204
  fascioliasis in, 41, 43
  liver fluke in, 43
Australian National Animal Disease
  Information System, 130
Autochthonous ecosystem, 86

*Babesia* spp., 51, 103
Badgers,
  density of setts, 42, 44
  role in bovine tuberculosis, 6, 20,
    44
  tuberculosis in, 191
Balance of nature, 78
  disease control and, 223
Bats, rabies in, 25
Beef cattle, health and productivity
  schemes, 213
Biocenosis, 86
Biomes, 77
*Biomphalaria glabrata*, 82
Biotopes, 86
Birth rates, 36
Blood flukes, 68
Blood splash, 12
Bluetongue, 41, 43, 53
  eradication, 216
  transmission of, 70
  virus, 52, 54, 64
Bovine ephemeral fever virus, 64
Bovine hypomagnesaemia, 25, 26
Bovine petechial fever, 29
Bovine tuberculosis, 6
  role of badgers, 20
Bovine virus diarrhoea, 55, 194

Breast cancer,
  hormonal factors, 51
  in dogs and man, 49, 50
*Brucella abortus*, 68, 181
  transmission, 220
*Brucella suis*, 120
Brucellosis, 6, 11, 68
  control and eradication, 13, 197,
    200, 223
  genetic resistance, 219
  human, 94
  prevalence, 183
  screening tests, 183
  in UK, 196
Budgerigars, goitre in, 37
Bulls, Leydig cell tumours in, 37, 38

Calorific energy flow, 85
*Campylobacter jejuni*, 67
Cancer,
  cause of, 60
  induction of, 60
  initiation by viruses, 61
Cancer eye, 12
Canine distemper, 4, 55, 66, 103, 220
Canine parvovirus infection, sentinels
    for, 16
Carcinogens, 61
Carrier state, 55, 229
Case-control studies, 17, 176
Case fatality rate, 35, 36
Cats,
  coat colour, skin cancer and, 52
  conjunctivitis in, 23
  dysautonomia, 8, 103
  leukaemia in, transmission, 100
  panleucopenia, 70, 72, 95
  urological syndrome, 59, 148, 168
Cattle,
  abortion in, 22
  anaplasmosis, 72
  anthrax, 41
  beef, health and productivity
    schemes, 213
  bovine virus diarrhoea virus, 55,
    194
  copper deficiency, 41
  dairy, health and productivity
    schemes, 208, 209
  disease eradication in, 219
  enzootic bovine leucosis, 169
  ephemeral fever virus, 64
  foot-and-mouth disease, 74, 75
    *See also* Foot-and-mouth disease
  *Haemonchus contortus* infection, 24
  helminthiasis, cost of, 202
  hypomagnesaemia, 25, 26, 46, 95
  Johne's disease, 34
  keratoconjunctivitis, 68
  ketosis in, 24
    milk yield and, 200
  Kikuyu grass poisoning, 29
  lameness in, 149, 208
  leptospirosis in, 26, 28, 29

Cattle (*cont.*)
  leucosis, 33
  malignant catarrhal fever of, 13
  mannosidosis in, 28, 218
  mastitis, 200, 223
    control of, 208, 216, 218, 220
    eradication, 219
    metabolic profiles, 209
    milk yield, ketosis and mastitis and,
      200
  optimum feeding, 208
  petechial fever, 29
  protoporphyria, 218
  respiratory disease, 58
  rhinotracheitis virus, 56
  size of herds, 32
  squamous cell carcinoma of eye, 12,
    27, 37
  Texas fever, 215
  ticks, 90
  trypanosomiasis, 198
    eradication, 215, 216
    tolerance to, 219
  tuberculosis in, 44, 220
  world productivity, 7
Cattle cultures, 2
Causal hypothesis,
  formulating, 27
  testing, 14
Causality of disease, 8
Causal models, 25
Causes, 61
  direct, 24
  indirect, 24
  necessary, 25
  sufficient, 25
Census, 153
Chemotherapy, therapeutic and
    prophylactic, 216
$x^2$-distribution, 144, 236
Chlamydiosis, 115
Choroplethic maps, 41
*Chrysomyia bezziana*, control of
    infestation, 204
Classification of disease, 101
Climate,
  as disease determinant, 56
  classification of, 77
  effects of, 76
  importance of, 13
  population dispersal and, 80
Clinical trials, 16
Coat colour, disease and, 52
Co-carcinogens, 61
*Coccidioides immitis*, 77, 79
Coccidioidomycosis, 51, 89
Cohort life tables, 39
Cohort studies, 17, 166
Coitus, infection via, 69
Coli septicaemia, 58
Colorado tick fever, 66
Commercial livestock enterprises, as
    sources of data, 119
Companion animals, health
    schemes, 213

Companion animal medicine, 224
Comparison of groups, 16
Competitive exclusion, principle of,
    81
Computers, 125
  auxiliary storage, 126
  basic components, 125
  changing attitudes towards, 127
  choice of language, 127
  handling capacity, 126
  languages, 126
  programs, 127
  structure of, 125
Computer System for Recording
    Events affecting Economically-
    important Livestock
    (COSREEL), 131
Concomitant variation, 28
Confounding, 26, 170, 229
Conjugation, 53
Contagion, 3
Contagious spatial pattern, 100
Contagium animatum, 3
Contagium vivum fluidum, 3
Copper deficiency, 41
Cost-benefit analysis, 200, 218, 219,
    231
  in disease control, 202
  example of, 204
  principles of, 202
  problems, 205
*Coxiella burnetti*, 68, 176
Cross-sectional studies, 17, 166
Cross-sectional surveys, 16
Crude measures of disease
    occurrence, 37
*Culicoides* spp., 216
*Culicoides imicola*, 70
Cyclical trends in disease, 94
Cyclic neutropenia, 218
*Cysticercus bovis*, 217
*Cysticercus pisiformis*, 64
*Cysticercus tenuicollis*, 117
*Cytoecetes ondiri*, 29

Dairy health,
  optimum feeding, 208
  schemes, 208
Dairy herds, metabolic profiles, 209
Danish swine slaughter inspection
    data bank, 130
Data,
  accuracy, 104, 117
  bias in, 106
  box and whisker plots, 138
  case-specific, 121
  categorical, 112
  codes and coding, 107–112
    alpha, 109, 110
    alphanumeric, 109
    check digits, 111
    choice of, 110
    components, 107
    consecutive and hierarchic, 107
    consistency, 111

Data (*cont.*)
  codes and coding (*cont.*)
    error detection, 111
    numeric, 107, 110
    structure, 107
    symbols, 110
  collecting information, 114, 159
    cooperation in, 114
    cost of, 115
    from abattoirs, 117
    from agricultural organizations,
      119
    from commercial livestock
      enterprises, 119
    from farm records, 119
    from government departments,
      119
    from knacker yards, 118
    from pharmaceutical sales, 119
    from poultry packing plants, 118
    from veterinary practices, 115
    from zoos, 119
    in developing countries, 115
    questionnaires, 159
    role of registries, 118
    trace-back, 114, 117
  continuous measurements, 112
  cusums, 139
  dilated pupil syndrome, 103
  discrete measurements, 112
  elements of, 101
  improvement in quality of, 224
  interpretative, 103
  measurements, 112
    bias in, 106
    continuous, 112
    discrete, 112
  nature of, 101–113, 114
  numerical presentation, 132–140
    confidence intervals and limits,135
    definitions, 132
    descriptive statistics, 133
    interval estimation, 134
    means, medians and quartiles,
      133, 134
    measures of position, 133
    measures of spread, 134
    parameters, 133
    standard deviation, 134
    statistical distributions, 135
    transformation, 137
    variables, 132, 133
  observational, 101, 103
  pie charts, 138
  qualitative, 104
  quantitative, 101
  records,
    case-specific, 121
    centre-punched (feature) cards, 125
    computerized techniques, 125
    day books, 123
    edge-punched (item) cards, 123
    in health and productivity
      schemes, 207
    longhand techniques, 122

Data (*cont.*)
  records (*cont.*)
    non-computerized, 122
    problem-orientated medical
      records, 123
    pro-formas, 123
    punched-card techniques, 123
    record cards, 123
  record-specific, 121
  representation of, 107
  sensitivity and specificity, 104
  Shewhart charts, 138
  sources of, 114–120
    bias in, 115
  specifier types, 121
  storage and retrieval, 121–131
    *See also* Data bases
    accessing computerized data, 128
    computer handling capacity, 126
    computer languages, 126, 127
    programming computers, 127
  variability of, 132
  verification of, 111
Data bases, 121
  approach to data storage, 128
  hierarchic model, 121
  macroscale projects, 129
  mesoscale projects, 129
  microscale projects, 129
  models, 121
  network model, 122
  project recording, 129
  record model, 121
  relational model, 122
  veterinary, 129
    examples of, 130
Day books, as sources of data, 123
Death rates, 36
Definitions of epidemiology, 11, 18
Demographic base maps, 44
Demography, 30
Demonic theory of disease, 2, 5
*Dermacentor andersoni*, 66
Descriptive epidemiology, 14
Determinants of disease, 46–62
  agent, 52
  associated with host, agent and
    environment, 46
  biological interaction, 59
  classification of, 46
  climate, 56
  environmental, 56
  genetic factors, 48, 51
  hormonal, 51
  host, 48
  husbandry factors, 57
  interactions, 58
  intrinsic and extrinsic, 46
  microbial colonization of host, 55
  occupational, 51
  primary and secondary, 46, 47
  sex, 49
  size and conformation, 52
  social and ethological, 51
  species and breed, 51

Determinants of disease (*cont.*)
  statistical interaction, 59
  stress, 57
Diabetes mellitus,
  incidence rates, 37
  sex incidence, 51
Diagnosis,
  bias in, 106
  criteria, 103
  performance related, 9
  precision, 105
  refinement, 105
  reliability, 105
  repeatability of tests, 105
  results of tests, 104
  sensitivity and specificity, 181
  validity of technique, 105
*Dictyocaulus viviparus*, 224
Diet, in disease, 57
*Diphyllobothrium* spp., 64
Disease,
  adjusted (standardized) measures
    of, 38
  age factors, 48
  animals' niches relating to, 82
  assessment of cost, 200
  cause,
    causal associations, 8, 22, 23, 29,
      101, 141–152
    *See also* Association
    causal postulates, 22
    changing attitudes towards, 5
    changing concepts of, 2
    confounding, 26
    enabling factors, 25
    Evans' postulates, 22
    formulating hypotheses, 27
    models, 25
    necessary, 25
    place and, 27
    population factors, 27
    precipitating factors, 25
    predisposing factors, 25
    response and explanatory
      variables, 23
    risk factors, 24
    statistical association, 24
    sufficient, 25
    timing, 27
    variables, 23
  classification of, 101
    levels of, 102
    significance in epidemiology,
      103
  control of, 17, 82, 215–224
    balance of nature and, 223
    biological vectors, 217
    cause, maintenance and
      transmission and, 220
    chemotherapy, 216
    compensation and, 223
    cost-benefit analysis, 218, 219
    definitions, 215
    diagnosis and, 221
    ecological consequences of, 223

Disease (*cont.*)
control of (*cont.*)
environment, husbandry and
feeding in, 217
factors in, 220
finance of, 223
fomites disinfection, 217
genetic improvement, 218
grazing and, 217
host/parasite relationship in, 220
host range in, 220
legislation, 223
minimal disease methods, 219
movement of hosts, 217
niche filling, 217
planning and monitoring of, 13
public health considerations, 222
public opinion in, 222
quarantine, 216
replacement stock in, 221
selecting campaigns, 203
slaughtering in, 216
strategies, 216
uncertainty in, 203
vaccination, 216, 220, 224
veterinary infrastructure and, 221
cumulative incidence, 33
cyclical trends, 94
crude measures of, 37
determinants of, 46–62
agents, 52
associated with host, agent and
environment, 46
biological interaction, 59
classification, 46
climatic factors, 56
environmental, 56
genetic, 48, 51
hormonal, 51
husbandry factors, 57
interactions, 58
intrinsic and extrinsic, 46
occupation, 51
primary and secondary, 46, 47
sex, 49
size and conformation, 52
social and ethological, 51
species and breed, 51
statistical interaction, 59
stress, 57
diagnosis, 103
ecology of,
*See under* Ecology
economics of, 8, 13, 199–205
assessment of cost, 200
cost-benefit analysis, 200, 202
discounting, 203
evaluation, 200
internal and external costs and
benefits, 203
nature of decisions, 199
shadow prices, 203
eradication of, 215, 224
*See also* Disease, control of
in the UK, 219
strategies, 216

Disease (*cont.*)
host determinants, 48
implications of population control,
81
incidence of, 31, 33
statistically significant, 23
multifactorial, 48
natural history of, 12, 14
nomenclature of, 101
significance in epidemiology, 103
non-infectious, 8
occurrence,
describing, 30–45
measures of, 31
of unknown origin, 8
patterns of, 91–100
prevalence, 31
prevention of, 206, 215
reinforcing factors, 25
relation between prevalence and
incidence, 33
reporting systems, 9
*See also* Data, collecting
information
seasonal trends in, 81, 94
serological diagnosis of, 175
spatial distribution, 30, 100, 136
specific measures of, 37
subclinical, 7
temporal distribution, 30, 94, 100, 136
temporal trends, 100
detection, 96
regression analysis, 98
rolling (moving) averages, 97
time-space clustering, 100
Disease vectors, 6
Distemper, 4, 55, 66, 103, 220
Distribution maps, 41
Divination, 3
Divine cause of disease, 2
Dogs, 1
anaemia in, 72
anthelmintics, 195
congenital incontinence, 144
conversion to human age equivalent,
49, 50
cyclic neutropenia, 218
distemper, 4, 55, 66, 103, 220
epilepsy in, 51
haemophilia, 51
health schemes, 214
heart disease in, 46, 51, 52, 146, 169
heartworm infection, 51
helminthiasis, 220
hip dysplasia, 218
lung disease in, 56
mastocytomas, 46, 52
oral tumours, 61
parvovirus infection, 21, 51
progressive retinal atrophy, 218
pruritus, 46, 47, 48
testicular neoplasia in, 38
urinary incontinence in, neutering
and, 144, 146, 171
Domestic animals, demography, 30
Domestication of animals, 1, 5

Echinococcosis, 222
*Echinococcus granulosus*, 84, 195
Ecological climax, 87
Ecological interfaces, 87
Ecological mosaics, 88
Ecology of disease, 12, 76–90
basic concepts, 76
information on, 12
Economics of disease, 8, 13, 199–205
assessment of cost, 200
cost-benefit analysis, 200, 202
example of, 204
internal and external costs and
benefits, 203
principles of, 202
problems of, 205
discounting, 203
eradication and, 223
evaluation, 200
nature of decisions, 199
shadow prices, 203
Ecosystems, 86–88
Edinburgh SAPTU recording system,
131
Embryo, transmission of infection to,
70
Enabling factors, 25
Endemic occurrence of disease, 20, 230
Enteric disease, 58
Environment,
importance of, 13
reproduction and, 48
Environmental determinants of
disease, 56
Environmental factors, in causation
of disease, 22
Environmental resistance, 78
Enzootic bovine leucosis, 33, 169
Enzootic pneumonia, 202
Epidemics, 20
common source, 92
epidemic waves, 93
models of, 190
point source, 93
propagating, 92, 93
Reed-Frost model, 190
Epidemic curves, 91
Epidemic occurrence of disease, 20
Epidemiological interference, 83
Epidemiological investigation, types
of, 14
Epidemiological rates, 35
Epidemiological ratios, 35, 39
Epidemiology,
components of, 14
definitions, 11, 18
interplay with other sciences, 17
quantitative and qualitative
investigations, 14
relation to diagnostic disciplines, 18
scope of, 11–19
uses of, 11
Epilepsy, in dogs, 51
Epizootics, 11
Epizootiology, 11
Epornitics, 11

Equine grass sickness, 8
Equine influenza, plagues, 4
Equine parasitic mange, 6
Eradication of disease,
    *See under* Disease, control of
*Escherichia coli*, 8, 47, 51, 103, 216,
    218
Ethiopia, trypanosomiasis in, 198
Evans' postulates, 22, 141
Evolution, convergent, 77
Experimental epidemiology, 14
Extrinsic incubation period, 66
Eye, squamous cell carcinoma of, 12,
    27, 37

Farms,
    economics of, 199
    profiles, 207
Farm hygiene, 5
Farm records, 119
*Fasciola hepatica*, 13, 188, 193, 217,
    220
Fascioliasis,
    in Australia, 41, 43
    models of, 188, 193
    seasonal aspects, 189
Fatality rate, 35, 36
Fertility rates, 36
Fetal death rate, 36, 39
Fetal death ratio, 36, 39
Fleas, host/parasite relationships, 74
Fluke, life-cycle of, 85
Fomites, 230
    disinfection, 217
Food,
    competition for, 80
Food chains, 83
    relationship between predator and
        prey, 86
    trophic levels, 83, 85
Food poisoning, 27, 93
Food webs,
    animal size and, 83
    significance to disease transmission,
        84
Foot-and-mouth disease, 18
    airborne spread of, 13, 56, 70, 189
    as propagating epidemic, 93
    cost-benefit analysis and, 203
    cyclical trend in, 94
    details of epidemic, 71
    epidemic in the USA, 196
    eradication, 219, 222
    in Paraguay, 99, 188
    pandemics, 21
    relationships with game species, 74,
        75
    seasonal periodicity, 87
    some plagues, 4
Foot rot, 58, 59
Forecasting systems, 188
Foxes,
    movement of, 83
    rabies in, 81, 86, 88, 92, 94, 191

Gastroenteritis, of pigs, 94, 95
Genetic determinants of disease, 51
Genetic improvement, in disease
    control, 218
Genetic screening, 218
Geographic base maps, 41
Glanders, 6, 215
Goats, domestication, 1
Goitre, 37
Goverment departments, as sources
    of data, 119
Gray collie syndrome, 218
Grazing, and disease control, 217
Gumboro disease, 194

*Haemonchus contortus*, 24
Haemophilia, in dogs, 51
*Haemophysalis spinigera*, 90
Hares, *Brucella suis* from, 120
Healers, primitive, 1, 2
Health and productivity schemes,
    206–214, 230
    action lists, 207
    components of, 206
    development of, 206
    for beef cattle, 213
    for companion animals, 213
    for dairy cattle, 208
    for pigs, 209, 210
    for sheep, 211, 212, 213
    justification of, 207
    objectives, 206
    structure of, 206
    targets of, 207
Heart disease, in dogs, 46, 51, 52,
    146, 169
Heartworm infection, 51
Helminthiasis,
    in cattle, 202
    in dogs, 220
Helminths, vaccines against, 224
Helminth infestation, environment
    and, 13
Hepatitis B, 53
Herd health programme, 1
Herpesvirus, 51
    causing malignant catarrhal fever,
        13
Home range of animals, 80
Hookworm, 68
Horses,
    grass sickness, 8
    health programmes, 214
    helminths in, 214
    influenza, 4
    parasitic mange, 6
    rhinopneumonitis, 65
Horse cultures, 2
Host, 12
    characteristics of, 65
    environment within, 72
    in infection, 64
    microbial colonization of, 55
    susceptibility, 65
    types of, 64

Host determinants of disease, 48–52
Host/parasite relationship, in disease
    control, 220
Humoral pathology, 3, 5
Hydatids, control in New Zealand, 194
Hyperendemic disease, 20
Hypocupraemia, in cattle, 41
Hypomagnesaemia, bovine, 25, 26,
    46, 95
Hypotheses,
    methods of formulating, 27
    testing, 14

Immunity, sterile, 55
Immunization, 1
    natural, 83
Immunological status, vertical
    transmission and, 72
Incidence of disease, 230
    calculation from prevalence, 33, 34
Incidence rate of disease, 33, 96
Incidence values, 34, 37
Incubation periods, 65
Infection,
    agents, 52
        antigens on, 179
        biomes affecting, 77
        classification, 188
        genotypic changes in, 53
        hazards to, 72
        resistant forms, 72
    ascending, 72
    at parturition, 72
    characteristics of pathogens, 66
    clinical, 54
    effective contact, 67
    extrinsic incubation period, 66
    generation time, 65
    gradient of, 53
    group types, 48
    host and vector, 64
    host/parasite relationships, 74
    inapparent (silent), 54
    incubation period, 65
    latent, 55
    maintenance of, 72
        environment in host, 72
        external environment, 73
        persistence in host, 73
        'rapidly-in, rapidly-out' strategy,
            73
        resistance and, 73
        strategies, 73
    mixed, 7, 58
    oral route of, 68
    outcome of, 54
    respiratory route of, 68
    routes of, 67
    salivarian transmission, 65
    subclinical, 54
    transmission, 63–72, 81
        biological, 65
        by ingestion, 69
        characteristics of hosts, 65
        coitus, 69

Infection (*cont.*)
  transmission (*cont.*)
    contact, 69
    cyclopropagative, 65
    developmental, 65
    direct, 63
    droplet muclei, 70
    epidemiological interference in, 83
    factors in, 65
    food webs and, 84
    germinative, 70
    horizontal, 63
    iatrogenic, 69
    inhalation, 69
    inoculation, 69
    long-distance, 70
    methods of, 69
    oral route of, 67
    propagative, 65
    respiratory route of, 68
    routes of, 67
    stercorarian, 65
    transovarial, 72
    trans-stadial, 72
    vectors, 89
    vertical, 63, 70
    via skin, cornea and mucous membranes, 68
  vectors, 65
  virulence, 67
Infectious disease, 48, 63
  *See also* Infection
  complex, 7
  diagnosis of, 175, 224
Infectivity, 66
Influenza, serological tests for, 180
Influenza A, 53, 179
Influenza viruses, 179
  classification, 180
  detection, 105
Inhalation, infection by, 69
Inoculation, infection by, 69
Insect vectors, 13
Interaction, 230
Interference level, 207
International Directory of Animal Health and Disease Data Banks, 115
Interepidemic period, 91
Intervention studies, 16
Intestinal carcinoma, in sheep, 37
Investigations, types of, 16
Isomorbs, 44
Isomorts, 44
Isoplethic maps, 44

Jaagziekte, 219
Jaw tumours, in sheep, 52
Johne's disease, 34, 69, 219

Kendall's Threshold Theorem, 92
Keratoconjunctivitis, bovine, 68

Ketosis, in cattle, 24, 200
Key-Gaskell syndrome, 8, 103
Kikuyu grass poisoning, 29
Knacker yards, as sources of data, 118
Koch's postulates, 3, 6, 8, 22
Kyasanur Forest disease, 89

Landscape epidemiology, 89
Lassa fever, 64, 94
Latent infection, 55
*Leptospira* spp., 59, 74, 176
*Leptospira interrogans*, 13, 22
Leptospires, 73
Leptospirosis, 11, 25
  epidemic, 93
  genetic resistance, 219
  in dairy cattle, 26, 28, 29
  landscape epidemiology, 89
  seasonal trends, 94, 95
Leukaemia, in cats, 100
Leydig cell tumours, in bulls, 37, 38
Life span, 49
Life tables, 39
Life zones, 77, 78
*Limnea truncatula*, 220
*Listeria* spp., 48
Live birth rate, 36
Liver fluke, in Australia, 43
Livestock,
  population of Great Britain, 7
  world populations of, 6
Livestock medicine, 223
Livestock production, as economic process, 199
Loiasis, 88
Longitudinal studies, 167
Longitudinal surveys, 16
Lotka-Volterra equations, 81
Louping ill, 34
Louse, infestations, 82
Lung disease, canine, 56
Lymphocytic choriomeningitis, 72

Macroparasites, 188
Magnesium,
  deficiency, 46, 95
  levels of, 26, 28
Mannosidosis, 218
  in cattle, 28
Maps,
  choroplethic, 41
  demographic base, 41, 44
  distribution, 41
  epidemiological, 27
  geographic base, 41
  isoplethic, 44
  point (dot or location), 41
*Marisa cornuarietis*, 82
Markov Chain, 196
Mastitis, 8, 200, 219, 223
  control of, 203, 208, 216, 218, 220
  environmental, 47
  summer, 58

Mastocytomas, in dogs, 46, 52
*Mastomys natalensis*, 64
Maternal mortality ratio, 36
Mathematics, notation and terms, 233
Measurements, 112–113
  continuous, 112
  discrete, 112
Medical records, as sources of data, 123
Megatherms, 77
Mesotherms, 77
Metaphysical medicine, 2
Miasma, 3, 5
Microeconomics, 199
Microparasites, 188
Milk yields, productivity schemes, 208
Mites, as vectors in infection, 80
Models and modelling, 17, 187–198, 224, 230
  causal, 25
  continuous time, 190
  definitions, 187
  density type, 187
  deterministic, 188
    using differential calculus, 190
  deterministic matrix, 192
  deterministic population, 189
  empirical, 188
  explanatory, 188, 189
  forecasting systems, 188
  prevalence type, 187
  sensitivity analysis, 188
  state-transition, 190
  state vectors, 192
  stochastic, 188
  stochastic network, 194
  stochastic population, 193
  types of, 187
  use of, 187
Monitoring, 9, 16, 230
*Moraxella bovis*, 68
Morbidity, 30, 230
  measures of, 31
  true and false changes in, 96
Mortality, 30, 230
Mortality rates, 35, 36
Mosquito, in yellow fever transmission, 87
Mouse, Lassa virus infection in, 94
Multifactorial disease, 26, 48, 230
Multivariate analysis, 151
Muscle, ecchymoses in, 12
Mutation, 53
*Mycobacterium johnei*, 73
*Mycobacterium tuberculosis*, 13, 82, 221
*Mycoplasma felis*, 23
*Mycoplasma mycoides*, 12
Myxomatosis, 65

*Naegleria fowleri*, 52
Natural history of disease, 12, 14
Natural law, universe of, 3
Nature, balance of, 78, 223

*Neisseria* spp., 53
Nematodiriasis, models of, 189
*Nematodirus* spp., 217
*Neorickettsia helminthoeca*, 85
Newcastle disease virus, 52
New Zealand,
  hydatid control in, 194
  intestinal carcinoma of sheep in, 37
  leptospirosis in dairy cattle, 26, 28, 29
Niche filling, disease control and, 217
Nidality, 88, 230
Nomenclature of disease, 101
North Amercia, life zones, 78
Nosoarea, 88
Nosogenic territory, 88
Nuthatches, 82
Nutrition, 48

Observational studies, 16, 166
Office International des Epizooties, 130
Oncogenes, 60
Opportunistic pathogens, 8, 48, 55
Oral tumours, canine, 61
Orbiviruses, antigenic change in, 53
*Ostertagia circumcincta*, 195, 217
*Ostertagia ostertagi*, 189
Ostertagiasis, 189, 194
Outbreaks of disease, 231
*Oxytrema silicula*, 85

Pandemic occurrence, 21, 231
*Paramecium* spp., 81, 82
Paraguay, foot-and-mouth disease in, 94, 99, 188
Parasites, modelling of, 188
Parasitism, intracellular, 82
Parturition, infection at, 72
Parvovirus infection, 21, 51
*Pasteurella haemolytica*, 8
Pathogenicity, 52, 231
Pathogens,
  characteristics of, 66
  endogenous, 55
  exogenous, 55
  opportunistic, 55
Performance-related diagnosis, 9
Petechial fever, bovine, 29
Pharmaceutical companies, as sources of data, 119
Piglets, mortality, 206
Pigs,
  adenomatosis, 7
  cost of disease in, 201, 202
  disease eradication, 219
  fattening unit, cost of disease in, 201, 202
  foot lesions in, 57
  gastroenteritis of, 56, 94, 95
  health and productivity schemes, 209, 210
  herd structure, 7

Pigs (*cont.*)
  intestinal adenomatosis, 139
  leptospirosis, 22
  lymphosarcoma, 61
  parvovirus, 7, 9, 48
  porcine stress syndrome, 58
  reproductive failure in, 48
  respiratory disease in, 27
  small litters, 7, 9
  stillbirths in, 28
  vaccination, feedback, 216
Plague, 3, 68
Plants, relationships between types, 83
*Plasmodium* spp., 65
Pleurisy, in sheep, 96, 97
Pleuropneumonia, 4, 5, 12, 200
  eradication of, 6, 215
    economic benefits of, 200
*Pneumococcus* spp., 73
Pneumonia,
  acute bacterial, 34
  causes of, 25
  enzootic, 68, 202
  in sheep, 58, 96, 97, 98
Poisson distribution, 136, 231
Poliovirus immunization, natural, 83
Population(s), 27, 30
  competitive exclusion, 81
  contiguous, 30
  control of, implications for disease, 81
  density-dependent competition, 79
  deterministic models, 189
  disease in, 11
  dispersal of, 80
  distribution of, 76
    biomes, 77
    vegetational zones, 76
  for surveys, 153
  group behaviour, 80
  home range, 80
  interspecific competition, 81
  intraspecific competition, 81
  life zones, 77
  niches, 81
  predator/prey relationship, 86
  regulation of size, 78
  separated, 31
  serological estimations and comparisons in, 178
  size,
    competition for food and, 80
    control by competition, 78
    logistic equation, 79
    predation and, 80
    Wynne-Edwards hypothesis, 80
  social dominance, 80
  stochastic models, 193
  structure of, 30
  sympatric species, 82
Portugal, bluetongue in, 41, 43
Postcapture myopathy syndrome, 58
Poultry, disease eradication, 219
Poultry packing plants, as sources of data, 118

Precipitating factors, 25
Predators, relation to prey, 86
Predisposing factors, 25
Pregnancy rate, 36
Prevalence, disease, 31, 96, 231
  calculation of incidence from, 34
  period, 34
  point, 31
  relation to incidence, 33
Prevalence rate, 35
Prevention of disease, 206, 215
Production,
  as an economic process, 199
  schemes,
    *See under* Health and productivity schemes
  shortfall in, 207
Progressive retinal atrophy, in dogs, 218
Prospective studies, 167
Prospective surveys, 16
*Proteus* spp., 53
Protoporphyria, bovine, 218
Pruritus, in dogs, 46, 47, 48
*Pseudomonas* spp., 53
*Pseudomonas aeruginosa*, 69
*Pulex irritans*, 74
Pulmonary disease, in dogs, 56

Q fever, 27, 37
Quarantine, 5, 70, 216

Rabies, 3, 222
  endemic occurence of, 89
  eradication, 215
  in foxes, 81, 86, 88, 92, 94, 191
  from bats, 25
  infection, 66
  legal aspects of, 223
  long-term trends in, 95
  in skunks, 44
  sporadic cases, 21
  transmission, 69
  in the USA, 96
Rates, 35
Ratios, 35
Rats,
  in synanthropic ecosystems, 87
  plague and, 3
  scrub typhus and, 80
Rat plague, 94
*Rattus norvegicus*, 87
Recombination, 53
Record cards, as sources of data, 123
Reed-Frost model of epidemics, 190
Registries, as sources of data, 118
Regression analysis, 98
Reinforcing factors, 25
Reporting systems, 9
Reproduction, environment and, 48
Retrospective studies, 167
Retrospective surveys, 16
Rhinotracheitis virus, 56

*Rhipicephalus appendiculatus*, 72
*Rhipicephalus sanguineus*, 89
Rickettsiae, 82
Rinderpest, 55, 88
  control of, 219
  economic aspects, 8, 200
  eradication of, 6, 200, 219
  pandemic, 21
  plague, 4, 5
Risk factors, 24
Risk indicators, 24
Rocky Mountain spotted fever, 89
Rolling (moving) averages, 97
Ross River virus, 67
Rotaviruses, 68

Salivarian transmission of infection, 65
*Salmonella* spp., 55, 74, 217
Salmonellosis, 12, 27, 89
*Schistosoma bovis*, 114
*Schistosoma mansoni*, 85
Schistosomiasis, 82
Scrapie, 73, 219
Screening, 16, 104, 231
Screw-worm fly, 70, 204
Scrub typhus, 80, 88
Seasonal trends in disease, 94
Selenium, 76
Sensitivity analysis, 188
Sentinel units, 16
Serological epidemiology, 175–186
  antibodies,
    comparison of levels of, 178
    detecting presence of, 178
  antibody assay, 175
    mean titres, 176
    multiple serial dilution assay, 177
    relative sensitivity of, 181
    single serial dilution assay, 177
    Spearman-Kärber titration, 177
  antibody prevalence, 184
  antigenic tolerance, 181
  interpreting tests, 179
  sensitivity of antigen and antibody assays, 181
  seroconverted animals, 175
  seronegative animals, 175
  seropositive animals, 175
  serum banks, 184
  tests,
    accuracy of, 180
    interpretation of, 179
    positive and negative results, 181
    possible results, 183
    predictive value of, 182
    refinement, 179
    relationship between sensitivity and specificity, 181
    repeatability of, 184
Serological estimations,
  in populations, 178
Serum,
  collection and storage, 185

Serum (*cont.*)
  constituents of, 175
  sources of, 185
Serum banks, 184, 185
  as sources of data, 118
Sex, as a disease determinant, 49
Sheep,
  disease eradication in, 219
  domestication, 1
  foot rot, 58, 59
  health and productivity schemes, 211, 212, 213
  intestinal carcinoma, 37
  jaw tumours of, 56
  pleurisy in, 96, 97
  pneumonia in, 96, 97, 98
Sheep pox, introduction of, 5
Sheep ticks, populations, 193
*Shigella* spp., 53
Shipping fever, 8, 58
Shock, 57
*Sitta neumayer*, 82
*Sitta tephronota*, 82
Skin, infection via, 68
Skin cancer, coat colour and, 52
Skunk, rabies in, 44
Slaughter, as a control measure, 216
Slow virus diseases, 73
SMEDI viruses, 48
Snails,
  as vectors, 220
  control of, 82
Spatial distribution of disease, 30, 100, 136
Special measures of disease, 37
Sporadic occurrence, of disease, 21
Standard Nomenclature of Veterinary Diseases and Operations, 107, 108
*Staphylococcus* spp., 48
State vector, 192
Statistics, 132–140
  basic definitions, 132
  binomial distribution, 135
    Normal approximations, 137
  confidence intervals and limits, 135
  constants, 233
  correlation, 149
  correlation coefficient, 237
  degrees of freedom, 143
  descriptive, 133
  distributions, 135
  errors of inference, 142
  interval estimation, 134, 142
  means, medians and quartiles, 133, 134
  measures of position, 133
  measures of spread, 134
  measuring interaction, 147
  multivariate analysis, 151
  non-parametric tests, 150
  Normal distribution, 135
  null hypothesis, 142
  one- and two-tailed tests, 142
  parameters, 133

Statistics (*cont.*)
  Poisson distribution, 136, 137
  probability, 132
  sample sizes, 240
    random numbers, 238, 239
    significance test, 141
    standard deviation, 134
    Student's *t*-test, 142, 235
    tests, 132
    transformations, 137
    variables, 132, 133, 141, 233
    variance-ratio (*F*) distribution, 245
    $x^2$-distribution, 144, 236
Sterile immunity, 55
*Streptobacillus moniliformis*, 68
*Streptococcus uberis*, 8, 47, 218
Stress, 57
Student's *t*-test, 142, 235
Studies, 16, 231
  *See also* Surveys
  observational, 166–174, 231
    bias in, 168
    case-control, 166, 167, 171, 172, 174
    cohort, 166, 167, 171, 172, 174
    comparison of types, 171, 172, 174
    confounding, 170
    controlling bias, 170
    cross-sectional, 166, 172, 174
    examples of, 172, 173
    frequency matching, 170
    individual matching, 170
    interpreting results, 168
    longitudinal, 167
    misclassification in, 169, 170
    multivariate techniques, 171
    nomenclature, 167
    prospective, 167
    retrospective, 167
    selection bias, 168
    selection of sample size, 171
    types of, 166, 171, 172, 174
  types of, 16–17
Summer mastitis, 58
Surveillance, 9, 16
Surveys, 16, 153–165, 232
  *See also* Studies
  collecting information, 159
    questionnaires, 159
  cost of, 159
  cross-sectional, 230
  designs of, 155
  detecting cases, 242, 244
  detecting presence of disease, 157
  estimation of disease prevalence, 156
  expected frequency of disease, 156
  precision of the estimate of prevalence, 156
  questionnaires, 159–165
    closed questions, 159
    coding, 159
    criteria for success, 164

Surveys (*cont.*)
  questionnaires (*cont.*)
    design of, 162
    interviews, 164
    mailed and self-completed, 164
    presentation and wording, 163
    questions, 163
    response rate, 164
    response to, 163
    structure, 159
    testing, 164
  sampling, 153, 240
    cluster, 155
    from large population, 156
    from small (finite) population,
      157
    multistage, 156
    non-probability, 154
    probability, 154
    purposive selection, 154
    selection of size, 156
    simple, 154, 155
    stratified random, 155
    systematic, 154
    types of, 154
    use of random numbers, 154, 240
  stratified random sampling, 155
  target population, 153
Swine dysentery, 58
Swine fever, eradication, 200
Synanthropic ecosystems, 87
Synergism, 60, 147, 232
*Syphacia obvelata*, 20, 21, 94

*Taenia hydatigena*, 195
*Taenia ovis*, 195
Tapeworm infections, 73
Temperature, 112
Temporal distribution of disease, 30,
  94, 100, 136
Testicular neoplasia, in dogs, 38
Texas fever, eradication, 215
Theileriosis, 72

Theoretical epidemiology, 14
Threshold level, 66, 92
Ticks,
  disease transmission by, 3, 13, 72,
    89, 90
  sheep, 193
Time series analysis, 96
Tobacco rattle virus, 53
*Toxoplasma gondii*, 73
Transduction, 53
Transformation, 53
Transition matrix, 193
Transmission of disease,
  horizontal, 230
  vertical, 70–72, 232
*Trichinella spiralis*, 54
Trophic levels of food chain, 83
*Trypanosoma* spp., 65
*Trypanosoma congolense*, 83
Trypanosomiasis, 6
  eradication, 215, 216
  in Ethiopia, 198
  tolerance to, 219
Tsetse fly, 198, 217
Tuberculosis, 6
  in badgers, 191
  in cattle, 44, 220
  eradication, 219, 223
Tularaemia, landscape epidemiology,
  89
Tumour-inducing viruses, 60
Tumour registry, 118

Union of Soviet Socialist Republics,
  leptospirosis epidemic in, 93
United Kingdom,
  brucellosis in dairy herds, 196
  disease eradication in, 219
  holdings by size of herd, 32
  livestock population, 7
  pig herd structure, 7
United States,
  epidemic foot-and-mouth disease
    in, 196

United States (*cont.*)
  human brucellosis in, 94
  leptospirosis in, 95
  rabies in, 95, 96
*Utricularia* spp., 85

Vaccination, 216, 220, 224
Variance-ratio (*F*) distribution, 245
Vegetional zones, 76
Vectors in infection, 63, 64, 65, 232
Veterinary Investigation Diagnosis
  Analyses, 131
Veterinary Medical Data Program,
  131
Veterinary medicine,
  contemporary, 6
  development of, 1–10
Veterinary schools, origin of, 1, 5
Virulence, 52, 67, 232
Viruses, 3, 48
  initiation of cancer by, 61
  particle-infectivity ratio, 66

Wales, pig herd structure, 7
Warble fly infestation, 219, 202
Wind-chill index, 56
Wooden tongue, 25
Wynne-Edwards hypothesis, 80

Xerophiles, 77

Yellow fever, transmission of, 87
*Yersinia enterocolitica*, 181

Zoonoses, 11, 232
Zoonosis incidence ratio, 36
Zoos, as sources of data, 119